KV-063-077

3

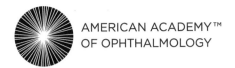

AMERICAN ACADEMY™
OF OPHTHALMOLOGY

Clinical Optics

Last major revision 2013–2014

2016–2017
BCSC
**Basic and Clinical
Science Course™**

Protecting Sight. Empowering Lives.™

EB○ Published after collaborative
review with the European Board
of Ophthalmology subcommittee

The American Academy of Ophthalmology is accredited by the Accreditation Council for Continuing Medical Education to provide continuing medical education for physicians.

The American Academy of Ophthalmology designates this enduring material for a maximum of 15 *AMA PRA Category 1 Credits*™. Physicians should claim only the credit commensurate with the extent of their participation in the activity.

Originally released June 2013; reviewed for currency September 2, 2015; CME expiration date: June 1, 2017. *AMA PRA Category 1 Credits*™ may be claimed only once between June 1, 2013, and the expiration date.

BCSC® volumes are designed to increase the physician's ophthalmic knowledge through study and review. Users of this activity are encouraged to read the text and then answer the study questions provided at the back of the book.

To claim *AMA PRA Category 1 Credits*™ upon completion of this activity, learners must demonstrate appropriate knowledge and participation in the activity by taking the posttest for Section 3 and achieving a score of 80% or higher. For further details, please see the instructions for requesting CME credit at the back of the book.

Cover image: From BCSC Section 10, *Glaucoma.* Typical gonioscopic appearance of angle recession. *Courtesy of Steven T. Simmons, MD.*

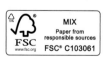

FSC
www.fsc.org

MIX
Paper from
responsible sources
FSC® C103061

Basic and Clinical Science Course

Louis B. Cantor, MD, Indianapolis, Indiana, *Senior Secretary for Clinical Education*
Christopher J. Rapuano, MD, Philadelphia, Pennsylvania, *Secretary for Ophthalmic Knowledge*
George A. Cioffi, MD, New York, New York, *BCSC Course Chair*

Section 3

Faculty

Dimitri T. Azar, MD, *Chair,* Chicago, Illinois
Nathalie F. Azar, MD, Chicago, Illinois
Scott E. Brodie, MD, PhD, New York, New York
Kenneth J. Hoffer, MD, Santa Monica, California
Tommy S. Korn, MD, San Diego, California
Thomas F. Mauger, MD, Columbus, Ohio
Leon Strauss, MD, PhD, Baltimore, Maryland
Edmond H. Thall, MD, Highland Heights, Ohio

The Academy wishes to acknowledge the following committees for review of this edition:

Committee on Aging: Hilary Beaver, MD, Houston, Texas

Vision Rehabilitation Committee: Mary Lou Jackson, MD, Boston, Massachusetts

Practicing Ophthalmologists Advisory Committee for Education: Robert E. Wiggins Jr, MD, *Primary Reviewer,* Asheville, North Carolina; William S. Clifford, MD, *Past Chair,* Garden City, Kansas; Hardeep S. Dhindsa, MD, Reno, Nevada; Robert Fante, MD, Denver, Colorado; Dasa Gangadhar, MD, Wichita, Kansas; Edward K. Isbey III, MD, Asheville, North Carolina; James Mitchell, MD, Edina, Minnesota; Sara O'Connell, MD, Overland Park, Kansas

European Board of Ophthalmology: Wolfgang Radner, MD, *EBO Chair,* Vienna, Austria; Tero Kivelä, MD, FEBO, *EBO Liaison,* Helsinki, Finland; Roderich Fellner, MD, Graz, Austria; Stefan Pieh, MD, Vienna, Austria; Klaus Rohrschneider, MD, FEBO, Heidelberg, Germany

Financial Disclosures

Academy staff members who contributed to the development of this product state that within the past 12 months, they have had no financial interest in or other relationship with any entity discussed in this course that produces, markets, resells, or distributes ophthalmic health care goods or services consumed by or used in patients, or with any competing commercial product or service.

The authors and reviewers state the following financial relationships:*

Dr D. Azar: ForSight Labs (C, O), Novartis Pharmaceuticals (C, O)

Dr N. Azar: None for self. Financial disclosure of spouse: ForSight Labs (C, O), Novartis Pharmaceuticals (C, O)

Dr Beaver: Genzyme (L)

Dr Clifford: Transcend Medical (S)

Dr Gangadhar: Inspire Pharmaceuticals (C, L)

Dr Hoffer: Haag-Streit (P), OCULUS (P), SLACK (P), Ziemer (P)

Dr Jackson: Optelec US (S)

Dr Mauger: Topcon Medical Systems (S)

Dr Rohrschneider: Heidelberg Engineering (L), Novartis Pharmaceuticals (C)

Dr Wiggins: Medflow/Allscripts (C), Ophthalmic Mutual Insurance Company (C)

The other authors and reviewers state that they have no significant financial interest or other relationship with the manufacturer of any commercial product discussed in this course or with the manufacturer of any competing commercial product.

*C = consultant fee, paid advisory boards, or fees for attending a meeting; L = lecture fees (honoraria), travel fees, or reimbursements when speaking at the invitation of a commercial sponsor; O = equity ownership/stock options of publicly or privately traded firms (excluding mutual funds) with manufacturers of commercial ophthalmic products or commercial ophthalmic services; P = patents and/or royalties that might be viewed as creating a potential conflict of interest; S = grant support for the past year (all sources) and all sources used for a specific talk or manuscript with no time limitation

Recent Past Faculty

> Penny A. Asbell, MD
> Neal H. Atebara, MD
> Forrest J. Ellis, MD
> Eleanor E. Faye, MD

In addition, the Academy gratefully acknowledges the contributions of numerous past faculty and advisory committee members who have played an important role in the development of previous editions of the Basic and Clinical Science Course.

American Academy of Ophthalmology Staff

Dale E. Fajardo, *Vice President, Education*
Beth Wilson, *Director, Continuing Professional Development*
Ann McGuire, *Acquisitions and Development Manager*
Stephanie Tanaka, *Publications Manager*
D. Jean Ray, *Production Manager*
Beth Collins, *Medical Editor*
Naomi Ruiz, *Editorial Assistant*

American Academy of Ophthalmology
655 Beach Street
Box 7424
San Francisco, CA 94120-7424

Contents

8   Physical Optics   285

General Introduction

The Basic and Clinical Science Course (BCSC) is designed to meet the needs of residents and practitioners for a comprehensive yet concise curriculum of the field of ophthalmology. The BCSC has developed from its original brief outline format, which relied heavily on outside readings, to a more convenient and educationally useful self-contained text. The Academy updates and revises the course annually, with the goals of integrating the basic science and clinical practice of ophthalmology and of keeping ophthalmologists current with new developments in the various subspecialties.

The BCSC incorporates the effort and expertise of more than 80 ophthalmologists, organized into 13 Section faculties, working with Academy editorial staff. In addition, the course continues to benefit from many lasting contributions made by the faculties of previous editions. Members of the Academy's Practicing Ophthalmologists Advisory Committee for Education, Committee on Aging, and Vision Rehabilitation Committee review every volume before major revisions. Members of the European Board of Ophthalmology, organized into Section faculties, also review each volume before major revisions, focusing primarily on differences between American and European ophthalmology practice.

Organization of the Course

The Basic and Clinical Science Course comprises 13 volumes, incorporating fundamental ophthalmic knowledge, subspecialty areas, and special topics:

1 Update on General Medicine
2 Fundamentals and Principles of Ophthalmology
3 Clinical Optics
4 Ophthalmic Pathology and Intraocular Tumors
5 Neuro-Ophthalmology
6 Pediatric Ophthalmology and Strabismus
7 Orbit, Eyelids, and Lacrimal System
8 External Disease and Cornea
9 Intraocular Inflammation and Uveitis
10 Glaucoma
11 Lens and Cataract
12 Retina and Vitreous
13 Refractive Surgery

In addition, a comprehensive Master Index allows the reader to easily locate subjects throughout the entire series.

References

Readers who wish to explore specific topics in greater detail may consult the references cited within each chapter and listed in the Basic Texts section at the back of the book.

These references are intended to be selective rather than exhaustive, chosen by the BCSC faculty as being important, current, and readily available to residents and practitioners.

Study Questions and CME Credit

Each volume of the BCSC is designed as an independent study activity for ophthalmology residents and practitioners. The learning objectives for this volume are given on page 1. The text, illustrations, and references provide the information necessary to achieve the objectives; the study questions allow readers to test their understanding of the material and their mastery of the objectives. Physicians who wish to claim CME credit for this educational activity may do so by following the instructions given at the end of the book.

Conclusion

The Basic and Clinical Science Course has expanded greatly over the years, with the addition of much new text and numerous illustrations. Recent editions have sought to place a greater emphasis on clinical applicability while maintaining a solid foundation in basic science. As with any educational program, it reflects the experience of its authors. As its faculties change and as medicine progresses, new viewpoints are always emerging on controversial subjects and techniques. Not all alternate approaches can be included in this series; as with any educational endeavor, the learner should seek additional sources, including such carefully balanced opinions as the Academy's Preferred Practice Patterns.

The BCSC faculty and staff are continually striving to improve the educational usefulness of the course; you, the reader, can contribute to this ongoing process. If you have any suggestions or questions about the series, please do not hesitate to contact the faculty or the editors.

The authors, editors, and reviewers hope that your study of the BCSC will be of lasting value and that each Section will serve as a practical resource for quality patient care.

Objectives

Upon completion of BCSC Section 3, *Clinical Optics,* the reader should be able to

- explain the principles of light propagation and image formation and work through some of the fundamental equations that describe or measure such properties as refraction, reflection, magnification, and vergence

- explain how these principles can be applied diagnostically and therapeutically

- describe the clinical application of Snell's law and the lensmaker's equation

- identify optical models of the human eye and describe how to apply them

- define the various types of visual perception and function, including visual acuity, brightness sensitivity, color perception, and contrast sensitivity

- summarize the steps for performing streak retinoscopy

- identify the steps for performing a manifest refraction using a phoropter or trial lenses

- describe the use of the Jackson cross cylinder

- describe the indications for prescribing bifocal lenses and common difficulties encountered in their use

- identify the materials and fitting parameters of both soft and rigid contact lenses

- explain the optical principles underlying various modalities of refractive correction: spectacles, contact lenses, intraocular lenses, and refractive surgery

- discern the differences among these types of refractive correction and describe how to apply them most appropriately to individual patients

- discuss the basic methods of calculating intraocular lens (IOL) powers and the advantages and disadvantages of the different methods

- explain the conceptual basis of multifocal IOLs and how the correction of presbyopia differs between IOLs and spectacles

- appraise the visual needs of low vision patients and determine how to address these needs through use of optical and nonoptical devices and/or appropriate referrals

- describe the operating principles of various optical instruments in order to use them more effectively

- compare and contrast physical and geometric optics

- describe the clinical and technical relevance of such optical phenomena as interference, coherence, polarization, diffraction, and scattering

- explain the basic properties of laser light and how they affect laser–tissue interaction

CHAPTER 1

Geometric Optics

Geometric optics is the study of light and images using geometric principles. In contrast, physical optics emphasizes the wave nature of light, and quantum optics (not covered in this text) emphasizes the particle nature of light and the interaction of light and matter. Geometric optics uses linear rays to represent the paths traveled by light.

This introductory chapter discusses the basic concepts of geometric optics that form the foundation for deeper understanding of the topics covered in subsequent chapters. Included are 6 Clinical Examples and 24 end-of-section and end-of-chapter exercises to reinforce these concepts. The chapter starts by discussing rays, refraction, and reflection; object and image characteristics; light propagation and the lensmaker's equation; vergence and reduced vergence; and ophthalmic lenses. After a set of exercises, the discussion continues with focal lengths and afocal systems, followed by another set of exercises. The final section discusses thick lenses, aberrations, mirrors, spherocylindrical lenses, and prisms. The end-of-chapter exercises are followed by 2 chapter appendixes with additional details.

Rays, Refraction, and Reflection

Introduction

Imagine a point source of light emitting light waves heading away from the point in all directions. If the medium in which the light travels is uniform, such that the wavefronts move at the same speed in all directions heading away from the source, then the expanding wavefronts are spherical. In geometric optics, we consider a ray to be an arrow denoting the direction of propagation of energy perpendicular to a wavefront surface (Fig 1-1). A ray is not a vector, as we do not attach any meaning to its length. If the medium is not uniform, such that light travels through regions of it at various speeds, then the expanding wavefronts become nonspherical and the rays will not form straight lines. This phenomenon explains how, for example, the regions of more and less dense air over a hot desert can form a mirage; to a thirsty observer, the image of a lake appears to come from a place other than where the lake is.

Let's assume that our light travels only in uniform media, so that we do have *spherical wavefronts* and *straight-line rays;* we will find that we can analyze the rays to understand what happens when the waves meet the *interface* between one uniform medium and

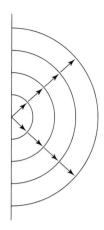

Figure 1-1 Rectilinear propagation of light through uniform medium. Here, the speed of light is constant with spherical wavefronts and straight rays. Note that in nonuniform medium, the speed of light is variable and rays are not straight. *(Illustration developed by Leon Strauss, MD, PhD.)*

another, and either travel into the new medium (refraction), bounce back into the first medium (reflection), or are lost as heat (absorption).

Refraction and reflection are called *diffuse* if the interface is so rough that the direction of the wavefronts is lost; they are called *specular* if there continues to be an identifiable direction of propagation of the wavefronts (Figs 1-2, 1-3).

If we study the behavior of these rays at refracting and reflecting surfaces, we can learn to determine how images are formed by optical systems, where they are located, and how large they are.

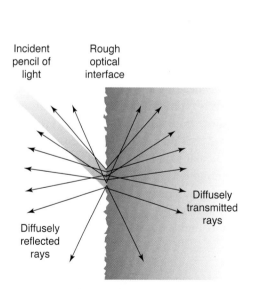

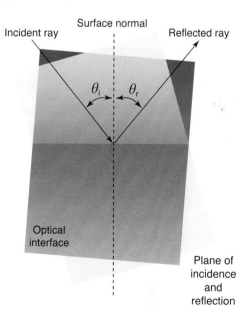

Figure 1-2 Light striking a rough surface is diffusely reflected and/or transmitted. *(Illustration developed by Kevin M. Miller, MD, and rendered by C. H. Wooley.)*

Figure 1-3 Light striking a smooth surface is specularly reflected and/or refracted. θ_i = angle of incidence; θ_r = angle of refraction. *(Illustration developed by Edmond H. Thall, MD, and Kevin M. Miller, MD, and rendered by C. H. Wooley.)*

Point Sources, Pencils, and Beams of Light

You can think of a distant star as a point source of light, as its apparent size is so small. If we cut off a portion of the bundle of rays of light that emanate from a point source by placing an aperture in their path, the light that passes through the hole is called a *pencil of rays* (Fig 1-4). The rays passing just inside the edges of the aperture are called *limiting rays*. The rays of a pencil of light are *divergent, parallel,* or *convergent* in the direction of travel of the light (Fig 1-5). Waves of light naturally diverge from their source but can become convergent if they are redirected, for instance, by passing through a convex lens.

A beam of light includes many pencils of light that arise from the points of an extended source (Fig 1-6). A light bulb and the sun are examples of extended sources of light, and the objects you see around you are extended sources of reflected light. A slide projector emits a mildly diverging beam of convergent pencils of light, each of which has been focused by a lens to converge to points on the screen across the room, forming a larger picture on the screen of the smaller picture on the slide. (See Clinical Example 1-1.)

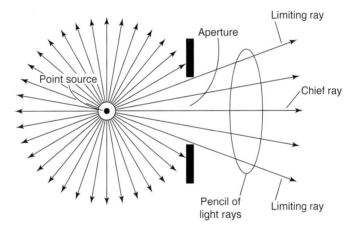

Figure 1-4 Point source of light and an aperture, creating a pencil of rays. *(Redrawn from Basic and Clinical Science Course Section 2: Optics, Refraction, and Contact Lenses. San Francisco: American Academy of Ophthalmology; 1986–1987:38. Fig 1.)*

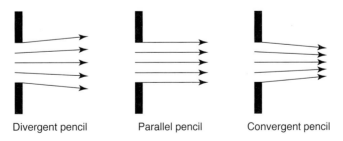

Figure 1-5 Divergent, parallel, and convergent pencils of light. *(Redrawn from Basic and Clinical Science Course Section 2: Optics, Refraction, and Contact Lenses. San Francisco: American Academy of Ophthalmology; 1986–1987:39. Fig 2.)*

Figure 1-6 A beam of light, consisting of pencils emanating from many point sources, that is being limited by an aperture. *(Redrawn from Basic and Clinical Science Course Section 2: Optics, Refraction, and Contact Lenses. San Francisco: American Academy of Ophthalmology; 1986–1987:39. Fig 3.)*

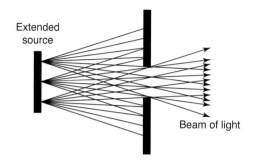

CLINICAL EXAMPLE 1-1

The concept of conjugate points is illustrated by retinoscopy. When performing retinoscopy, the examiner observes light emanating from the patient's retina and passing through the patient's pupil. Because the examiner is observing the light at the patient's pupil, the examiner's retina is conjugate with the patient's pupil (Fig 1-7A). At the point of neutrality in the refraction, the patient's retina is conjugate with the peephole of the retinoscope (Fig 1-7B). Adjustment for the distance between the examiner and the patient (working distance) makes the patient's retina conjugate with optical infinity (Fig 1-7C). (Retinoscopy is covered in detail in Chapter 3, Clinical Refraction.)

Another example of conjugacy is demonstrated by direct ophthalmoscopy. When the ophthalmoscope is focused to compensate for the refractive error of the examiner and that of the patient, the 2 retinas are

Figure 1-7   A, In retinoscopy, the examiner's eye is conjugate with the patient's pupil. **B,** At the point of neutrality, the patient's retina is conjugate with the retinoscope peephole. **C,** With the working distance subtracted, the patient's retina is conjugate with optical infinity. *(Illustration developed by Kevin M. Miller, MD, and rendered by C. H. Wooley.)*

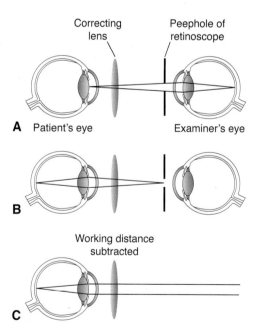

conjugate (Fig 1-8). An image of the patient's retina is present on the examiner's retina and vice versa. However, the patient does not "see" the examiner's retina, because it is not illuminated by the ophthalmoscope light and because this light is so bright.

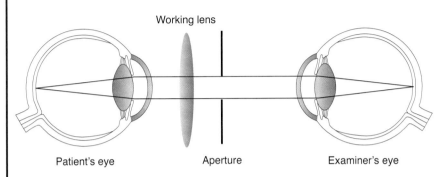

Figure 1-8 Conjugacy in direct ophthalmoscopy. *(Illustration developed by Kevin M. Miller, MD, and rendered by C. H. Wooley.)*

Object Characteristics

Objects may be characterized by their location with respect to the imaging system and by whether they are luminous. If an object point such as a candle flame produces its own light, it is called *luminous*. If it does not produce its own light, it can be imaged only if it is *reflective* and *illuminated*.

Image Characteristics

Images are described by characteristics such as magnification, location, quality, and brightness. Some of these features will be discussed briefly.

Magnification

Three types of magnification are considered in geometric optics: *transverse, angular,* and *axial.* The ratio of the height of an image to the height of the corresponding object is *transverse magnification* (Fig 1-9):

$$\text{Transverse Magnification} = \frac{\text{Image Height}}{\text{Object Height}}$$

To calculate transverse magnification, we compare the height of an object (ie, the distance an object extends above or below the optical axis) to that of its conjugate image (ie, the distance its image extends above or below the axis). *Object* and *image heights* are measured perpendicularly to the optical axis and, by convention, are considered positive when the object or image extends above the optical axis and negative when below the axis.

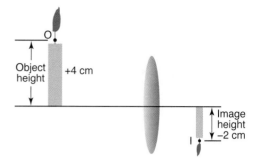

Figure 1-9 Object height (O) and image height (I) may be measured from any pair of off-axis conjugate points. *(Illustration developed by Edmond H. Thall, MD, and Kevin M. Miller, MD, and rendered by C. H. Wooley.)*

An image is a scale model of the object. If the object or image is upright (extending above the optical axis), a positive (+) sign is used; an object or image that is inverted (extending below the optical axis) is indicated by a minus (–) sign. The transverse magnification represents the size of the image in relation to that of the object. For instance, in Figure 1-9, the object height is +4 cm and the image height –2 cm; thus, the transverse magnification is –0.5, meaning that the image is inverted and half as large as the object. A magnification of +3 means the image is upright and 3 times larger than the object.

Transverse magnification can be confused with linear magnification. Linear magnification refers to the magnification of the *area* of an image relative to that of an object located perpendicular to the optical axis. For example, a 4 cm × 6 cm object imaged with a magnification of 2 produces an 8 cm × 12 cm image. Both width and length double, yielding a fourfold increase in image area. The reader should also not confuse transverse magnification with axial magnification, which is measured along the optical axis and is discussed at the end of this section. Generally, the multiplication sign, ×, is used to indicate magnification. The transverse magnification of microscope objectives, for example, is sometimes expressed by this convention.

The word *power* is sometimes used synonymously with *transverse magnification*. This is unfortunate because *power* has several different meanings, and confusion often arises. Other uses of the word include the terms *refracting power, resolving power, prism power,* and *light-gathering power.*

Most optical systems have a pair of *nodal points* (Fig 1-10). Occasionally, the nodal points overlap, appearing as a single point, but technically they remain a pair of overlapping nodal points. The nodal points are always on the optical axis and have an important property. From any object point, a unique ray passes through the anterior nodal point. This ray emerges from the optical system along the line connecting the posterior nodal point to the conjugate image point. These rays form 2 angles with the optical axis. The essential property of the nodal points is that these 2 angles are equal for any selected object point. Because of this feature, nodal points are useful for establishing a relationship among transverse magnification, object distance, and image distance. (See Appendix 1.1, Quick Review of Angles, Trigonometry, and the Pythagorean Theorem, at the end of the chapter.)

Regardless of the location of an object, the object and the image subtend equal angles with respect to their nodal points.

Optical system

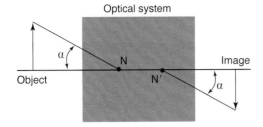

Figure 1-10 The anterior and posterior nodal points (N and N', respectively) of an optical system. The angle subtended by the object (α) is equal to the angle subtended by the image. *(Illustration developed by Kevin M. Miller, MD, and rendered by C. H. Wooley.)*

Therefore,

$$\text{Transverse Magnification} = \frac{\text{Image Height}}{\text{Object Height}} = \frac{\text{Image Distance } (i)}{\text{Object Distance } (o)}$$

Angular magnification is the ratio of the angular height subtended by an object viewed by the eye through a magnifying lens to the angular height subtended by the same object viewed without the magnifying lens. By convention, the standard viewing distance for this comparison is 25 cm. For small angles, the angular magnification *(M)* provided by a simple magnifier *(P)* is independent of the actual object size:

$$M = \frac{1}{4}P \quad \text{or} \quad M = \frac{P}{4}$$

More will be said about simple magnifiers later.

Axial magnification, also known as *longitudinal magnification,* is measured along the optical axis. For small distances around the image plane, axial magnification is the square of the transverse magnification.

$$\text{Axial Magnification} = (\text{Transverse Magnification})^2$$

For example, if an object 4 cm in height (perpendicular to the optical axis) and 0.5 cm in length along the optical axis is imaged with a transverse magnification of 2×, the axial magnification is 4×. This produces an 8 cm × 2 cm image (4 × 2 = 8 cm height perpendicular to the optical axis and 0.5 × 4 = 2 cm length along the optical axis). This concept will be discussed in greater detail in Chapter 7.

Image Location

Another important characteristic of an image is its location. Refractive errors result when images formed by the eye's optical system are in front of or behind the retina. Image location is specified as the distance (measured along the optical axis) between a reference point associated with the optical system and the image.

The reference point depends on the situation. It is often convenient to use the back surface of a lens as a reference point. The back lens surface is usually not at the same location as the posterior nodal point, but it is easier to locate.

Frequently, image distance is measured from the posterior principal point to the image. The principal points (discussed later in the chapter), like the nodal points, are a pair of useful reference points on the optical axis. The nodal points and principal points often overlap.

Whatever reference point is used to measure image distance, the sign convention is always the same:

By convention, when the image is to the right of the reference point, image distance is positive; when the image is to the left of the reference point, the distance is negative.

Depth of Focus

If we perform a basic imaging demonstration with a lens and focus an image of a light source on a paper, we notice that if the paper is moved forward or backward within a range of a few millimeters, the image remains relatively focused. With the paper positioned outside this region, the image appears blurred. The size of this region represents the *depth of focus,* which may be small or large depending on several factors. (See Clinical Example 1-2.) In the past, depth of focus was of concern only in the management of presbyopia. However, it is an important concept in refractive surgery as well.

Depth of focus applies to the image. *Depth of field* is the same idea applied to objects. If a camera or other optical system is focused on an object, nearby objects are also in focus. Objects within the range of depth of field will be in focus, whereas objects outside the depth of field will be out of focus.

Image Quality

Careful examination reveals that some details in an object are not reproduced in the image. Images are imperfect facsimiles, not exact scaled duplicates of the original object.

Consider an object 50 cm in front of a pinhole 1 mm in diameter. Paper is placed 50 cm behind the pinhole, so the magnification is –1×. A small pencil of rays from each object point traverses the pinhole aperture (Fig 1-11A, B).

Each object point produces a 2-mm-diameter spot in the image. These spots are called *blur circles.* This term is somewhat misleading because off-axis object points technically produce elliptical spots in the image. In addition, this analysis ignores diffraction effects that make the spot larger and more irregular. Regardless, each object point is represented by a blur circle in the image. The farther the image is from the pinhole, the larger the blur circle in the image. To the extent that these blur circles overlap, the image detail is reduced (blurred).

CLINICAL EXAMPLE 1-2

Pinholes are often placed in front of the naked eye to screen for uncorrected refractive error. Positioned over existing glasses and contact lenses, a pinhole screens for residual refractive errors. What is the depth of focus of a pinhole?

When an object is distant from a pinhole aperture, the image formed is relatively focused and remains so over a relatively long range. Thus, a pinhole creates a very long depth of focus.

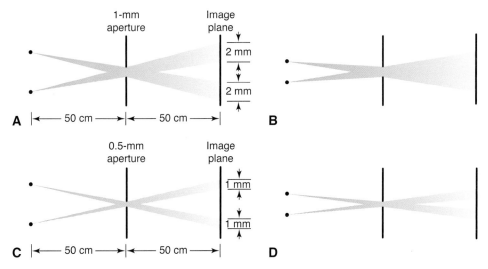

Figure 1-11 **A,** In pinhole imaging, a small pencil of rays from each object point traverses the aperture, producing a small spot in the image. **B,** If the object points are too close to each other, their images overlap. **C,** A smaller pinhole restricts light from a single object point to a smaller spot in the image. **D,** Object points can be closer together before their images overlap, and thus the image contains more detail. This analysis ignores diffraction effects. *(Illustrations developed by Kevin M. Miller, MD, and rendered by C. H. Wooley.)*

To some extent, the loss of detail is mitigated with the use of a smaller pinhole (Fig 1-11C, D). A smaller pinhole gives a dimmer, but more detailed, image. However, the smaller the pinhole, the more that diffraction reduces image quality.

Although a smaller blur circle preserves more detail, the only way to avoid any loss of detail is to produce a perfect point image of each object point. Theoretically, if a perfect point image could be produced for every point of an object, the image would be an exact duplicate of the object. A perfect point image of an object point is called a *stigmatic image. Stigmatic* is derived from the Greek word *stigma,* which refers to a sharply pointed stylus.

Loss of detail occurs in lens and mirror imaging as well, because light from an object point is distributed over a region of the image rather than being confined to a perfect image point (Fig 1-12). Generally, lenses focus light from a single object point to a spot 10–100 μm across. This is better than a typical pinhole, but the shape of the spot is very irregular. The term *blur circle* is especially misleading when applied to lenses and mirrors. A better term is *point spread function (PSF),* which describes the way light from a single object point is spread out in the image.

To summarize, a stigmatic image is a perfect point image of an object point. However, in most cases, images are not stigmatic. Instead, light from a single object point is distributed over a small region of the image known as a blur circle or, more generally, a PSF. The image formed by an optical system is the spatial summation of the PSF for every object point. The amount of detail in an image is related to the size of the blur circle or PSF for each object point. The smaller the PSF, the better the resemblance between object and image.

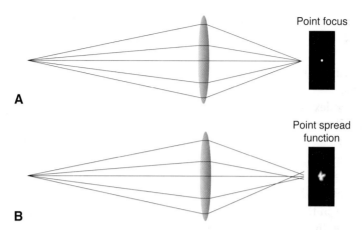

Point focus

A

Point spread
function

B

Figure 1-12   A, Textbooks often illustrate images produced by lenses as stigmatic. **B,** In most cases, however, the images are not stigmatic. The point spread function reveals how faithfully an imaging system reproduces each object point. *(Illustration developed by Kevin M. Miller, MD, and rendered by C. H. Wooley.)*

Light Propagation

An intensive investigation of light propagation was begun in the late 1500s. Numerous experiments measuring light deviation were conducted, and the data were collected and summarized as laws. These laws are described in the following sections.

Optical Media and Refractive Index

Light travels through a variety of materials, such as air, glass, plastics, liquids, crystals, some biological tissues, the vacuum of space, and even some metals. A *medium* is any material that transmits light.

Light travels at different speeds in different media. Light moves fastest in a vacuum and slower through any material. The refractive index of an optical medium is the ratio of the speed of light in a vacuum to the speed of light in the medium and is usually denoted in mathematical equations by the lowercase letter n. The speed of light in a vacuum is 299,792,458 m/s. This speed is approximately equal to 300 million meters per second, or 186,000 miles per second. In 1983, the Système International defined a meter as the distance light travels in a vacuum during 1/299,792,458 of a second. (This concept is discussed in greater detail in Chapter 8.) Refractive index is always greater than or equal to 1. In computations, it is often easier to work with the refractive index of a material than directly with the speed of light.

The refractive index,

$$n = \frac{\text{Speed of Light in Vacuum}}{\text{Speed of Light in Medium}}$$

is quite sensitive to a material's chemical composition. A small amount of salt or sugar dissolved in water changes its refractive index. Because refractive index is easy to measure accurately, chemists use it to identify compounds or determine their purity. Glass manufacturers alter the refractive index of glass by adding small amounts of rare earth elements. Until recently, clinical laboratories screened for diabetes mellitus by measuring the refractive index of urine. Table 1-1 lists the refractive indices of various tissues and materials of clinical interest.

Refractive index varies with temperature and barometric pressure, but these changes are usually small enough to be ignored. One exception is for silicone polymer. The refractive index of polymerized silicone at room temperature (20°C) differs enough from its index at eye temperature (35°C) that manufacturers of silicone intraocular lenses (IOLs) have to account for the variation.

Refractive index also varies with wavelength. As discussed in Chapter 8, physical optics regards light in the spectrum of electromagnetic waves. The visual system perceives different wavelengths of light as different colors. Long wavelengths appear red, intermediate wavelengths appear yellow or green, and short wavelengths appear blue. In a vacuum, all wavelengths travel at the same speed. In other mediums, short wavelengths usually travel more slowly than long wavelengths. This phenomenon is called *dispersion.*

In the human eye, chromatic dispersion leads to *chromatic aberration.* If yellow wavelengths are focused precisely on the retina, blue light will be focused in front of the retina and red light will be focused behind the retina. (See Clinical Example 1-3.)

Some media, such as quartz, are optically inhomogeneous. That is, the speed of light through the material depends on the direction of light propagation through the material.

Law of Rectilinear Propagation

The law of rectilinear propagation states that light in a homogeneous medium travels along straight-line paths called *rays.* The light ray is the most fundamental construct in geometric optics. Of particular note, rays traversing an aperture continue in straight lines in geometric optics. As stated earlier, a bundle of light rays traveling close to each other in the same direction is known as a *pencil of light.*

The law of rectilinear propagation is inaccurate insofar as it does not account for the effect of diffraction as light traverses an aperture (see Chapter 8). The basic distinction between physical and geometric optics is that geometric optics ignores diffraction because it is based on the law of rectilinear propagation. For clinical purposes, diffraction effects

Table 1-1 Refractive Index (Helium D Line) for Some Materials of Clinical Interest

Material	Refractive Index
Air	1.000
Water	1.333
Aqueous and vitreous humor	1.336
Cornea	1.376
Silicone	1.438
Acrylic	1.460
Polymethylmethacrylate (PMMA)	1.492
Spectacle crown glass	1.523

CLINICAL EXAMPLE 1-3

You may notice that red objects appear nearer than blue objects when they are displayed against a black background (Fig 1-13). This effect stands out in slide presentations that are rich in red and blue text and is known as *chromostereopsis*. It occurs because the human eye has approximately 0.5 D of chromatic aberration. Even individuals with red-green color blindness can observe the effect. To bring red print into focus, the eye must accommodate. To bring blue print into focus, the eye must relax accommodation. As a result, red print appears closer than blue print. The accommodative effort required to bring the various pieces of a chromatic image into focus imparts a 3-dimensional quality to the image.

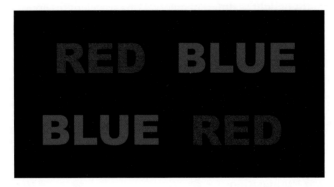

Figure 1-13 Chromostereopsis is demonstrated by this illustration of red and blue print on a black background. The illustration is not very dramatic unless rendered on a computer monitor or projected onto a screen. *(Illustration developed by Kevin M. Miller, MD, and rendered by C. H. Wooley.)*

are rarely important. However, in situations for which diffraction effects are significant, geometric optics does not fully describe the image.

Optical Interfaces

The boundary between 2 different optical media is called an *optical interface*. Typically, when light reaches an optical interface, some light is transmitted through the interface, some is reflected, and some is absorbed, or converted to heat, by the interface. The amount of light transmitted, reflected, and absorbed depends on several factors.

Law of Reflection (Specular Reflection)

In specular reflection, the direction of the reflected ray bears a definite relationship to the direction of the incident ray. To express a precise relationship between incident rays and reflected rays, it is necessary to construct an imaginary line perpendicular to the optical interface at the point where the incident ray meets the interface. This imaginary line is a *surface normal* (Fig 1-14). The surface normal and the incident ray together define an

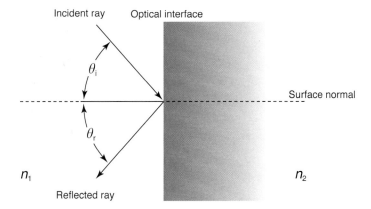

Figure 1-14 The law of specular reflection. The angle of reflection (θ_r) is equal to the angle of incidence (θ_i) and lies in the same plane (in this case the plane of the paper) that contains the incident ray and the "normal" perpendicular to the surface. n_1 = refractive index of initial medium; n_2 = refractive index of reflecting medium. *(Illustration developed by Edmond H. Thall, MD, and Kevin M. Miller, MD, and rendered by C. H. Wooley.)*

imaginary plane known as the *plane of incidence and reflection.* The angle formed by the incident ray and surface normal is the *angle of incidence,* θ_i. This is not the angle between the incident ray and the optical interface. The reflected ray and the surface normal form the *angle of reflection,* θ_r.

The law of reflection states that the reflected ray lies in the same plane as the incident ray and the surface normal (ie, the reflected ray lies in the plane of incidence) and that $\theta_i = \theta_r$.

The amount of light reflected from a surface depends on θ_i and the plane of polarization of the light. The general expression for reflectivity is derived from the Fresnel equations, which are beyond the scope of this text. The reflectivity at normal incidence is simple and depends only on the optical media bounding the interface. The *reflection coefficient* for normal incidence is given by

$$R = \left(\frac{n_2 - n_1}{n_2 + n_1} \right)^2$$

The reflection coefficient is used to calculate the amount of light transmitted at an optical interface if absorption losses are minimal.

Law of Refraction (Specular Transmission)

In specular transmission, the transmitted ray's direction bears a definite relation to the incident ray's direction. Again, a surface normal is constructed, and the angle of incidence and the plane of incidence and transmission are defined just as they were for reflection (Fig 1-15). The angle formed by the transmitted ray and the surface normal is the *angle of refraction,* also known as the *angle of transmission.* The angle of transmission, θ_t, is preferred by some authors because the symbol for angle of refraction, θ_r, might otherwise be confused with that of the angle of reflection, θ_r.

At the optical interface, light undergoes an abrupt change in speed that, in turn, usually produces an abrupt change in direction. The law of refraction, also known as *Snell's*

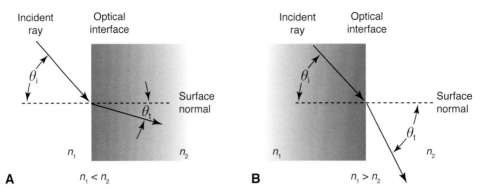

Figure 1-15 Light moving from a lower index to a higher one bends toward the surface normal **(A),** and that from a higher to a lower index bends away from the surface normal **(B).** *(Illustration developed by Edmond H. Thall, MD, and Kevin M. Miller, MD, and rendered by C. H. Wooley.)*

law in honor of its discoverer, states that the refracted, or transmitted, ray lies in the same plane as the incident ray and the surface normal and that

$$n_i \sin \theta_i = n_t \sin \theta_t$$

where

n_i = refractive index of incident medium
θ_i = angle of incidence
n_t = refractive index of transmitted medium
θ_t = angle of transmission (or refraction)

When light travels from a medium of lower refractive index to a medium of higher refractive index, it bends toward the surface normal. Conversely, when light travels from a higher to a lower refractive index, it bends away from the surface normal (Clinical Example 1-4; see Fig 1-15).

Normal Incidence

Normal incidence occurs when a light ray is perpendicular to the optical interface. In other words, the surface normal coincides with the ray. If the interface is a refracting surface, the ray is undeviated. Light changes speed as it crosses the interface but does not change direction. If the surface reflects specularly, rays and pencils of light will be reflected back along a 90° angle to the surface.

Total Internal Reflection

Total internal reflection (TIR) occurs when light travels from a high-index medium to a low-index medium and the angle of incidence exceeds a certain *critical angle*. Under these circumstances, the incident ray does not pass through the interface; all light is reflected back into the high-index medium. The law of reflection governs the direction of the reflected ray.

CLINICAL EXAMPLE 1-4

Imagine you are fishing from a pier and you spot a "big one" in front of you a short distance below the surface of the water. You don't have a fishing rod, but instead you are armed with a spear (Fig 1-16). How should you throw the spear to hit the fish?

From your knowledge of Snell's law, you know that the fish is not where it appears to be. If you throw the spear at the fish, you will certainly miss it. What you have to do is throw the spear in front of the virtual fish, the one you see, to hit the real fish.

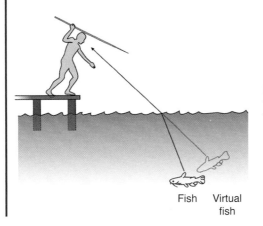

Figure 1-16 The fisherman must throw the spear in front of the virtual fish to hit the actual fish. *(Illustration developed by Kevin M. Miller, MD, rendered by Jonathan Clark, and modified by Neal H. Atebara, MD.)*

Fish   Virtual
        fish

Figure 1-17A shows a light ray traveling from a high-index medium (spectacle crown glass) into a low-index medium (air). In this situation, the transmitted ray bends away from the surface normal, and thus the angle of transmission exceeds the angle of incidence. As the angle of incidence increases, the angle of transmission increases to a greater degree. Eventually, the angle of transmission equals 90°. At this point, the ray grazes along the optical interface and is no longer transmitted (Fig 1-17B).

The critical angle is the angle of incidence that produces a transmitted ray 90° to the surface normal. The critical angle, θ_c, is calculated from Snell's law:

$$n_i \sin \theta_c = n_t \sin 90°$$

The sine of 90° is 1; thus,

$$n_i \sin \theta_c = n_t$$

Rearranging gives

$$\sin \theta_c = \frac{n_t}{n_i}$$

So, the angle of transmission is 90° when the angle of incidence is

$$\theta_c = \arcsin \frac{n_t}{n_i}$$

In the current example, $n_i = 1.000$ and $n_t = 1.523$, so the critical angle is 41.0°.

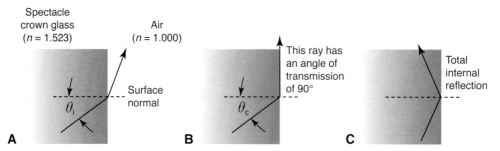

Figure 1-17 A, When light travels from a high-index medium to a low-index medium, it bends away from the surface normal. **B,** At the critical angle, θ_c, the refracted light travels in the optical interface. **C,** Beyond the critical angle, all light is reflected by the interface. In **A** and **B,** light is also reflected by the interface (not shown). *(Illustration developed by Kevin M. Miller, MD, and rendered by C. H. Wooley.)*

What happens when the angle of incidence exceeds the critical angle? As Figure 1-17C shows, the angle of transmission increases as the angle of incidence increases, but the angle of transmission cannot exceed 90°. Consequently, refraction cannot occur. Indeed, Snell's law has no valid mathematical solution (in real numbers) when the critical angle is exceeded. Instead, the incident ray is 100% reflected.

TIR is a rather curious phenomenon. Consider light traveling from spectacle crown glass to air. If the angle of incidence is 10°, the light transmits easily as it crosses the interface. However, if the angle of refraction is 45°, the interface becomes an impenetrable barrier! The interface is transparent to some rays and opaque to others. Physicists have devoted considerable attention to this phenomenon.

TIR has great practical value. In the early 1600s, it was difficult to make a good mirror. The best surfaces could specularly reflect only about 80% of incident light, and the rest was diffusely reflected, which made these surfaces nearly useless as imaging devices. However, TIR is just that—total. When TIR occurs, 100% of the light is reflected. In the past, often the only way to make a practical mirror was to use internally reflecting prisms. Today, TIR is still used in prisms within binoculars, slit lamps, and operating microscopes, for example. Clinically, TIR is a nuisance when clinicians are trying to examine the anterior chamber angle. (See Clinical Example 1-5.)

CLINICAL EXAMPLE 1-5

Total internal reflection (TIR) makes it impossible to view the eye's anterior chamber angle without the use of a contact lens. Light from the angle undergoes TIR at the air–cornea interface (technically, the air–tear-film interface) (Fig 1-18A). Light from the angle never escapes the eye. Using a contact lens to eliminate the air at the surface of the cornea (Fig 1-18B) overcomes the problem. Light travels from the cornea (or coupling gel) to the higher-index contact lens. TIR never occurs when light travels from a medium of lower index to one of higher index, so light enters the contact lens and is

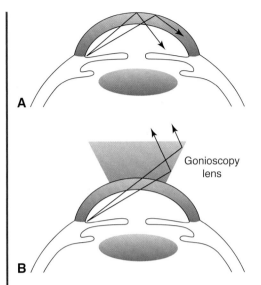

Figure 1-18 **A,** Light from the anterior chamber angle undergoes total internal reflection (TIR) at the air–tear-film interface. **B,** A contact lens prevents TIR and allows visualization of the angle structures. *(Illustration developed by Kevin M. Miller, MD, and rendered by C. H. Wooley.)*

reflected from the mirror. TIR does not occur at the front surface of the contact lens because the angle of incidence is less than the critical angle.

Assuming the refractive index of the tear film on the front surface of the cornea is 1.333, the critical angle for the air–tear-film interface is

$$\theta_c = \arcsin \frac{1}{1.333} = 48.6°$$

From trigonometry, we can estimate the angle at which light rays from the trabecular meshwork strike the air–tear-film interface. The situation is illustrated in Figure 1-19 using average anatomical dimensions. We ignore the effect of the back surface of the cornea because this surface has relatively little power and we are performing only a rough calculation. From basic trigonometry,

$$\theta_i = \arctan \frac{5.5}{3.5} = 57.5°$$

Interestingly, this rough calculation shows that θ_c is exceeded by only a few degrees. When the cornea is ectatic (as in some cases of keratoconus), the angle of incidence is less than θ_c and the angle structures are visible without a gonioscopy lens.

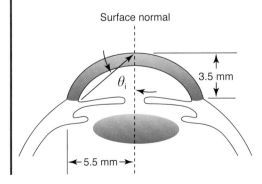

Surface normal

3.5 mm

θ_i

←5.5 mm→

Figure 1-19 Average anatomical dimensions of the anterior segment. *(Illustration developed by Kevin M. Miller, MD, and rendered by C. H. Wooley.)*

Dispersion

With the exception of a vacuum, which always has a refractive index of 1.000, refractive indices are not fixed values. They vary as a function of wavelength. In general, refractive indices are higher for short wavelengths and lower for long wavelengths. As a result, blue light travels more slowly than red light in most media, and Snell's law predicts a greater angle of refraction for blue light than for red light (Fig 1-20).

The *Abbe number,* also known as the *V-number,* is a measure of a material's dispersion. Named for the German physicist Ernst Abbe (1840–1905), the Abbe number V is defined as

$$V = \frac{n_D - 1}{n_F - n_C}$$

where n_D, n_F, and n_C are the refractive indices of the Fraunhofer D, F, and C spectral lines (589.2 nm, 486.1 nm, and 656.3 nm, respectively). Low-dispersion materials, which demonstrate low chromatic aberration, have high values of V. High-dispersion materials have low values of V. Abbe numbers for common optical media typically range from 20 to 70.

Reflection and Refraction at Curved Surfaces

For the sake of simplicity, the laws of reflection and refraction were illustrated at flat optical interfaces. However, most optical elements have curved surfaces. To apply the law of reflection or refraction to curved surfaces, the position of the surface normal must be determined because the angles of incidence, reflection, and refraction are defined with respect to the surface normal. Once the position of the surface normal is known, the laws of refraction and reflection define the relationship between the angle of incidence and the angles of refraction and reflection, respectively.

Although there is a mathematical procedure for determining the position of the surface normal in any situation, the details of it are beyond the scope of this text. For selected geometric shapes, however, the position of the surface normal is easy to determine. In particular, the surface normal to a spherical surface always intersects the center of the sphere.

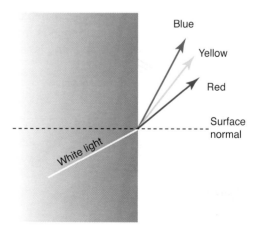

Figure 1-20 Chromatic dispersion. *(Illustration developed by Kevin M. Miller, MD, and rendered by C. H. Wooley.)*

For example, Figure 1-21 shows a ray incident on a spherical surface. The incident ray is 2 cm above, and parallel to, the optical axis. The surface normal is found with the extension of a line connecting the center of the sphere to the point where the incident ray strikes the surface. The angle of incidence and the sine of the angle of incidence are determined by simple trigonometry.

The Fermat Principle

The mathematician Pierre de Fermat posited that light travels from one point to another along the path requiring the least time. Both Snell's law of refraction and the law of reflection can be mathematically derived from the Fermat principle. This principle is summarized below and further detailed in Appendix 1.2 at the end of this chapter.

Suppose that the law of refraction were unknown, and consider light traveling from a point source in air, across an optical interface, to some point in glass (Fig 1-22). Unaware of Snell's law, we might consider various hypothetical paths that light might follow as it moves from point A to point B. Path 3 is a straight line from A to B and is the shortest total distance between the points. However, a large part of path 3 is inside glass, where light travels more slowly. Path 3 is not the fastest route. Path 1 is the longest route from A to B

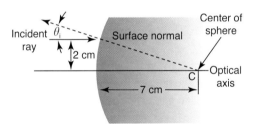

Figure 1-21 A ray 2 cm above and parallel to the optical axis is incident on a spherical surface. The surface normal is found by connecting the point where the ray strikes the surface to the center of the sphere (point C). The angle of incidence is found using similar triangles and trigonometry (arctan 2/7 = 16.6°). *(Illustration developed by Edmond H. Thall, MD, and Kevin M. Miller, MD, and rendered by C. H. Wooley.)*

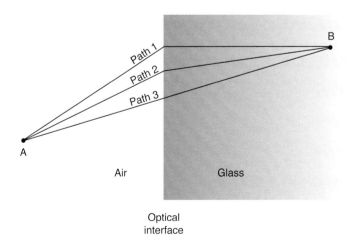

Figure 1-22 Light traveling from points A to B follows only path 2 because it requires the least time. Light does not travel along either path 1 or path 3. *(Illustration developed by Edmond H. Thall, MD, and Kevin M. Miller, MD, and rendered by C. H. Wooley.)*

but has the shortest distance in glass. Nevertheless, the extreme length of the overall route makes this a fairly slow path. Path 2 is the best compromise between distance in glass and total path length, and this is the path light will actually follow.

Using mathematics beyond the scope of this text, it can be shown that the optimal path is the one predicted by Snell's law. Thus, Snell's law is a consequence of the Fermat principle.

Figure 1-23 shows light from an object point traveling along 2 different paths to the image point. According to the Fermat principle, the time required to travel from object to image point (or, alternatively, the *optical path length, OPL*) must be exactly identical for each path or the paths will not intersect at the image point.

Pinhole Imaging

The pinhole camera is the earliest (c. 400 BC) known imaging device. Creating your own pinhole camera is an easy and worthwhile exercise. You can make a viewing screen by taping a piece of waxed paper to a simple frame cut out of poster board or the backing of a pad of paper. Another method is to create a pinhole near the middle of a fairly large opaque material such as a large index card.

In a dark room, light a candle, hold the pinhole about 30 cm (≈1 foot) from the candle, and place the screen about 30 cm behind the pinhole. You should observe an inverted image of the flame on the screen.

There is an image anywhere behind the pinhole, so a pinhole camera requires no focusing. However, the image is often too faint to be observed. Increasing pinhole size brightens but also blurs the image.

If you replace the pinhole with a +8.00 D spherical convex trial lens, the image is much brighter but appears in only one location behind the lens. In fact, you will probably have to adjust the distance between the lens and screen to get a clear image. Lenses overcome the main disadvantage of pinhole imaging—faint images—but sacrifice the main advantage—no need to focus. For lenses, image location is crucial.

Locating the Image: The Lensmaker's Equation

Increase the distance between the candle and lens to about 1 m (≈1.1 yard). You must move the screen closer to the lens to see a brighter, smaller image. Move the lens closer to the candle and the image is farther away from the lens.

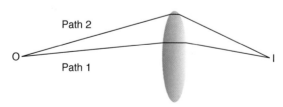

Figure 1-23 Light traveling the shorter distance from object (O) to image (I) point traverses a thick part of the lens. Light traveling the longer path 2 goes through less glass. If the lens is properly shaped, the greater distance in air is perfectly compensated for by the shorter distance in glass, and the time required to travel from object to image is identical for both paths. *(Illustration developed by Edmond H. Thall, MD, and Kevin M. Miller, MD, and rendered by C. H. Wooley.)*

The situation is shown schematically in Figure 1-24. The optical axis is an imaginary but well-defined line determined by rotational symmetry of the lens. The vertices V and V′ are the intersections of the axis with the lens surfaces. More important, the principal points P and P′ are major reference points used to define several other variables. Point P is the object principal point and P′ the image principal point. Object distance, o, is measured from P to the object, and image distance, i, is measured from P′ to the image (Fig 1-25). Note that the principal points are not the same as the vertices and do not even have to be "inside" the lens.

The image location can be calculated using the lensmaker's equation (discussed below):

$$\frac{1}{o} + P = \frac{1}{i'}$$

By convention, light travels from left to right, which is the positive direction. Suppose an object is 0.50 m in front of a +6.00 D lens. Because object distance is measured from P to the object, its direction is right to left, or negative. According to the lensmaker's equation,

$$\frac{1}{-0.50 \text{ m}} + (+6.00 \text{ D}) = \frac{1}{i'}$$

The unit diopter is a reciprocal meter, so $\dfrac{1}{-0.50 \text{ m}} = -2.00$ diopters

$$(-2.00 \text{ D}) + (+6.00 \text{ D}) = \frac{1}{i'}$$

$$+4.00 \text{ D} = \frac{1}{i'}$$

$$i' = \frac{1}{+4.00 \text{ D}}$$

Again, because a diopter is a reciprocal meter, $\dfrac{1}{+4.00 \text{ D}} = +0.25$ meter

$$i' = +0.25 \text{ m}$$

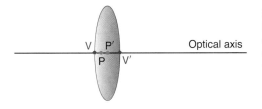

Figure 1-24 The optical axis is an imaginary but well-defined line defined by the lens's symmetry. The vertices V and V′ are the points of intersection of the axis with the lens surfaces. In general, the principal points P and P′ do not coincide with the vertices. *(Illustration developed by Edmond H. Thall, MD.)*

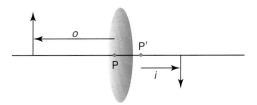

Figure 1-25 Definition of the variables in the lensmaker's equation. Object distance, o, is measured along the axis from P to the object, and image distance, i, is measured along the axis from P′ to the image. The positive direction is left to right. *(Illustration developed by Edmond H. Thall, MD.)*

The lensmaker's equation

The lensmaker's equation (LME) is as follows:

$$\frac{n}{o} + P = \frac{n'}{i} \quad \text{or} \quad U + P = V$$

where the ratio n/o is the *reduced object vergence (U)* and the ratio n'/i is the *reduced image vergence (V)*. The concepts of *vergence* and *reduced vergence* are discussed in detail in the section Ophthalmic Lenses.

The LME is one of the most important equations in ophthalmology. Unfortunately, it is also one of the most misused equations in ophthalmology.

Fundamentally, the LME says 2 things. First, the location of the image depends on the location of the object. Consider a specific example wherein the refractive index of a glass rod is 1.5 and the radius of curvature is 0.1 m. Suppose an object is in air with $n = 1.0$. The LME becomes

$$\frac{1}{o} + \frac{1.5 - 1.0}{0.1\,\text{m}} = \frac{1.5}{i}$$

or

$$\frac{1}{o} + 5\,\text{m}^{-1} = \frac{1.5}{i}$$

Note the units of reciprocal, or inverse, meters. Suppose the object is 1 m in front of the lens. Object distances are negative, so

$$\frac{1}{-1\,\text{m}} + 5\,\text{m}^{-1} = 4\,\text{m}^{-1} = \frac{1.5}{i}$$

$$i = \frac{1.5}{4\,\text{m}^{-1}} = 0.375\,\text{m}$$

Thus, the image is 37.5 cm behind the refracting surface.

Second, the LME establishes a relationship between the shape of the refracting surface and its optical function. The radius of the spherical refracting surface affects the image characteristics. The *refractive power* (or simply *power*) of a spherical refracting surface is

$$P = \frac{n' - n}{r}$$

To demonstrate the significance of power, consider 2 spherical refractive surfaces, both constructed from glass rods ($n = 1.5$). Suppose that 1 refracting surface has a radius of 10 cm, as in the previous example, and the other has a radius of 20 cm. If an object is 1 m in front of each surface, where is the image? As shown in the previous example, the first surface has a power of 5.0 D and produces an image 37.5 cm behind the surface. The second surface has a power of 2.5 D and forms an image 1 m behind the refracting surface. Notice that the second surface has half the power, but the image is more than twice as far behind the refracting surface.

Refractive power, strictly speaking, applies to spherical surfaces, but the cornea is not spherical. In general, every point on an aspheric surface is associated with infinitely many curvatures. There is no such thing as a single radius of curvature. The sphere is a very special case: a single radius of curvature characterizes the entire sphere. A single radius can characterize no other shape, and refractive power should not be applied to a nonspherical surface.

In addition, power is a paraxial concept; thus, it applies only to a small area near the optical axis. Power is not applicable to nonparaxial regions of the cornea. In the paraxial region, imaging is stigmatic (ie, paraxial rays focus to a common point). Even for spherical surfaces, rays outside the paraxial region do not focus to a single point. That is, away from the paraxial region, rays do not focus as predicted when the LME is used.

For further information about first-order optics and the lensmaker's equation, see Appendix 1.2 at the end of the chapter.

Ophthalmic Lenses

In this section, we build upon the basic principles of first-order optics to show how both simple lenses and complex optical systems are modeled. We also demonstrate how imaging problems are solved.

Vergence

We begin by considering the concept of vergence. Light rays emanating from a single object point spread apart and are referred to as *divergent*. Light rays traveling toward an image point, after passing through an optical lens, come together and are referred to as *convergent*. If rays are diverging, the vergence is negative; if rays are converging, the vergence is positive. Consider a lens placed close to an object point (Fig 1-26A). The lens collects a large fraction of the light radiating from the object point. When the lens is moved away from the object point, it collects a smaller portion of the light radiated by the object

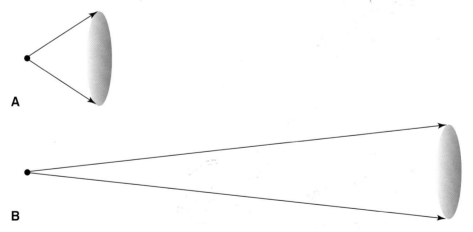

Figure 1-26 **A,** Close to an object point, light is strongly divergent, so a lens placed close to the object point collects a large fraction of the light radiated from the point. **B,** Farther from an object point, light is much less divergent, so a lens collects a much smaller portion of the light radiated by the object point. *(Illustration developed by Kevin M. Miller, MD, and rendered by C. H. Wooley.)*

point. The rays that reach the lens are less divergent than they were when the lens was closer to the object (Fig 1-26B). Close to the object point, the light is more divergent; farther from the object point, the light is less divergent. Similarly, close to an image point, light is more convergent; farther from the image point, light is less convergent.

Vergence is inversely proportional to distance from the object or image point. Vergence is the reciprocal of the distance. The distances used most often in ophthalmology are 4 m, 2 m, 1 m, 0.5 m, 0.33 m, 0.25 m, and 0.2 m. For convenience, the reciprocal meter (m^{-1}) is given another name, the *diopter (D)*. The reciprocals of these distances are, respectively, 0.25 m^{-1} (or 0.25 D), 0.5 m^{-1} (or 0.5 D), 1 m^{-1} (or 1 D), 2 m^{-1} (or 2 D), 3 m^{-1} (or 3 D), 4 m^{-1} (or 4 D), and 5 m^{-1} (or 5 D).

As light travels away from an object point or toward an image point, its vergence constantly changes. To calculate the vergence of light at any point, one must know the location of the object or image point. Conversely, if one knows the vergence at a selected point, the position of the object or image point can be determined.

Reduced Vergence

Reduced vergence is vergence multiplied by the refractive index of the medium. This term is confusing because reduced vergence is numerically larger than vergence. For example, 1 m in front of an image point, light traveling in glass ($n = 1.5$) has a vergence of +1.0 D but a reduced vergence of +1.5 D. Confusing or not, however, the term *reduced vergence* is too well entrenched to be changed.

The LME can be interpreted in terms of reduced vergence. Light from an object point diverges, but the degree of divergence decreases as the light moves farther from the object point. Eventually, the light encounters the refracting surface, and just as it reaches the surface, it has a reduced vergence of n/o. The refracting surface suddenly changes the light's vergence by an amount equal to its power. As the light leaves the refracting surface, it has a reduced vergence of $(n/o) + P$, but because the light is converging to an image point, this must equal n'/i.

Calculations using the LME are inconvenient because they involve reciprocal distances. Vergence is a way to simplify the calculations. By means of reduced vergence, the LME,

$$\frac{n}{o} + P = \frac{n'}{i}$$

can be written in a very simple form:

$$U + P = V$$

where U is *reduced object vergence* and V is *reduced image vergence.*

Consider an object in air 50 cm in front of a +5 D refracting surface with $n = 1.5$. Where is the image? Light diverging from the object has a negative vergence. When the light reaches the lens, it has a reduced vergence of –2 D. The lens adds +5 D, for a final reduced vergence at the lens of +3 D. The plus sign indicates that the light converges as it leaves the lens. Dividing the reduced vergence by the index of the glass gives a vergence of +2 D, so the image is 50 cm behind the refracting surface.

The most common mistake in working with vergence calculations is ignoring the negative sign for divergent light. One way to avoid this mistake is to deal with the signs first, rather than with the numbers. For example, to solve the previous problem, many people would begin by converting distance to diopters—that is, the object is 50 cm from the lens, so the vergence is 2 D. After this conversion has been performed, it is easy to forget about the minus sign. It is better to deal with the sign first. In this problem, begin by noting that light diverges from the object and has a negative value; then write down the negative sign and convert distance to vergence (–2 D). Always write the sign in front of the vergence, even when the sign is positive, as in the preceding example (+5 D and +3 D). If you encounter difficulties with a vergence calculation, check the signs first. The problem is most likely a dropped minus sign. (See Clinical Example 1-6.)

Thin-Lens Approximation

The LME concerns a single refracting surface, but, of course, lenses have 2 surfaces. According to the LME, when light from an object strikes the front surface of a lens, its (reduced) vergence changes by an amount equal to the power of the front surface, P_f. The vergence continues to change as the light moves from the front to the back surface; this is known as the *vergence change on transfer*, P_t. The back lens surface changes the vergence by an amount equal to the back-surface power, P_b. Thus,

$$\frac{n}{o} + P_f + P_t + P_b = \frac{n'}{i}$$

The powers of the front and back lens surfaces are easily calculated, but the vergence change on transfer is difficult to calculate. However, because the vergence change on

---

CLINICAL EXAMPLE 1-6

Imagine you are having a difficult time outlining the borders of a sub-retinal neovascular membrane on a fluorescein angiogram. You pull out a 20 D indirect ophthalmoscopy lens and use it as a simple magnifier. If you hold the lens 2.5 cm in front of the angiogram, where is the image?

Light from the angiogram enters the 20 D lens with a reduced vergence of

$$U = -\frac{1}{0.025 \text{ m}} = -40 \text{ D}$$

It exits the lens with a reduced vergence of

$$-40 \text{ D} + 20 \text{ D} = -20 \text{ D}$$

The light is divergent as it exits the lens; thus, the virtual image you see is on the same side of the lens as the angiogram. It is located (1/20 D) = 0.05 m = 5 cm in front of the lens. Because the image is twice as far from the lens as is the object, the transverse magnification is 2×.

transfer is small in a thin lens, it is ignored to arrive at the thin-lens approximation. The total lens power is the sum of the front- and back-surface powers. Thus,

$$\frac{n}{o} + P = \frac{n'}{i}$$

This is the *thin-lens equation (TLE)*. Although the TLE and LME appear to be the same, there is an important difference. In the LME, P is the power of a single surface; in the TLE, P is the combined power of the front and back surfaces.

For example, if a +5 D thin lens has water ($n = 1.33$) in front and air in back and an object is 33 cm in front of the lens, where is the image? Light from the object strikes the lens with a reduced vergence of ($-1.33/0.33$ m) = -4 D. The lens changes the vergence by +5 D, so light leaves the lens with a vergence of +1 D, forming an image 1 m behind the lens.

The transverse magnification is the ratio of reduced object vergence to reduced image vergence. In the preceding example, the magnification is $-4\times$, indicating that the image is inverted and 4 times as large as the object.

Lens Combinations

Most optical systems consist of several lenses. For instance, consider an optical system consisting of 2 thin lenses in air. The first lens is +5 D, the second lens is +8 D, and they are separated by 45 cm. If an object is placed 1 m in front of the first lens, where is the final image and what is the transverse magnification?

In paraxial optics, the way to analyze a combination of lenses is to look at each lens individually. The TLE shows that the first lens produces an image 25 cm behind itself with a magnification of -0.25. Light converges to the image and then diverges again. The image formed by the first lens becomes the object for the second lens. The image is 20 cm in front of the second lens; thus, light strikes the second lens with a vergence of -5 D and forms an image 33 cm behind the second lens. The transverse magnification for the second lens alone is (-5 D/3 D) = -1.66. The total magnification is the product of the individual magnifications $-1.66 \times -0.25 = 0.42$.

It is absolutely essential to calculate the position of the image formed by the first lens. Only after locating the first image is it possible to calculate the vergence of light as it reaches the second lens.

Any number of lenses can be analyzed in this way. Locate the image formed by the first lens and use it as the object for the second lens. Repeat the process for each subsequent lens. The overall transverse magnification is the product of the transverse magnifications produced by each individual lens.

Virtual Images and Objects

Many people find the subject of virtual images and virtual objects to be the most difficult aspect of geometric optics. Virtual images and objects can be understood with the use of a few simple rules. The trick is to not "overthink" the subject.

Consider an object 10 cm in front of a +5 D thin lens in air (Fig 1-27A). Light strikes the lens with a vergence of -10 D and leaves with a vergence of -5 D. In this case, unlike in

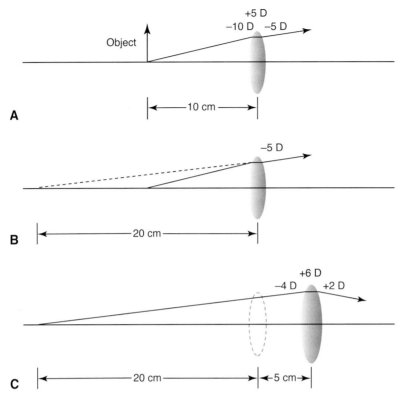

Figure 1-27 Light exits the +5 D lens with a vergence of –5 D **(A)**, producing a virtual image 20 cm in front of the lens **(B)**. The virtual image becomes the object for the +6 D lens, which in turn produces a real image 50 cm to the right of the lens **(C)**. *(Illustration developed by Kevin M. Miller, MD, and rendered by C. H. Wooley.)*

all the previous examples, light emerges with a negative vergence, which means that light is still diverging after crossing the lens. No real image is produced. The reader can easily verify this by repeating the basic imaging demonstration with a +5 D spherical convex trial lens. Notice that an image does not appear, no matter where the paper is held.

Now, suppose a +6 D thin lens is placed 5 cm behind the first lens. Will an image form? If so, what are its characteristics? Light has a vergence of –5 D, but as the light crosses the 5 cm to the second lens, its vergence changes (the vergence change on transfer). In order to determine the vergence at the second lens, it is necessary to find the location of the image formed by the first lens. However, if the first lens does not form an image, how can the vergence at the second lens be calculated?

The solution is to use a mathematical trick. Light leaving the first lens has a vergence of –5 D. The same vergence would be produced by an object 20 cm away if the first lens were not present (Fig 1-27B).

So, light leaving the second lens appears to be coming from an object 20 cm away from the first lens and 25 cm away from the second lens. The virtual image formed by the first lens is a real object for the second lens. When this imaginary object is used as a reference point, it is easy to see that the vergence at the second lens is –4 D. When light leaves the second lens, it has a vergence of +2 D, forming a real image 50 cm behind the second lens (Fig 1-27C).

In this example, an imaginary reference point was used to determine the vergence at the second lens. In geometric optics, this reference point is commonly called the *virtual image* formed by the first lens. A virtual image is a mathematical convenience that allows all of the formulas developed thus far (ie, the LME, TLE, and transverse magnification formulas) to be used even when a lens does not form a real image.

Mathematically, virtual images are used in exactly the same way as real images. In Figure 1-27, the first lens forms a virtual image 20 cm to the left. The transverse magnification for the first lens is (−10 D/−5 D) = 2×. Thus, the virtual image is upright and twice as large as the original object. This virtual image now becomes the object for the second lens. The vergence at the second lens is −4 D, and after the light traverses the second lens, the vergence is +2 D. The image now formed is real and 50 cm to the right of the second lens. The transverse magnification for the second lens is −2. The total magnification is therefore 2 × −2 = −4×. The final image is inverted and 4 times larger than the original. Again, this is verified with trial lenses.

Objects may also be virtual. Consider an object 50 cm in front of a +3 D thin lens in air. A +2 D thin lens in air is placed 50 cm behind the first lens. The first lens forms a real image 1 m to the right. However, before the light can reach this image, it strikes a second lens. The image formed by the first lens is the object for the second lens, but this object is on the wrong side of the lens. Thus, it is called a *virtual object* (Fig 1-28).

Here, unlike in all the previous examples, light is convergent when it strikes the second lens (vergence = +2 D). The second lens increases the vergence to +4 D, forming a real image 25 cm behind the second lens. The transverse magnification for the first lens is −2 and for the second lens +0.5, for a total magnification of −1×.

A common misconception is that inverted images are real and upright images are virtual. This is not the case. The correct rule is very simple: For any individual lens, the object is virtual when light striking the lens is convergent, and the object is real when light striking the lens is divergent. When light emerging from the lens is convergent, the image is real, and when light emerging from a lens is divergent, the image is virtual.

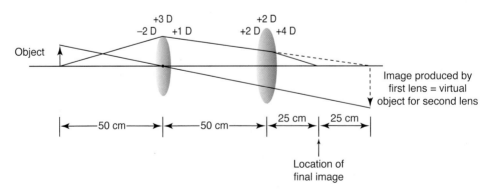

Figure 1-28 The real image formed by the +3 D lens is the virtual object for the +2 D lens. *(Illustration developed by Kevin M. Miller, MD, and rendered by C. H. Wooley.)*

Focal Points and Planes

The +5 D lens in Figure 1-29A has an *anterior (primary) focal point,* F_a, that is (1/5 D) = 0.2 m = 20 cm in front of the lens. By definition, light emanating from F_a exits the lens collimated and comes to a focus at plus optical infinity. The same is true of light emanating from any point in the *anterior focal plane* (Fig 1-29B). Collimated light entering a lens from minus optical infinity images to the *posterior (secondary) focal point,* F_p (Fig 1-29C). Collimated off-axis rays from minus infinity focus to the *posterior focal plane* (Fig 1-29D). For a thin lens immersed in a uniform optical medium such as air or water, F_a and F_p are equidistant from the lens. For a convex (plus-power) spherical lens, F_a is located anterior to the lens and F_p is located posterior to the lens. For a concave (minus-power) spherical lens, the points are reversed: F_a is posterior to the lens and F_p, anterior to the lens. To avoid confusion, some authors prefer the terms F and F′ instead of F_a and F_p.

Paraxial Ray Tracing Through *Convex* Spherical Lenses

From any object point, 3 simple rays are drawn through a thin lens to locate a corresponding point in the image. Only 2 rays are actually needed. The same rays are used to find

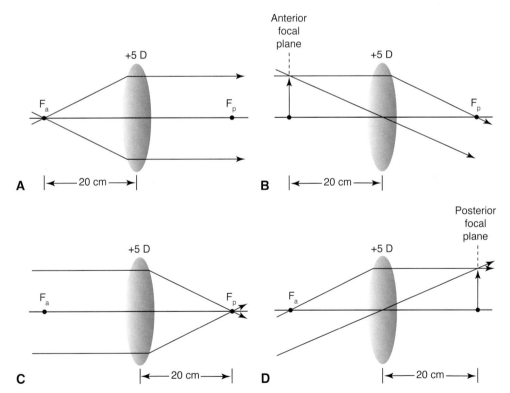

Figure 1-29 **A,** Light that emanates from the anterior focal point, F_a, leaves the lens collimated. **B,** All object points in the anterior focal plane focus to plus optical infinity. **C,** Collimated on-axis light from minus optical infinity focuses to the posterior focal point, F_p. **D,** Collimated off-axis rays focus to the posterior focal plane. *(Illustration developed by Kevin M. Miller, MD, and rendered by C. H. Wooley.)*

corresponding points if a thick lens or a multi-element lens system is modeled by first-order optical principles. The first 2 rays traverse F_a and F_p. The final ray, known as the *central ray* or *chief ray*, traverses the nodal points. For a thin lens immersed in a medium with a uniform refractive index, the nodal points overlap at the optical center of the lens. The central ray traverses the nodal point undeviated; that is, it does not change direction with respect to the optical axis as it passes through the lens.

It is customary to represent objects as arrows to show size and orientation. The tip of an arrow represents a single object point. Suppose an object is placed 20 cm in front of a +10 D lens immersed in air (Fig 1-30).

A ray is drawn from the tip of the object through F_a. This ray emerges from the lens parallel to the optical axis and heads off to plus infinity. A second ray is drawn that parallels the optical axis until it enters the lens. It emerges from the lens and passes through F_p on its way to plus infinity. The intersection of these 2 rays defines the corresponding image point. Note that the image in this example is inverted. The location of the image is determined by vergence calculations. The vergence of light entering the lens is (–1/0.2 m) = –5 D. By the LME, the vergence of light exiting the lens is –5 D + 10 D = +5 D. The image is located (1/5 D) = 0.2 m = 20 cm to the right of the lens. Because the object and image are equidistant from the lens, the transverse magnification is –1×. The central ray can also be drawn through the optical center of the lens to confirm the location of the image.

Now suppose the object in the previous example is moved closer so that it is 5 cm in front of the lens instead of 20 cm in front (inside F_a), as shown in Figure 1-31A. The ray that leaves F_a and passes through the object point emerges from the lens parallel to the optical axis. The ray that enters the lens parallel to the optical axis exits through F_p. Finally, the central ray traverses the optical center of the lens undeviated. On the back side of the lens, these 3 rays are divergent. So where is the image? If you are looking at the back side of the lens, you see the image point as the backward extension of all 3 rays (Fig 1-31B).

By the LME, the vergence of light exiting the lens is –10 D. The image is located (1/–10 D) = 10 cm to the left of the lens. The image is upright and virtual, and by similar triangles, its transverse magnification is +2×. This is the optical basis of a simple, handheld plus-lens magnifier. An object positioned inside the focal point of a plus spherical lens will produce a magnified, upright, virtual image. Try this simple experiment with the lens you use for indirect ophthalmoscopy.

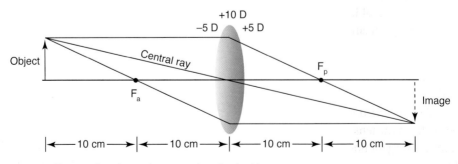

Figure 1-30 Ray tracing through a convex spherical lens. *(Illustration developed by Kevin M. Miller, MD, and rendered by C. H. Wooley.)*

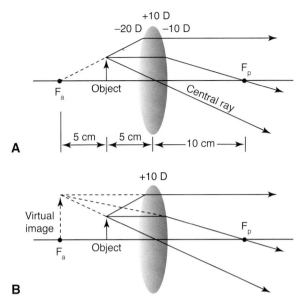

Figure 1-31 Ray tracing through a convex spherical lens. **A,** This time, the object is located inside the anterior focal point. **B,** The image is magnified, upright, and virtual and is located to the left of the object. *(Illustration developed by Kevin M. Miller, MD, and rendered by C. H. Wooley.)*

Paraxial Ray Tracing Through *Concave* Spherical Lenses

In the examples we have used thus far, the lenses have been convex, or positive. Light emerges from a convex lens more convergent—or at least less divergent—than it entered. By contrast, a concave, or negative, lens makes light more divergent.

The principles of paraxial ray tracing are the same for concave spherical lenses as for convex spherical lenses. Consider a –2 D lens. Its F_a is (1/–2 D) = 50 cm behind the lens. By definition, a ray of light directed through F_a will exit the lens parallel to the optical axis (Fig 1-32A). Similarly, a virtual object in the anterior focal plane of a concave lens will image to plus infinity. A ray of light entering the lens parallel to the optical axis will pass through F_p after exiting the lens (Fig 1-32B). Similarly, a real object at minus optical infinity will produce a virtual image in the posterior focal plane of a concave lens.

Now consider an object placed 100 cm in front of the lens. The 3 usual rays are drawn (Fig 1-33). A virtual image is formed 33 cm in front of the lens. By similar triangles, the transverse magnification is +0.33×. No matter where a real object is placed in front of a minus lens, the resulting image is upright, minified, and virtual.

Objects and Images at Infinity

If an object is placed 50 cm in front of a +2 D thin lens in air, where is the image? Light emerges from the lens with a vergence of zero. A vergence of zero means that light rays are neither convergent nor divergent but parallel; thus, the light is collimated. In this example, light rays emerge parallel to one another, neither converging to a real image nor diverging from a virtual image. In this case, the image is said to be at *infinity*.

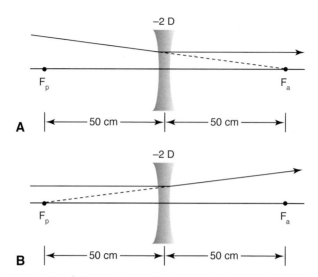

Figure 1-32 **A,** Incoming light directed through the anterior focal point, F_a, of a concave spherical lens exits the lens collimated. **B,** Collimated incoming light parallel to the optical axis leaves the lens as if it had come through the posterior focal point, F_p. *(Illustration developed by Kevin M. Miller, MD, and rendered by C. H. Wooley.)*

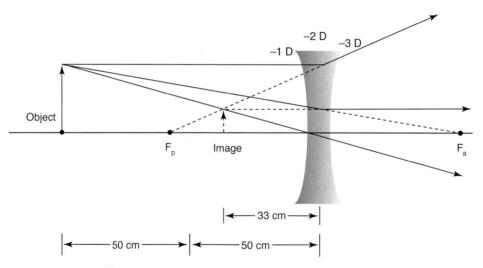

Figure 1-33 No matter where a real object is placed in front of a concave (negative) spherical lens, the image is upright, minified, and virtual. *(Illustration developed by Kevin M. Miller, MD, and rendered by C. H. Wooley.)*

Objects can be located at infinity as well. If a second lens is placed anywhere behind the first one, light striking the second lens has a vergence of zero; the object is at infinity. As a practical matter, a sufficiently distant object may be regarded as being at infinity. Clearly, an object like the moon, which is 400 million meters away, has a vergence of essentially zero. For clinical work, objects more than 20 ft (6 m) distant may be regarded as being at optical infinity. An object 20 ft away has a vergence of about −0.17 D; clinically, this is small enough to be ignored. When a refractive correction is being determined, few patients can notice a change of less than 0.25 D.

Some people think that objects in the anterior focal plane are imaged in the posterior focal plane. This is not true. Objects in the anterior focal plane image at plus infinity; objects at minus infinity image in the posterior focal plane.

Principal Planes and Points

If an object's position changes in front of a lens, both the location and magnification of the image change. Most optical systems have one particular object location that yields a magnification of 1. In other words, when an object is located in the correct position, the image will be upright and the same size as the object. The principal planes are perpendicular to the optical axis and identify the object and image locations that yield a magnification of 1. The principal planes are also called the *planes of unit magnification* and are geometric representations of where the bending of light rays occurs.

Consider an optical system consisting of 2 thin lenses in air (Fig 1-34). The first lens is +6 D, the second lens is +15 D, and the 2 lenses are separated by 35 cm. An object located 50 cm in front of the first lens is imaged 25 cm behind the first lens with a magnification of –0.5. The real image becomes a real object for the second lens, which produces a real image 20 cm behind the second lens with a magnification of –2. The *anterior principal plane* of this system is 50 cm in front of the first lens; the *posterior principal plane* is 20 cm behind the second lens. Often, both the anterior and posterior principal planes are virtual; in some cases, the posterior principal plane is in front of the anterior principal plane.

The intersection of the anterior and posterior principal planes with the optical axis defines the corresponding *anterior* and *posterior principal points*. Like the nodal points, the principal points are an important pair of reference points.

Collectively, the nodal points, focal points, and principal points are called the *cardinal points*, because these 3 pairs of points completely describe the first-order properties of an optical system. Notice that 2 pairs of cardinal points are conjugate. The posterior principal

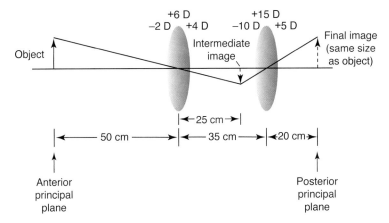

Figure 1-34 These 2 thin lenses in air produce an image that is upright, real, and the same size as the object. *(Illustration developed by Kevin M. Miller, MD, and rendered by C. H. Wooley.)*

point is the image of the anterior principal point, and the same relationship holds for the nodal points. The focal points, however, are not conjugate. Two pairs of cardinal points are associated with planes: the focal points and the principal points, but there is no such thing as a nodal plane associated with a nodal point.

Section Exercises

Questions

1.1. An object is 25 cm to the left of point P for a +9.00 D lens. Where is the image?

1.2. An object is 1 m to the left of point P for a +9.00 D lens. Where is the image?

1.3. An object is 20 cm to the left of point P for a +9.00 D lens. Where is the image?

1.4. An object is 50 cm to the left of point P for a +5.00 D lens. Where is the image?

1.5. An object is 25 cm to the left of point P for a +5.00 D lens. Where is the image?

1.6. Suppose the object is 1.00 m to the right of point P, and the lens has a power of +4.00 D (Fig 1-35). Where is the image?

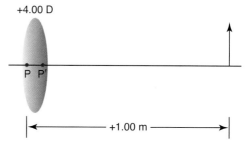

Figure 1-35 In this case, the object is to the right of point P. Since by convention light moves from left to right, how does light from the object reach the lens? *(Illustration developed by Edmond H. Thall, MD.)*

1.7. A (virtual) object is 50 cm to the right of P for a +2.00 D lens. Where is the image?

1.8. A (virtual) object is 1 m to the right of P for a +1.00 D lens. Where is the image?

1.9. A (virtual) object is 40 cm to the right of P for a +2.50 D lens. Where is the image?

1.10. Locate the image of an object 1 m to the left of P for a –4.00 D lens.

1.11. Suppose an object is 50 cm to the left of a +10.00 D lens. A +9.00 D lens is 32.5 cm to the right of the first lens (Fig 1-36). Where is the image?

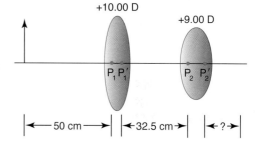

Figure 1-36 Example of imaging using 2 lenses. *(Illustration developed by Edmond H. Thall, MD.)*

1.12. An object in air is 50 cm to the left of P and the lens power is +6.00 D. On the other side of the lens is water ($n = 1.33$). Where is the image?

Answers

1.1. The image is 20 cm to the right of point P′.
1.2. The image is 12.5 cm to the right of point P′.
1.3. The image is 25 cm to the right of point P′.
1.4. The image is 33 cm to the right of point P′.
1.5. The image is 1.00 m to the right of point P′.
1.6. This situation does not seem to make sense. If light starts at the object and moves to the right, how does it ever reach the lens? Putting that rather important question aside for the moment, apply the LME:

$$\frac{1}{+1.00 \text{ m}} + (+4.00 \text{ D}) = \frac{1}{i'}$$

$$+5.00 \text{ D} = \frac{1}{i'}$$

$$i' = \frac{1}{+5.00 \text{ D}}$$

$$i' = +0.20 \text{ m}$$

Although this situation seems unrealistic, it does have practical value, as discussed later. For now, it is enough to understand that even in this case, the LME can be used to calculate an image location (Fig 1-37). To distinguish this case from those of the previous questions, the object is called virtual. The rule is that an object to the left of P is real, whereas an object to the right of P is virtual.

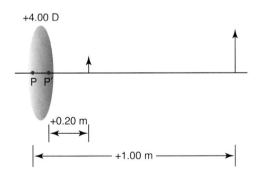

+4.00 D

P P′

+0.20 m

+1.00 m

Figure 1-37 Although the situation seems unrealistic, an image location can still be calculated using the lensmaker's equation. If you try this using trial lenses, however, you will not observe an image 20 cm to the right of P′. See text for explanation. *(Illustration developed by Edmond H. Thall, MD.)*

1.7. The image is 25 cm to the right of P′.
1.8. The image is 50 cm to the right of P′.
1.9. The image is 20 cm to the right of P′.
1.10. Note that the lens power was positive in all previous questions. Again, apply the LME. Skipping some intermediate steps,

$$i' = \frac{1}{-5.00 \text{ D}}$$

$$i' = -0.20 \text{ m}$$

A negative image distance means the image is to the left of point P (Fig 1-38). This is another confusing situation: how can the image form before the light gets to the lens? In this case, the object is real, but the image is virtual. The rule is that the image is real if it is to the right of P' and virtual if to the left of P'.

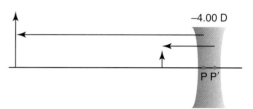

Figure 1-38 Example of imaging by a lens with negative power. The object is real, but the image is virtual. *(Illustration developed by Edmond H. Thall, MD.)*

If you try to do this experiment using a candle and trial lens, you will find that no matter where you locate the viewing screen, you will not see an image. The significance of virtual objects and images will become clear in the next section.

1.11. The procedure is to start with the first lens and completely ignore the second lens for the moment. From the standpoint of the first lens, the object is real and the first lens produces a real image. According to the LME, the first lens produces an image 12.5 cm to the right of P_1' (Fig 1-39):

$$\frac{1}{-0.5} + (+10.00 \text{ D}) = \frac{1}{i'}$$

$$i' = 12.5 \text{ cm}$$

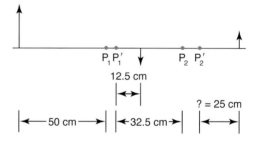

Figure 1-39 The first lens produces an image 12.5 cm to the right of P_1'. Note that the outlines of the lenses have been omitted. Because all distances are measured from principal points, the lens outlines provide no additional information, and the diagram is less cluttered without them. *(Illustration developed by Edmond H. Thall, MD.)*

Now, from the standpoint of the second lens, the real image formed by the first lens becomes a real object for the second lens. The image formed by the first lens is 20 cm to the left of P_2. Applying the LME to the second lens shows the final image is 25 cm to the right of P_2'.

In this case, the image formed by the first lens became the object for the second lens, which in turn produced a final image. Any number of lenses can be analyzed in the same way. The image produced by the first lens becomes the object for the second lens; the image formed by the second lens becomes the object for the third lens; and so forth. Note in this case that the intermediate, inverted image can be observed by placing a screen 12.5 cm to the right of P_1'.

Consider a second 2-lens example (Fig 1-40). An object is 12.5 cm to the left of a +10.00 D lens, and 10 cm to the right of the first lens is a +7.50 D lens. Where is the final image? Applying the LME, the first lens produces an image 50 cm to the right of P_1'. The first lens produces a real image because it is to the right of P_1'.

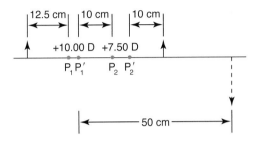

Figure 1-40 Another 2-lens example. In this case, light never reaches the image produced by the first lens *(inverted dashed arrow)* because it is intercepted by the second lens. Placing a screen 50 cm behind the first lens will not show an image. *(Illustration developed by Edmond H. Thall, MD.)*

The first image becomes the object for the second lens. Because the first image is to the right of P_2, it is a virtual object for the second lens. For the second lens, the object is 40 cm to the right of P_2, so the object distance is +0.40 m. Thus,

$$\frac{1}{+0.40 \text{ m}} + (+7.50 \text{ D}) = \frac{1}{i'}$$

$$+10.00 \text{ D} = \frac{1}{i'}$$

$$i' = \frac{1}{+10.00 \text{ D}} = 10 \text{ cm}$$

The final image is 10 cm to the right of P_2' and therefore real. In this case, you cannot observe the intermediate virtual image, but the final real image can be observed on a screen placed 10 cm behind the second lens.

The significance of virtual objects and images is that they allow us to analyze systems of multiple lenses. Simply apply the LME to each lens in a serial fashion. The image formed by 1 lens becomes the object for the next lens. The concept of virtual objects and images is necessary for this approach to work. Granted, the procedure becomes quite tedious when applied to systems of several lenses, but conceptually the method is straightforward.

1.12. Optically, the cornea acts as a lens with air on one side and aqueous on the other. All of the questions thus far have had the same material (air) on both sides of the lens. When the refractive index on either side of the lens is not 1.00, the LME must be modified. The appropriate equation is

$$\frac{n}{o} + P = \frac{n'}{i'}$$

$$\frac{1.00}{-0.50 \text{ m}} + (+6.00 \text{ D}) = \frac{1.33}{i'}$$

$$+4.00\,\text{D} = \frac{1.33}{i'}$$

$$i' = \frac{1.33}{+4.00\,\text{D}}$$

$$i' = +0.33\,\text{m}$$

Note that if air were on both sides of the lens, the image distance would have been +0.25 m.

Focal Lengths

For any optical system, the distance from the anterior principal point to the anterior focal point is the *anterior focal length (AFL)*. Similarly, the *posterior focal length (PFL)* is the distance from the posterior principal point to the posterior focal point.

Following the sign convention, focal lengths are negative when the focal point is to the left of the principal point and positive when the focal point is to the right of the principal point. For instance, a +5 D thin lens in air has an *AFL* of –20 cm and a *PFL* of +20 cm.

For any optical system, focal lengths and refractive power *P* are related by

$$AFL = \frac{n_o}{P} \qquad PFL = \frac{n_i}{P}$$

For any optical system, the distance from the anterior principal point to the anterior nodal point is always equal to the distance from the posterior principal point to the posterior nodal point. The distance between principal point and nodal point follows the sign convention and is given by

$$\text{Distance} = AFL + PFL$$

For instance, for a +5 D thin lens in air, *AFL* + *PFL* = –20 cm + 20 cm = 0. Thus, the nodal points and principal points overlap. For a +5 D thin lens with water (*n* = 1.33) in front and air in back, the *AFL* = –26.6 cm and the *PFL* = 20 cm. Thus, the nodal points are 6.6 cm to the left of the principal points.

Gaussian Reduction

Thus far, we have discussed the properties of a single optical system. The treatment of refractive errors usually involves adding a lens to an existing optical system, the patient's eye. Gaussian reduction describes what happens when 2 optical systems (such as a correcting lens and the eye) are combined.

When 2 optical systems—each with its own cardinal points—are combined, a totally new optical system is created that is described by a new set of cardinal points. The thick-lens equation is used to reduce the 2 individual systems to a single system with its own set of cardinal points. Typically, the combined system's cardinal points and power differ from those of either of the individual systems. Clinically, Gaussian reduction is most important when used in conjunction with the correction of ametropias (discussed in Chapter 3) and in the calculation of IOL power (see Chapter 5).

Knapp's Law, the Badal Principle, and the Lensmeter

One problem in treating refractive errors is that the correcting lens often changes the size of the retinal image. If the retinal image in 1 eye differs in size from that in the other eye, the difference is usually tolerated by the patient unless this difference is large. The adult brain can fuse retinal images that differ in size by as much as 8%; the child's brain can handle an even greater disparity. According to Knapp's law, the size of the retinal image does not change when the center of the correcting lens (to be precise, the posterior nodal point of the correcting lens) coincides with the anterior focal point of the eye (Fig 1-41).

For example, if eyes have identical refractive power and differ only in axial length, then placing a lens at the anterior focal point of each eye will produce retinal images identical in size. However, it is rare that the difference between eyes is purely axial. In addition, the anterior focal point of the eye is approximately 17 mm in front of the cornea (see Chapter 2). Although it is possible to wear glasses so the spectacle lens is 17 mm in front of the eye, most people prefer to wear them at a corneal vertex distance of 10–15 mm. Because the clinician is rarely certain that any ametropia is purely axial, Knapp's law has limited clinical application.

Manual lensmeters make use of the same principle, although for an entirely different reason. When applied to lensmeters, Knapp's law is called the *Badal principle*. One type of optometer used for performing objective refraction is based on a variation of Knapp's law wherein the posterior focal plane of the correcting lens coincides with the anterior nodal point of the eye. The effect is the same. Retinal image size remains constant. In this application, the law is called the *optometer principle*. Optical engineers use

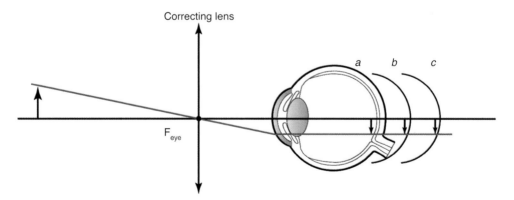

Figure 1-41 Illustration of Knapp's law. If the refractive power of eyes is the same but the axial length varies *(a, b, c)*, a correcting lens placed at the anterior focal point of each eye (F_{eye}) will produce an identical retinal image size regardless of the axial length. In this example, the power of the correcting lens will change depending on the axial length of the eye. However, the retinal image size will remain constant. *(Illustration by C. H. Wooley.)*

a variation of Knapp's law called *telecentricity* to improve the performance of telescopes and microscopes. Regardless of the name, the principle remains the same.

Afocal Systems

Consider an optical system consisting of 2 thin lenses in air (Fig 1-42). The lens powers are +2 D and –5 D, respectively. Where is F_p for this system? The posterior focal point is where incoming parallel rays focus. However, as ray tracing demonstrates, rays entering the system parallel to the optical axis emerge parallel to the axis. This system has no focal points; in other words, it is an afocal system.

If an object is 2 m in front of the first lens, where is the image and what is the transverse magnification? Vergence calculations show that the image is virtual, that it is 44 cm to the left of the second lens (14 cm to the left of the first lens), and that the transverse magnification is 0.4×. If an object is 4 m in front of the first lens, vergence calculations show that the image is virtual, that it is 76 cm to the left of the second lens, and that the transverse magnification is exactly 0.4. In afocal systems, the transverse magnification is the same for every object regardless of location.

Where are the principal planes for this system? Actually, it has no principal planes. Remember, the principal planes are the unique conjugates with a transverse magnification of 1. In this system, the transverse magnification is always 0.4 and never 1. If the transverse magnification were equal to 1, it would be 1 for every pair of conjugates. Consequently, there would be no unique set of planes that could be designated principal planes. In general, afocal systems do not have cardinal points.

Afocal systems are used clinically as telescopes or low vision aids. The 2 basic types of refracting telescopes are the *Galilean telescope* (named for, but not invented by, Galileo) and the *Keplerian,* or *astronomical telescope* (invented by Johannes Kepler). The Galilean telescope consists of 2 lenses. The first lens, the *objective lens,* is always positive and usually has a low power, whereas the second lens, the *eyepiece,* or *ocular,* is always negative and usually has a high power. The lenses are separated by the difference in their focal lengths. The afocal system depicted in Figure 1-42 is a Galilean telescope. The Galilean telescope is also used in some slit-lamp biomicroscopes.

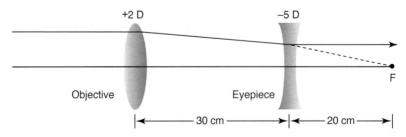

Figure 1-42 The Galilean telescope, an afocal system. The lenses are separated by the difference in focal lengths. F is simultaneously the posterior focal point of the plus lens and the anterior focal point of the minus lens. *(Illustration developed by Kevin M. Miller, MD, and rendered by C. H. Wooley.)*

The Keplerian telescope also consists of 2 lenses, a low-power objective and a high-power ocular, but both are positive and separated by the sum of their focal lengths. The image is inverted. For comparison, construct a Keplerian telescope using +2 D and +5 D trial lenses.

For each telescope,

$$\text{Angular Magnification} = -\frac{P_{eye}}{P_{obj}} = -\frac{f_{obj}}{f_{eye}}$$

where

P_{eye} = power of the eyepiece or ocular
P_{obj} = power of the objective lens
f_{obj} = focal length of the objective lens
f_{eye} = focal length of the eyepiece (negative for concave lenses)

For afocal telescopes like the Galilean and the Keplerian telescopes, the focal point of the objective lens and the focal point of the ocular lens are in the same position.

Each form of telescope has advantages and disadvantages. The advantage of a Galilean telescope is that it produces an upright image and is shorter than a Keplerian telescope. These features make the Galilean telescope popular as a spectacle-mounted visual aid or in surgical loupes.

Conversely, the Keplerian telescope uses light more efficiently, making faint objects easier to see (Fig 1-43). In the Keplerian design, all the light from an object point collected by the objective lens ultimately enters the eye. In the Galilean design, some of the light collected by the objective is lost. Because astronomical observation is largely a matter of making faint stars visible, all astronomical telescopes are of the Keplerian design. The inverted image is not a problem for astronomers, but inverting prisms are placed inside the telescope. Common binoculars and handheld visual aids are usually of the Keplerian design.

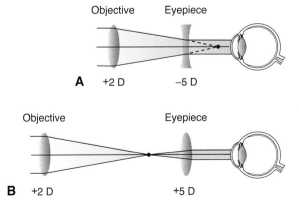

Figure 1-43 Comparison of Galilean and Keplerian telescopes. In the Galilean telescope **(A)**, some of the light collected by the objective is lost. In the Keplerian telescope **(B)**, all the light collected enters the eye. *(Illustration developed by Kevin M. Miller, MD, and rendered by C. H. Wooley.)*

Section Exercises

Questions

1.13. Calculate the magnification if an image is located 20 cm behind the lens and the object is located 40 cm in front of the lens (Fig 1-44).

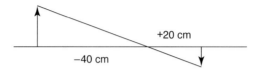

Figure 1-44 Magnification calculation. Image is located 20 cm behind the lens. Object is located 40 cm in front of the lens. The image is minified and inverted.

1.14. Calculate the magnification of a Galilean telescope with a +3 D objective and a −12 D eyepiece (Fig 1-45).

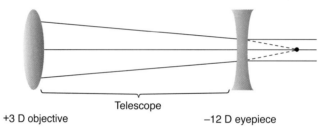

Figure 1-45 Galilean telescope. *(Illustration developed by Dimitri T. Azar, MD, and rendered by Joelle Hallak.)*

1.15. Calculate the length of the Galilean telescope shown in Figure 1-45.
1.16. Calculate the magnification of a Keplerian telescope with a +3 D objective and a +12 D eyepiece (Fig 1-46).

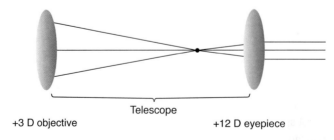

Figure 1-46 Keplerian telescope. *(Illustration developed by Dimitri T. Azar, MD, and rendered by Joelle Hallak.)*

1.17. Calculate the length of the Keplerian telescope shown in Figure 1-46.

Answers

1.13. $\text{Magnification} = \dfrac{\text{Image}}{\text{Object}} = \dfrac{\text{Image Distance}}{\text{Object Distance}}$. Thus,

$$\text{Magnification} = \frac{+20}{-40} = -0.5\times$$

1.14. $\text{Magnification} = -\dfrac{P_{\text{eye}}}{P_{\text{obj}}} = -\dfrac{-12}{3} = +4\times$; the plus sign implies an upright image.

1.15. Here,

$$f_{\text{obj}} = 1/3 \text{ m} = 33.33 \text{ cm}$$
$$f_{\text{eye}} = 1/120 \text{ m} = 8.33 \text{ cm}$$

This implies

$$\text{Length of Telescope} = 33.33 \text{ cm} - 8.33 \text{ cm} = 25 \text{ cm}$$

1.16. The magnification is $-4\times$; the minus sign implies an inverted image.

1.17. Here,

$$f_{\text{obj}} = 33.33 \text{ cm}$$
$$f_{\text{eye}} = 8.33 \text{ cm}$$
$$\text{Length of Telescope} = 41.66 \text{ cm}$$

Power of a Lens in a Medium

Looking at the expression for the power of a spherical surface, we see that power is proportional to the difference in refractive index between the lens and the medium. It makes sense that if a lens is put into a medium with almost the same refractive index, it will not have much power there.

Therefore, to find the power of a 20 D IOL in air instead of aqueous, we have the following equation:

$$\frac{\text{Power in Air}}{\text{Power in Aqueous}} = \frac{\text{Index of IOL} - \text{Index of Air}}{\text{Index of IOL} - \text{Index of Aqueous}}$$

Thus, the power in air of a 20 D IOL is 63 D.

Spherical Interface and Thick Lenses

Recall that we have been discussing a "thin" lens, which has a "power" to alter vergence. To follow rays passing into, through, and out of a thick lens, we need to see how vergence changes at a curved interface between 2 media, which we have not done yet. To take into account the different speeds of light in the 2 media, each vergence in the LME, $U + P = V$, is replaced by reduced vergence, which is vergence multiplied by the refractive index of the medium in which the light travels:

$$\frac{n}{o} + P = \frac{n'}{i}$$

One finds that the power, P, in diopters, of a spherical interface of radius r between 2 media with refractive indices of n and n' is (Fig 1-47):

$$P = \frac{n' - n}{r}$$

Does refraction at a spherical interface add plus or minus to the vergence? To determine whether the power of the surface is plus or minus, draw a rectangle containing the curved surface, and shade in the side with the higher refractive index. Look at the shaded lens to see whether it is thicker (+) or thinner (−) at its center.

Thick Lens

To calculate the change of vergence that occurs when rays pass through a thick lens, we must take into account what happens at each surface, in the manner just described, as well as the change in vergence when they move through the lens from one surface to the other. Fortunately, we can skip the calculations and model the thick lens in a way that looks quite familiar. In fact, we can go through a series of thick lenses, and still have an elegantly simple model, whose 6 cardinal points tell us everything (Fig 1-48).

Light emerges from the optical system as though refraction occurs at the principal planes, which intersect the axis at the principal points P and P'. The focal lengths are measured from the principal points. Starting from an object point, its central ray goes to the primary nodal point, N, and emerges from the secondary nodal point, N', heading parallel to the direction it was traveling when it arrived at N. If the lens is surrounded by uniform media, the nodal points, N and N', are located on the optical axis exactly at the principal planes P and P'. Suppose, however, that a thick lens has a more dense refractive medium on one side; for instance, the cornea has air on one side and

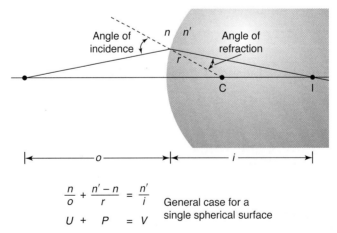

$$\frac{n}{o} + \frac{n' - n}{r} = \frac{n'}{i}$$ General case for a

$$U + P = V$$ single spherical surface

Figure 1-47 Refraction at a single spherical interface between 2 media, assuming small angles of incidence. C = center of curvature; i = image distance in meters; I = image; n = refractive index of the first medium; n' = refractive index of the second medium; r = radius of curvature in meters; o = object distance in meters; P = power in diopters; U = reduced object vergence; V = reduced image vergence. *(Redrawn from Basic and Clinical Science Course Section 2: Optics, Refraction, and Contact Lenses. San Francisco: American Academy of Ophthalmology; 1986–1987:63. Fig 36.)*

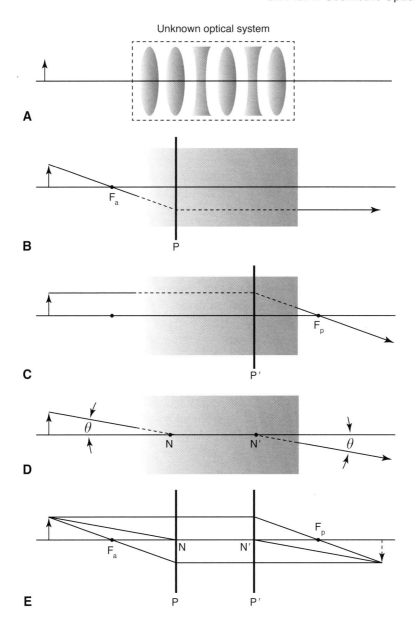

Figure 1-48 A multiple-lens system. **A,** An unknown "black box" optical system may contain any number of optical elements. **B,** A ray of light from an object point is traced that leaves the system parallel to the optical axis. The intersection of this ray with the optical axis defines the anterior focal point, F_a. The intersection of rays entering and leaving the optical system defines the location of the anterior principal plane, P. **C,** Another ray of light from the same object point enters the optical system parallel to the optical axis and exits through the posterior focal point, F_p. The intersection of the 2 rays entering and leaving the system defines the posterior principal plane, P'. **D,** The nodal points are defined by entering and exiting rays that intersect the optical axis at the same angle. If the refractive indices of the media bounding the optical system are the same on both sides, the nodal points correspond to the principal points. **E,** The final model simplifies the complex unknown optical system. *(Illustration developed by Kevin M. Miller, MD, and rendered by C. H. Wooley.)*

aqueous on the other. Then the nodal points are displaced from the principal planes, along the axis, toward the medium (toward the retina). In practice, we do not know where the principal points are, unless they are found empirically using an optical bench or through calculations.

Back Vertex Power Is Not True Power

Placement of a meniscus spectacle lens in a lensmeter measures not the true power of the lens but rather the "back vertex" power—the reciprocal of the distance from the back surface of the lens to its focal point. If glasses are placed in the lensmeter facing the wrong way, the lens measures as a less-strong plus or minus lens (Fig 1-49).

Aberrations of Ophthalmic Lenses

We began this discussion with the simplest situation: a single thin lens in air with paraxial pencils. Next, we considered multiple lenses, thick lenses, and lenses not in air. What about rays that are not paraxial? Ophthalmic lenses cause higher-order (monochromatic) aberrations and chromatic aberrations. The important higher-order aberrations that concern us are the third-order Seidel aberrations. Chromatic aberrations are discussed later.

Third-Order Seidel Aberrations

When we consider only paraxial rays, we ignore all but the first term of the Taylor series for the sine of an angle, measured in radians. We may call this approximation "first-order" optics. Considering the second term of the series,

$$\sin x = x - x^3 + x^5 \dots$$

so that we have third-order calculations, reveals the 5 primary so-called Seidel aberrations: *spherical aberration, coma, oblique astigmatism, field curvature,* and *distortion.* In

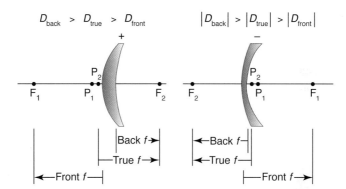

Figure 1-49 True vertex power vs back vertex power. Principal (P_1, P_2) and focal (F_1, F_2) points of plus and minus meniscus lenses. D = vertex power; f = focal length. *(Redrawn from Basic and Clinical Science Course Section 2: Optics, Refraction, and Contact Lenses. San Francisco: American Academy of Ophthalmology; 1986–1987:69. Fig 41.)*

recent years, with the development of laser refractive surgical techniques, it has become useful to describe wavefronts and classify their aberrations, including the effects of diffraction, in other ways, such as by means of Zernicke polynomials.

Spherical aberration

A spherical-surfaced lens focuses almost exactly the bundles of rays that travel close to the lens's axis. More peripheral rays, on the other hand, are bent more strongly and cross the optical axis closer to the lens than the paraxial rays do (Fig 1-50). Thus, there is no clear image point for all the rays passing through a lens, and as the aperture of a lens is increased, the "average" focal point moves toward the lens. Therefore, a patient's vision may become slightly more myopic when the pupil dilates. A smaller pupil aperture blocks passage of the rays that are farther from the axis and therefore reduces spherical aberration. In the eye, spherical aberration is reduced by the cornea having a flatter peripheral curve than central curve, and by the natural lens having a higher refractive index in the central region of the nucleus.

Spherical aberration occurs for on-axis as well as off-axis object points. The remaining 4 of the third-order monochromatic aberrations occur when pencils of light from off-axis object points pass through a lens.

Astigmatism of oblique incidence

As an object is located farther off-axis, another aberration becomes prominent: oblique astigmatism. The effect of tilting a +10 D spectacle lens, such that the wearer views off-axis through the lens, is shown below:

10° tilt	20° tilt	30° tilt
+10.10 +0.31 × 180°	+10.41 +1.38 × 180°	+10.95 +3.35 × 180°

Note that tilting a plus lens adds plus sphere and plus cylinder along the same axis as the tilt. Tilting a minus lens adds minus sphere and minus cylinder along the same axis as the tilt.

Distortion

Distortion and curvature of field differ from the other aberrations, in that they distort rather than blur the image. With distortion, straight lines that pass through the optical axis are unbent, but the images of other lines are distorted. Because the transverse magnification of an image varies with distance from the optical axis, the type and extent of distortion depends on lens characteristics and the presence (and position) of any aperture. For example, when we look at an object through a strong minus lens and our eye's pupil,

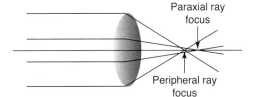

Paraxial ray focus

Peripheral ray focus

Figure 1-50 Spherical aberration. *(Redrawn from Basic and Clinical Science Course Section 2: Optics, Refraction, and Contact Lenses. San Francisco: American Academy of Ophthalmology; 1986–1987:76. Fig 46.)*

we experience barrel distortion, and a person with hyperopia looking through a strong plus lens will experience pincushion distortion (Fig 1-51).

Coma and field curvature

Coma and field curvature are aberrations of less interest to us here. Coma is produced when the object is off-axis, so that the principal "planes" become curved surfaces. Images have a blur that looks like the tail of a comet. Field curvature occurs because spherical lenses generally focus images on a curved (Petzval) surface, rather than on a flat plane (Fig 1-52). This completes our tour of third-order monochromatic aberrations.

Chromatic Aberrations

Chromatic aberration, referred to earlier, is the spreading apart of the colors of white light by a prism. Just as a prism bends blue light more sharply than it does red light, so a convex lens has its secondary focal point closer for blue light than it does for red light. Chromatic aberration of the eye itself gives us the "red-green" test (see Chapter 3). Chromatic aberration causes blur of off-axis viewing through spectacle lenses, more so with higher powers and lens materials of higher refractive index, which tend to have lower Abbe numbers.

Avoiding Aberrations

In the design of optical instruments, including spectacle lenses, engineers can try to minimize the blur that results from monochromatic and chromatic aberrations, as well as diffraction. Spectacle lenses are therefore usually of meniscus design. The curvatures for various powers are chosen to minimize the blur of the third-order aberrations. In multilens telescopes and microscopes, optical pathways are designed using techniques such as combining lenses of various materials and shapes, using apertures to block undesirable rays and mirrors to fold long optical pathways, and applying antireflective coatings.

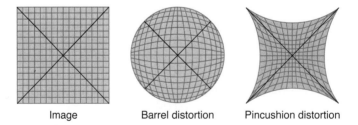

Image   Barrel distortion   Pincushion distortion

Figure 1-51   Barrel and pincushion distortion of an image. *(Illustration developed by Leon Strauss, MD, PhD.)*

Figure 1-52 Curvature of field. *(Redrawn from Basic and Clinical Science Course Section 2: Optics, Refraction, and Contact Lenses. San Francisco: American Academy of Ophthalmology; 1986–1987:76. Fig 47.)*

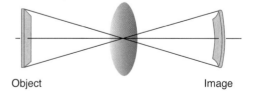

Object   Image

Aspheric lens design

Given that the peripheral part of a spherical lens refracts more strongly than the central part, how do we adjust for that? Indeed, there are aspheric designs in which the more peripheral part of the lens may be less steeply curved to accommodate for the spherical aberration. Descartes studied conic-section shapes for this purpose using Snell's law. Such designs are used in various optical instruments, including spectacles and implant lenses.

Mirrors

The angle of specular reflection of light rays from an interface is independent of the refractive index of the materials on each side of the interface, as the reflected light is not entering the second material. Obeying the Fermat principle of least time, the angle of reflection, as measured from the normal to the surface, is equal to the angle of incidence. Also, as with Snell's law of refraction, the reflected ray must lie in the same plane as the incident ray and the normal to the surface (see Fig 1-3).

Reflection From a Plane Mirror

The image of a real object in front of a mirror is located equally far behind the mirror, erect, and virtual. Looking into a mirror, you see an image that is laterally inverted—that is, what appears to be your right hand in the mirror is the virtual image of your left hand. To see yourself from head to toe in a plane mirror, you need the mirror to extend from the top of your head only halfway to the floor (Fig 1-53).

Spherically Curved Mirrors

The focal length (*f*) of a mirror is half its radius (*r*) of curvature. The power of a mirror is 1/focal length (1/*f*). Convex mirrors add negative vergence (like minus lenses). Looking in the convex rear-view mirror of an automobile, you see a virtual, erect, minified image

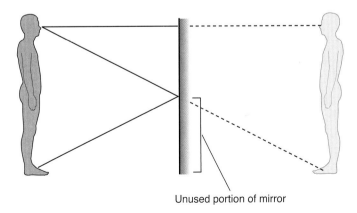

Unused portion of mirror

Figure 1-53 A half-length mirror gives a full-length view. *(Illustration developed by Edmond H. Thall, MD, and Kevin M. Miller, MD, and rendered by C. H. Wooley.)*

of the car behind you. Concave mirrors add positive vergence (like plus lenses). When you look in a convex cosmetic mirror, the image you see depends on how far you are from the mirror. If you are within the focal length, you will see a virtual, erect, magnified image of yourself. As you move farther away, rays cross, and the image becomes real, inverted, and magnified, and then it becomes minified (Fig 1-54).

Reversal of the Image Space

The basic vergence relationship, $U + P = V$, can be applied to mirrors, except that the mirror folds the optical path, reversing the image space. In our diagrams, light travels from left to right as it approaches the mirror and from right to left after reflection. Converging image rays have positive vergence and will form a real image to the left of the mirror, and diverging image rays with negative vergence will appear to come from a virtual image to the right of the mirror.

The Central Ray for Mirrors

The central ray for mirrors (see Fig 1-54), which passes through the center of curvature of the mirror, is as useful as the central ray for lenses, for if the image location is determined by vergence calculation, the central ray then immediately indicates the orientation and size of the image. Note that in using the ratio of image distance to object distance to calculate the size of the image, the image and object distances are measured from the center of curvature of the mirror, where we find the similar triangles to compare, just as we did for lenses.

Vergence Calculations for Mirrors

Plane mirrors create upright virtual images from real objects, with the virtual image located as far behind the mirror as the real image is in front. For example, light from an object 1 m to the left of a plane mirror has a vergence of –1 D at the mirror. On reflection, the vergence will still be –1 D, but by tracing imaginary extensions of the reflected image rays to the far side of the mirror (into virtual image space), we see the virtual image is located 1 m to the right of the mirror.

Concave mirror

A concave mirror adds positive vergence to incident light. It therefore has positive, or converging, power. If parallel rays strike the mirror, they will be reflected and converged toward a focal point halfway to the center of curvature. Note that the focal point of a concave mirror is not unique, for any central ray can serve as an optical axis. Note further that the primary and secondary focal points of a concave mirror are the same point. A central ray is constructed to pass through an object and the center of curvature.

As an example, we are given an object 1 m to the left of a concave mirror with a radius of curvature of 50 cm. Where is the image? The power of the mirror is equal to $1/f$, where $f = -r/2$, so the power is 4 D. Using $U + P = V$, we have $-1 + 4 = 3$. Therefore, the image is located 1/3 m, or 33 cm, to the left of the mirror, in real image space. It is also minified and inverted.

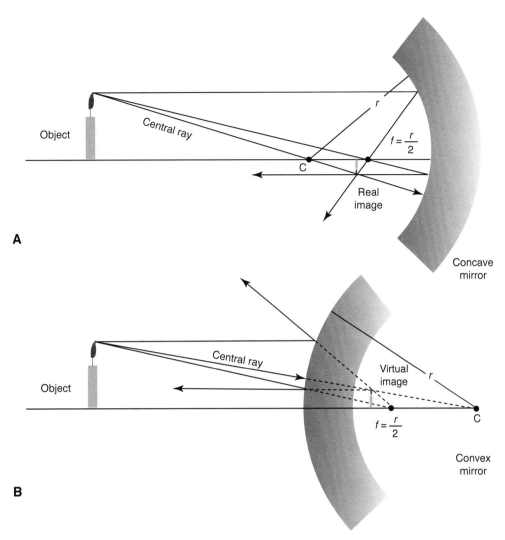

Figure 1-54 Ray tracing for concave **(A)** and convex **(B)** mirrors. The central ray for mirrors is different from the central ray for lenses in that it passes through the center of curvature (C) of the mirror, not through the center of the mirror. *(Illustration developed by Kevin M. Miller, MD, and rendered by C. H. Wooley.)*

Convex mirror

A convex mirror adds minus vergence to incident light. It therefore has negative, diverging power. The primary and secondary focal points, which coincide, are virtual focal points located halfway back to the center of curvature.

Using a convex, rather than a concave, mirror in the previous example, with the same radius of curvature, the power of the mirror will be –4 D:

$$U + P_\mathrm{m} = V$$
$$-1 + (-4) = V$$
$$V = -5 \text{ D}$$

In this case, the image rays are diverging, and a virtual image will appear to be located 20 cm to the right of the mirror. The image is minified and erect.

Consider another example: What is the reflecting power of the anterior surface of the cornea if this surface has a radius of 8 mm? The focal length is 8/2 = 4 mm, the inverse of which is –250 D power. Thus, an object at infinity would appear as an image slightly behind the iris plane, 4 mm posterior to the anterior corneal surface. This example shows why a camera focused on light reflections in the cornea is approximately in focus in the plane of the iris.

Spherocylindrical Lenses

The lenses and mirrors discussed thus far have been radially symmetric about an optical axis, so a flat diagram has sufficed. Now, however, we need to think in 3 dimensions in order to discuss the lenses used to correct regular astigmatism of the eye.

A cylinder has no curvature in one direction and has spherical curvature in the meridian perpendicular to that direction. A spherocylindrical lens has the shape of a torus. That is, its shape is similar to that of the outer surface of a bicycle tire or barrel, with a greater and a lesser circular curvature meeting at right angles where the tire (or the barrel lying on its side) touches the ground—at the point where we would find the optical center of a spherocylindrical spectacle lens (Fig 1-55).

We could describe such a spherocylindrical lens as having a power of –3 D at 30° and –5 D at 120°. Alternatively, we could describe the same lens by saying it is a –3 D sphere combined with a –2 D cylinder lens with the axis of the cylinder placed at 120° (–3.00 –2.00 × 120), or as a –5 D spherical lens combined with a +2 D cylinder lens with its axis held at 30° (–5.00 +2.00 × 30). The "spherical equivalent" lens, halfway between the 2 powers in diopters, is –4 D. To find that, we add half the cylinder amount to the sphere (Fig 1-56).

To convert a prescription from positive cylinder form to negative cylinder form (or conversely), consider the following points:

- The new sphere is the algebraic sum of the old sphere and cylinder.
- The new cylinder has the same value as the old cylinder but with opposite sign.
- The axis needs to be changed by 90°.

Combination of Spherocylindrical Lenses

If we hold 1 of these lenses just in front of a second lens, with the axes at any angle with respect to each other, the result will be another spherocylindrical lens; again the greatest and least curvature will be 90° apart. Determining the new axis and power is simple if the 2 old axes are aligned but is generally too much trouble to calculate by hand otherwise.

The Conoid of Sturm

A pencil of light rays is not brought to a point focus by passing perpendicularly through the center of a spherocylindrical lens; rather, 2 focal lines are formed, 1 for each of the

A torus has 2 different radiuses of curvature at any point on its surface.

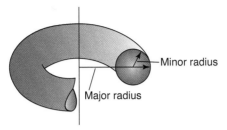

If we "slice off" a section of either of these toruses we will obtain a spherocylindric lens. The nontoric surface may be flat, or it may have positive or negative spherical power.

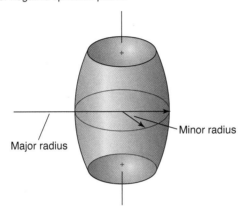

Figure 1-55 Toric surfaces. *(Redrawn from Duane TD, ed. Clinical Ophthalmology. Vol 1. Hagerstown, MD: Harper & Row; 1985:47, Fig 32-53, with permission from Lippincott Williams & Wilkins.)*

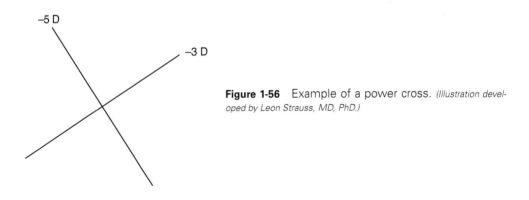

Figure 1-56 Example of a power cross. *(Illustration developed by Leon Strauss, MD, PhD.)*

2 powers of the power cross. The geometric envelope of a pencil of light rays refracted by a circular-aperture spherocylindrical lens is called the *conoid of Sturm.* This envelope of light rays traveling along the conoid of Sturm of a lens, for which both powers are positive, has an elliptical cross section that collapses first to 1 focal line and later to the other. The average of the 2 diopter lens powers is the spherical equivalent, and only at its place along

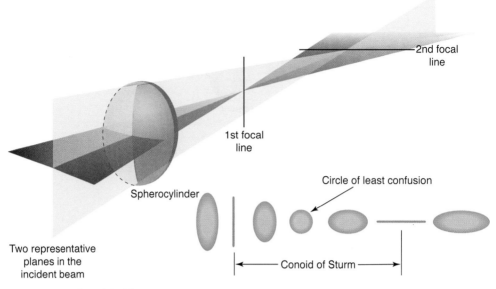

Figure 1-57 Conoid of Sturm. *(Illustration developed by Kevin M. Miller, MD, and rendered by Jonathan Clark.)*

the conoid of Sturm is the cross section circular, at which point it is called the *circle of least confusion* (Fig 1-57).

The Jackson Cross Cylinder

The Jackson cross cylinder is a spherocylindrical lens used in clinical refraction (see Chapter 3). It is the combination of a plus cylinder and a minus cylinder having axes 90° apart and equal power.

The cross-cylinder lens itself is usually ground in the spherocylindrical form. It has a cylindrical surface on one side and a spherical surface on the other side that has half the power and is of opposite sign to those of the cylindrical surface; thus, its spherical equivalent is zero.

Use of the Jackson cross cylinder to determine both the power and axis of the astigmatic correction for an eye is discussed in Chapter 3. The specific power (eg, ±0.25 D, ±0.37 D, ±0.50 D) of cross cylinder selected for use in clinical testing depends on the patient's visual acuity. For 20/30 and better, the ±0.25 D cross cylinder is appropriate. The ±0.50 D cross cylinder is useful for visual acuities between 20/40 and 20/70, and so forth.

Prisms

Prism Diopter

Prism power is defined by the amount of deviation produced as a light ray traverses the prism. The deviation is measured as the number of centimeters of deflection measured at a distance of 100 cm from the prism (Fig 1-58) and expressed in prism diopters (Δ).

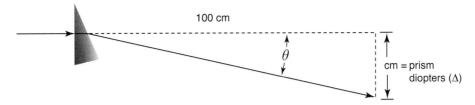

Figure 1-58 Definition of prism diopter. The power of the prism, when held in this particular position, is defined to be the number of centimeters of deflection of a ray, measured 100 cm after passage through the prism and expressed in prism diopters. *(Illustration developed by Edmond H. Thall, MD, and Kevin M. Miller, MD, and rendered by C. H. Wooley.)*

For angles less than 100Δ (45°), each change in deviation by 2 prism diopters is approximately equal to a change of 1°. For larger angles, increasingly more prism diopters are required for an equivalent change by 1°.

Glass prisms are calibrated to be held in the Prentice position, that is, with one of the faces of the prism perpendicular to the light rays. A glass prism, then, is correctly held with the back face parallel to the plane of the iris—the direction the eye is turned. All of the refraction occurs at the opposite face and is greater than the minimum deviation for that prism. This is the manner in which prism in spectacle lenses of any material is measured on a lensmeter, with the back surface of the spectacle lens flat against the nose cone of the lensmeter. If the rear surface of a 40Δ glass prism is erroneously held in the frontal plane of the subject's face, only 32Δ of effect will be achieved.

Plastic prisms and prism bars, on the other hand, are calibrated according to the angle of minimum deviation. To approximate this angle clinically, these prisms are held with the rear surface in the frontal plane of the subject's face (Fig 1-59).

The path of a pencil of rays passing through a prism is bent toward the base of the prism to form a real image, which is shifted in the direction of the base of the prism. If you put a prism in front of your vision chart projector with the apex pointed toward the left side of the room, the letters on the screen will be shifted in the direction you are pointing the base of the prism—that is, to the right (Fig 1-60).

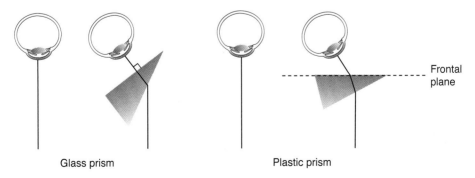

Glass prism   Plastic prism

Frontal plane

Figure 1-59 Correct positions for holding orthoptic glass and plastic prisms. *(Illustration developed by Edmond H. Thall, MD, and Kevin M. Miller, MD, and rendered by C. H. Wooley.)*

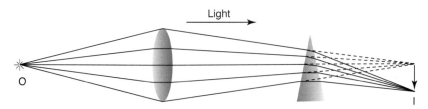

Figure 1-60 Real images are displaced by the prism toward the base of the prism. *(Illustration developed by Edmond H. Thall, MD, and Kevin M. Miller, MD, and rendered by C. H. Wooley.)*

On the other hand, if I am looking at a letter on the chart, a real object, and you interpose in front of my eye the same prism with its apex pointed toward the left side of the room, the prism will create a virtual image, which is displaced with respect to the original object, toward the apex of the prism. My eye sees those diverging rays as coming from an optically real object, which my eye brings to focus as a real image on my retina. To me, the letter will appear to have jumped to the left (Fig 1-61).

Prismatic Effect of Lenses and the Prentice Rule

A spherical lens obviously has prismatic power at every point on its surface that bends light rays toward the optical axis (plus lenses) or away from the optical axis (minus lenses). Prismatic power is zero at the optical center of the lens and increases away from the center, proportional to both the dioptric power of the lens and the distance from the center of the lens. This relationship is expressed by the Prentice rule, which states that the prismatic power of a lens (in prism diopters, Δ) at any point on its surface is equal to the distance from the optical center (in centimeters) times the power of the lens (in diopters) (Fig 1-62).

The prismatic effect of lenses becomes clinically important for patients with anisometropia (unequal lens power) in the vertical meridian, as different prismatic effects are produced for the 2 eyes in the reading position, and a vertical misalignment of the visual axes is produced. Thus, the effects of prismatic image displacement and prismatic image "jump" are taken into account in the design of bifocal lens segments.

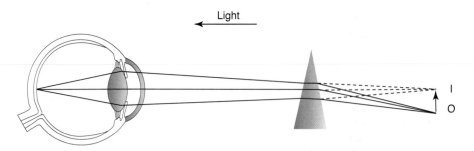

Figure 1-61 The prism forms a virtual image of a real object, and that virtual image is displaced, compared with the original object, toward the apex of the prism. *(Illustration developed by Edmond H. Thall, MD, and Kevin M. Miller, MD, and rendered by C. H. Wooley.)*

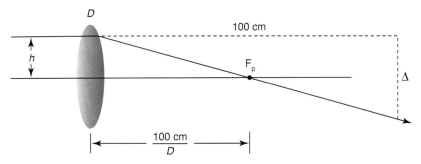

Figure 1-62 The Prentice rule. See text for explanation. D = power of the lens in diopters; F_p = focal point; h = distance from the optical center, in centimeters. *(Illustration developed by Kevin M. Miller, MD, and rendered by C. H. Wooley.)*

A prism may be effectively "added" to a spectacle lens simply by decentering the lens in the frame so that the patient's visual axis in primary position passes through an off-center portion of the lens. Whether the desired amount of prism can be added by such decentration depends on the power of the lens and the size of the lens blank. For example, adding 5Δ of base-out prism to a +1.00 D spherical spectacle lens would require decentering the lens temporally by 5 cm, which is farther than the edge of the lens blank; in this case, prism would need to be ground into the lens.

How can one quickly tell with a lensmeter whether a spectacle lens has been decentered or prism has been ground into the lens? The determination can be made simply by locating the optical center by moving the lens around until the lensmeter target is centered. If the greatest distance from the optical center to the edge of the lens is more than half the 60-mm diameter of the usual lens blank, then prism must have been ground into the lens.

Remember that prism in a spectacle lens is read at the position of the wearer's visual axis in primary position. A washable felt-tip pen is helpful in marking this position before transferring the glasses from the subject's face to the lensmeter. The lensmeter target, being a real image, is displaced in the direction of the base of the prism being measured. Therefore, if the optical centers appear in the lensmeter to be laterally displaced, for instance, the glasses have base-out prism.

If we need a certain amount of vertical prism and another of horizontal prism, we can add the 2 as vectors to find the obliquely angled prism that accomplishes both requirements (Fig 1-63). However, if we hold 2 loose prisms together, we will not have a prism whose power is equal to the sum of the 2, as the light path is already bent before it hits the second prism. For our purpose, we can add the powers by holding 1 prism in front of each eye.

When prescribing an oblique prism, it is important to specify the direction of the base clearly, by writing, for instance, "base up and out, in the 37° meridian" or "base down and in, in the 37° meridian."

A rotary prism (Risley prism), mounted on the front of most refractors, consists of 2 prisms of equal power that are counter-rotated with respect to one another to produce prismatic powers, varying from zero (prisms neutralizing each other) to the sum of the

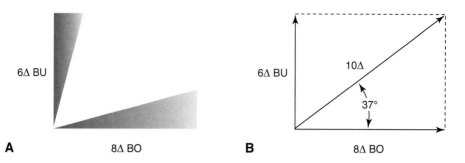

Figure 1-63 Vector addition of 2 prisms. **A,** The magnitude of the sum vector is $\sqrt{8^2 + 6^2}$. **B,** The angle of the sum vector is arctan (6/8). BU = base up; BO = base out. *(Illustration developed by Kevin M. Miller, MD, and rendered by C. H. Wooley.)*

2 powers (prisms aligned in the same direction). The Risley prism is particularly useful for measuring phorias (often in conjunction with the Maddox rod) and fusional vergence amplitudes.

Prism Aberrations

In addition to chromatic aberration (which produces colored fringes at the edges of objects viewed through the prism), prisms have other aberrations, such as asymmetric magnification and curvature of field. These aberrations can occasionally produce symptoms even with low-power ophthalmic prisms.

Fresnel Prisms

To avoid the weight and some of the aberrations of conventional prisms, clinicians may use Fresnel (pronounced *fre·nell'*) prisms, which are composed of plastic sheets of side-by-side long, narrow, thin prisms (Fig 1-64).

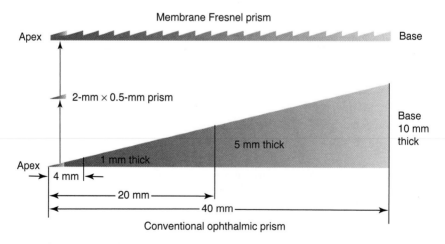

Figure 1-64 Comparison of a Fresnel prism with a conventional prism. *(Redrawn from Duane TD, ed. Clinical Ophthalmology. Vol 1. Hagerstown, MD: Harper & Row; 1976:chap 52, fig 52-2.)*

One form of Fresnel prism, the Press-On membrane prism, is applied with water to the back surface of a spectacle lens. Visual acuity suffers somewhat from the chromatic aberration and the presence of many edges.

Chapter Exercises

Questions 1.18 through 1.23 concern Figure 1-65.

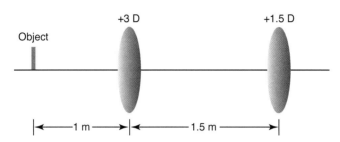

Figure 1-65   For Chapter Exercises 1.18 through 1.23. An object is placed 1 m in front of a +3 D spherical lens. The +3 D lens, in turn, is positioned 1.5 m in front of a +1.5 D spherical lens.

Questions

1.18. Where does the +3 D lens form an intermediate image?
   a. at optical infinity
   b. 2 m in front of the lens
   c. 1 m in front of the lens
   d. 0.5 m behind the lens
   e. 2 m behind the lens

1.19. The intermediate image would be described as
   a. upright, real, magnified
   b. inverted, real, minified
   c. upright, virtual, magnified
   d. upright, virtual, minified
   e. inverted, virtual, minified

1.20. What is the size of the intermediate image relative to the object?
   a. intermediate
   b. one-fourth the size
   c. half the size
   d. same size
   e. twice the size

1.21. What is the location of the final image?
   a. 1 m in front of the second lens
   b. 2 m behind the second lens
   c. 4 m behind the second lens
   d. 10 m behind the second lens
   e. at optical infinity

1.22. Compared with the intermediate image, the final image is
   a. real, magnified
   b. real, minified
   c. virtual, magnified
   d. virtual, minified

1.23. What is the size of the final image relative to the object?
   a. intermediate
   b. one-fourth the size
   c. half the size
   d. same size
   e. twice the size

1.24. An object is placed 25 cm in front of a concave spherical mirror with a radius of curvature of 1 m (Fig 1-66). The image is
   a. virtual with a transverse magnification of 2×
   b. virtual with a transverse magnification of –0.56×
   c. real with a transverse magnification of –1.77×
   d. real with a transverse magnification of 0.56×

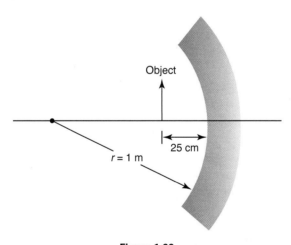

Figure 1-66

Answers

1.18. **d.** Light from the object, which is 1 m in front of the first lens, has a vergence of –1 D as it enters the lens. Vergence (diopters) = n/distance (meters) = –1/1 = –1 D. The lens adds an additional +3 D of vergence. Light leaving the lens, therefore, has a vergence of +2 D. Lights rays with a vergence of +2 D converge at a point 0.5 m behind the lens (Fig 1-67).

1.19. **b.** A ray traversing the nodal point of the lens, which corresponds to the optical center of the lens, will exit the lens undeviated. The image is real because it is on the opposite side of the lens from the object. If a screen were placed at the location of the image, an image would form. The central ray-tracing diagram shows that the image is minified.

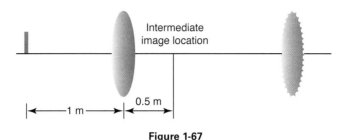

Figure 1-67

1.20. **c.** By similar triangles, the height of the intermediate image is one-half the height of the object. The transverse magnification is −0.5× (minus: inverted; 0.5 < 1: minified) (Fig 1-68).

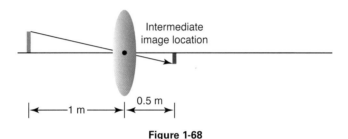

Figure 1-68

1.21. **b.** To answer this question, one makes the intermediate image the new object and forgets the first lens. The intermediate image is 1 m in front of the second lens. The vergence of light entering the second lens is, therefore, −1 D. Light rays with a vergence of +0.5 D come to a focus 2 m behind the second lens (Fig 1-69).

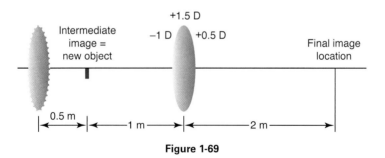

Figure 1-69

1.22. **a.** The intermediate image is an inverted new object. A ray traversing the nodal point of the lens, which corresponds to the optical center of the lens, will exit the lens undeviated (Fig 1-70). The image of the new object is real because it is on the opposite side of the lens from the object. A screen placed at this location would form a real image. The central ray-tracing diagram shows that the image is magnified and relative to the intermediate image.

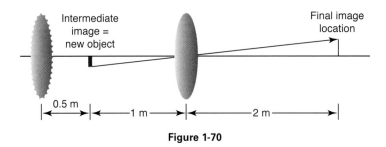

Figure 1-70

1.23. **d.** By similar triangles, the height of the final image is twice the height of the intermediate image (see Fig 1-70). Because the intermediate image is one-half the height of the object, the final image is the same height as the object. The final transverse magnification is 1×.

1.24. **a.** Light from the object has a vergence of –4 D when it strikes the mirror. The mirror adds +2 D, so light exiting the mirror has a vergence of –2 D. Because the mirror reverses image space, the image appears 50 cm to the right of the mirror. The image can be drawn by tracing rays, as shown in Figure 1-71A.

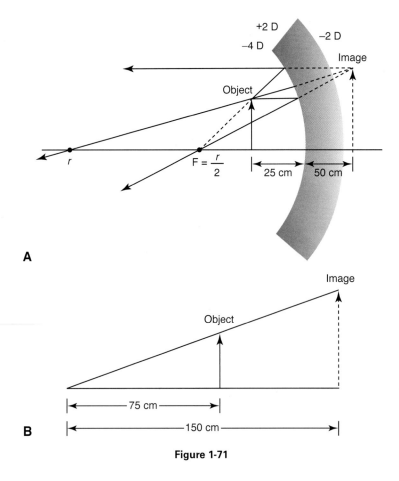

Figure 1-71

The image is upright. Image height can be determined by similar triangles, as shown in Figure 1-71B. The transverse magnification is 150/75 = 2×. A negative transverse magnification would indicate an inverted image.

Appendix 1.1

Quick Review of Angles, Trigonometry, and the Pythagorean Theorem

It is useful to review a few basic principles of geometry and trigonometry to help with our understanding of image magnification. Recall that a circle is divided angularly into 360°, which corresponds approximately to 6.28 radians. Converting between degrees and radians is frequently necessary when optics problems are being solved. A degree is subdivided into 60′ (minutes); each minute is subdivided into 60″ (seconds).

The sum of the angles in a triangle equals 180°, or π radians. For any right, or right-angled, triangle with sides a, b, and c (Fig 1-72) and angle θ between sides b and c, the trigonometric function is defined as follows:

$$\tan \theta = \frac{a}{b}$$

The Pythagorean theorem states that $c^2 = a^2 + b^2$; as a result, therefore, $c = \sqrt{a^2 + b^2}$. Triangles are said to be similar when their angles are equal. When 2 triangles have identical angles, their sides are proportional. The triangles in Figure 1-73 are similar.

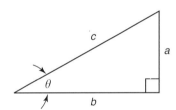

Figure 1-72 Right-angled triangle. *(Illustration developed by Kevin M. Miller, MD, and rendered by C. H. Wooley.)*

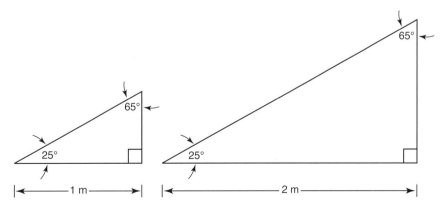

Figure 1-73 These 2 triangles are similar because their angles are equal. *(Illustration developed by Kevin M. Miller, MD, and rendered by C. H. Wooley.)*

Appendix 1.2

Light Properties and First-Order Optics

The Fermat principle

As discussed earlier in the chapter, the mathematician Pierre de Fermat believed that natural processes occur in the most economic way. The Fermat principle, as applied to optics, implies that light travels from one point to another along the path requiring the least time. Historically, the laws of reflection and refraction were discovered by careful experimental measurements before Fermat's time. However, both the law of refraction and the law of reflection can be mathematically derived.

The Fermat principle is an important conceptual and practical tool. The concept of *optical path length (OPL)* enhances the practical utility of this principle. *OPL* is the actual distance light travels in a given medium multiplied by the medium's refractive index. For instance, if light travels 5 cm in air (n = 1.000) and 10 cm in spectacle crown glass (n = 1.523), the *OPL* is (5 cm × 1.000) + (10 cm × 1.523) = 20.2 cm. According to the Fermat principle, light follows the path of minimum *OPL*.

Figure 1-23 shows light from an object point traveling along 2 different paths to the image point. Light traveling path 1 from object to image point traverses a relatively thick part of the lens. Light traveling the longer path 2 goes through less glass. If the lens is properly shaped, the greater distance in air is perfectly compensated for by the shorter distance in glass. In other words, the time required for light to travel from object to image—and, thus, the *OPL*—is identical for both paths.

Stigmatic imaging using a single refracting surface

By the early 1600s, the telescope and microscope had been invented. Although the images produced by these early devices were useful, their quality was not very high because the lenses did not focus stigmatically.

At the time, lensmakers were not very particular about the shape of the surfaces that were ground on the lens. It seemed that any curved surface produced an image, so lens surfaces were carefully polished but haphazardly shaped. However, as ideas such as stigmatic imaging and Snell's law developed, it became clear that the shape of the lens surfaces determined the quality of the image, and so, during the seventeenth century, lensmakers began to carefully shape the lens surface.

The following question arose: what surface produces the best image? Descartes applied the Fermat principle to the simplest situation possible—a single refracting surface. Consider a single object point and a long glass rod (Fig 1-74). Descartes realized that if the end of the rod were configured in a nearly elliptical shape, a stigmatic image would form in the glass. This shape became known as a Cartesian ellipsoid, or Cartesian conoid.

Some readers may be troubled by the fact that the image forms in the vitreous cavity, and in an emmetropic eye the image forms on the retina. Once a stigmatic image is produced, the rod is cut and a second Cartesian ellipsoid placed on the back surface (Fig 1-75). The final image is also stigmatic. The Cartesian ellipsoid produces a stigmatic image of only 1 object point. All other object points image nonstigmatically.

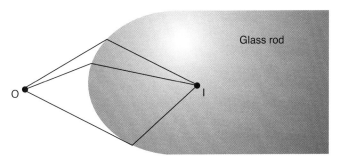

Figure 1-74 The Cartesian conoid is a single refracting surface that produces a stigmatic image for a single object point. *(Illustration developed by Edmond H. Thall, MD, and Kevin M. Miller, MD, and rendered by C. H. Wooley.)*

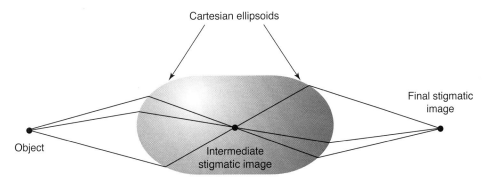

Figure 1-75 A combination of Cartesian ellipsoids also gives a stigmatic image. *(Illustration developed by Edmond H. Thall, MD, and Kevin M. Miller, MD, and rendered by C. H. Wooley.)*

Until about 1960, it was impossible to manufacture a Cartesian ellipsoid. The only surfaces that could be accurately configured were spheres, cylinders, spherocylinders, and flats. Now, aspheric surfaces are relatively easy to manufacture.

Descartes established that a single refracting surface could, at best, produce a stigmatic image of only 1 object point. By means of mathematics, it has been demonstrated that an optical system can produce a stigmatic image for only as many object points as there are "degrees of freedom" in the optical system. A single lens has 3 degrees of freedom *(df)*: the front surface, the back surface, and the lens thickness. A combination of the 2 lenses has *7 df*: the 4 lens surfaces, the 2 lens thicknesses, and the distance between the lenses. Optical systems utilizing multiple lenses improve image quality.

First-order optics

For centuries, the sphere was the only useful lens surface that could be manufactured. Descartes proved that lenses with spherical surfaces do not produce stigmatic images, but common experience shows that such lenses can produce useful images. Consequently, the properties of spherical refracting surfaces have been carefully studied.

The currently accepted approach for studying the imaging properties of any lens is through the method called *exact ray tracing*. In this technique, Snell's law is used to trace the paths of several rays, all originating from a single object point. A computer carries out the calculations to as high a degree of accuracy as necessary, usually between 6 and 8 significant figures.

Figure 1-76 shows an exact ray trace for a single spherical refracting surface. Because the image is not stigmatic, the rays do not converge to a single point. However, there is one location where the rays are confined to the smallest area, and this is the location of the image. The distribution of rays at the image location indicates the size of the blur circle, or point spread function (PSF). From the size of the blur circle, the image quality is determined. From the location of the image, other properties, such as magnification, are determined. Ultimately, all image properties may be determined with exact ray tracing.

Beginning in the 1600s, methods of analyzing optical systems were developed that either greatly reduced or eliminated the need for calculation. These methods are based on approximations—that is, these methods do not give exact answers. Nevertheless, carefully chosen approximations can yield results that are very close to the exact answer while greatly simplifying the mathematics.

The trick is to choose approximations that provide as much simplification as possible while retaining as much accuracy as possible. In this regard, the mathematician Carl Gauss (1777–1855) made many contributions to the analysis of optical systems. Gauss's work, combined with that of others, developed into a system for analyzing optical systems that has become known as *first-order optics.*

Ignoring image quality

Determining image quality requires knowledge of how light from a single object point is distributed in the image (ie, the PSF). To determine the PSF, hundreds of rays must be accurately traced. In Gauss's day, manufacturing techniques rather than optical system design limited image quality. Accordingly, there was little interest in theoretically analyzing image quality. Interest lay instead in analyzing other image features, such as magnification and location.

To determine all image characteristics except image quality requires tracing only a few rays. In fact, if image quality is ignored, analysis of optical systems is reduced from tracing

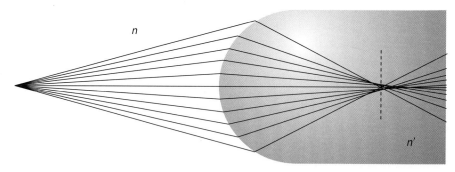

Figure 1-76 An exact ray trace for a single refracting surface. The image is not stigmatic. However, at one particular location, indicated by the *dotted line,* the rays are confined to the smallest area. This is the image location. *(Illustration developed by Edmond H. Thall, MD, and Kevin M. Miller, MD, and rendered by C. H. Wooley.)*

hundreds of rays to tracing just 2 rays. In Gauss's time, however, tracing even 2 rays exactly was a daunting task, especially if the optical system consisted of several lenses.

Paraxial approximation

To trace a ray through a refracting surface exactly, we need to establish a coordinate system. By convention, the origin of the coordinate system is located at the vertex, the point where the optical axis intersects the surface. Also by convention, the y-axis is vertical, the z-axis coincides with the optical axis, and the x-axis is perpendicular to the page (Fig 1-77). An object point is selected, and a ray is drawn from that object point to the refracting surface.

The first difficulty in making an exact ray trace is determining the precise coordinates (y,z) where the ray strikes the refracting surface. The formula for finding the intersection of a ray with a spherical surface requires fairly complicated calculations involving square roots.

Instead of tracing a ray through an optical system, it is easier to work with rays extremely close to the optical axis, the so-called *paraxial rays*. The portion of the refracting surface near the optical axis may be treated as flat. Just as the earth's surface seems flat to a human observer, a refracting surface "seems" flat to a paraxial ray (Fig 1-78). For a ray to be paraxial, it must hug the optical axis over its entire course from object to image. A ray from an object point far off-axis is not paraxial even if it strikes the refracting surface near the axis (Fig 1-79).

Small-angle approximation

To trace a paraxial ray, begin with an object point at or near the optical axis. Then extend a ray from the object point to the refracting surface, which is represented by a flat vertical plane (Fig 1-80). The next step is to determine the direction of the ray after refraction.

To determine the direction of the refracted ray, apply Snell's law. The angle of incidence is θ, and the angle of transmission is θ_t. Thus,

$$n \sin \theta = n' \sin \theta_t$$

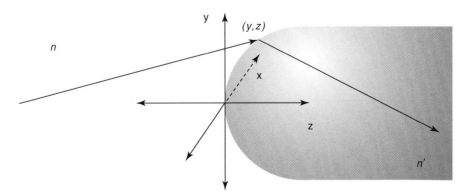

Figure 1-77 To trace a ray through a refracting surface exactly, it is necessary to establish a coordinate system (the x-, y-, and z-axes) and then find the precise coordinates (y,z) of the point where the ray intersects the surface. *(Illustration developed by Edmond H. Thall, MD, and Kevin M. Miller, MD, and rendered by C. H. Wooley.)*

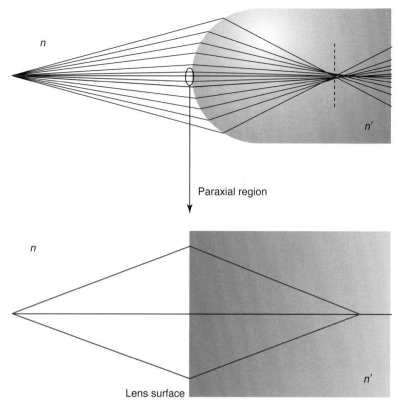

Figure 1-78 The paraxial region. The enlargement *(bottom)* shows the paraxial region with the vertical scale greatly increased but the horizontal dimensions unchanged. Notice that in the paraxial region, the lens is essentially flat. The paraxial rays are shown in *red. (Illustration developed by Edmond H. Thall, MD, and Kevin M. Miller, MD, and rendered by C. H. Wooley.)*

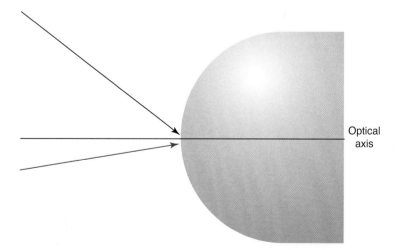

Figure 1-79 Both rays strike the refracting surface in the paraxial region. Only the lower *(red)* ray is a paraxial ray, however, because it is close to the optical axis over its entire path. *(Illustration developed by Edmond H. Thall, MD, and Kevin M. Miller, MD, and rendered by C. H. Wooley.)*

Now the polynomial expansion for the sine function is

$$\sin \theta = \theta - \frac{\theta^3}{3!} + \frac{\theta^5}{5!} - \frac{\theta^7}{7!} \cdots$$

where the angle θ is expressed in radians. If the angle θ is small, the third-order term, $\theta^3/3!$, and every term after it become insignificant, and the sine function is approximated as

$$\sin \theta \approx \theta$$

This is the mathematical basis of the (essentially equivalent) terms *small-angle approximation, paraxial approximation,* and *first-order approximation.* Only the first-order term of the polynomial expansion needs to be used when the analysis is limited to paraxial rays, which have a small angle of entry into the optical system.

The angles appear large in the bottom part of Figure 1-78 because of the expanded vertical scale, but the upper part shows that in the paraxial region these angles are quite small.

Using the small-angle approximation, Snell's law becomes

$$n\,\theta_i = n'\,\theta_t$$

Now, using geometry and Figure 1-80, the angle of incidence, θ_i, is

$$\theta_i = \alpha + \gamma$$

and the angle of transmission, θ_t, is

$$\theta_t = \gamma - \beta$$

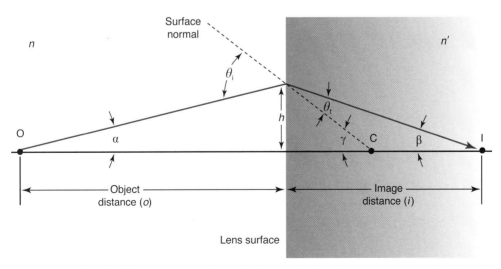

Figure 1-80 Detail of the paraxial region with the vertical scale greatly enlarged relative to the horizontal scale. The lens is spherical but appears flat in the paraxial region. The center of the lens is indicated by point C. The points O and I represent the object point and its image, respectively. θ_i and θ_t indicate the angles of incidence and transmission, respectively. *(Illustration developed by Edmond H. Thall, MD, and Kevin M. Miller, MD, and rendered by C. H. Wooley.)*

Thus, Snell's law becomes

$$n(a + \gamma) = n'(\gamma - \beta)$$

or

$$na + n'\beta = \gamma(n' - n)$$

Now, the small-angle approximation also works for tangents:

$$\tan a \approx a \qquad \tan \beta \approx \beta \qquad \tan \gamma \approx \gamma$$

and

$$\tan a \approx -\frac{h}{o}$$

The negative sign is used because the object distance *(o)*, which extends backward from the lens to the object point, is considered a negative distance.

$$\tan \beta \approx -\frac{h}{i} \qquad \tan \gamma \approx \frac{h}{r}$$

Thus,

$$-\frac{nh}{o} + \frac{n'h}{i} = \frac{h(n' - n)}{r}$$

Canceling the common factor *h* gives

$$-\frac{n}{o} + \frac{n'}{i} = \frac{n' - n}{r}$$

Rearranging yields

$$\frac{n}{o} + \frac{n' - n}{r} = \frac{n'}{i}$$

Finally, we define the refractive power of the surface, $P = [(n' - n)/r]$. Thus,

$$\frac{n}{o} + P = \frac{n'}{i} \qquad \text{or} \qquad U + P = V$$

This equation is the lensmaker's equation. The ratio *n/o* is the *reduced object vergence (U)*, and the ratio *n'/i* is the *reduced image vergence (V)*. Vergence is discussed in detail in the section Ophthalmic Lenses.

CHAPTER **2**

Optics of the Human Eye

The Human Eye as an Optical System

This chapter presents conceptual tools ("schematic eyes") that were developed to help us understand the inner workings of the optics of the human eye. In addition, it covers the various methods used to measure the eye's ability to "see" and reviews the types of refractive errors of the eye. Treatment of refractive errors is discussed in Chapter 3.

Schematic Eyes

The major challenges to understanding the optics of the human eye lie in the complexities and "imperfections"—compared with mathematical ideals—of some of the eye's optical elements. Simplifications and approximations make models easier to understand but detract from their ability to explain all the subtleties of the inner workings of the eye's optical system. As an example, the anterior surface of the cornea is assumed to be spherical, but the actual anterior surface tends to flatten toward the limbus. Also, the center of the crystalline lens is usually decentered with respect to the cornea and the visual axis of the eye.

Many mathematical models of the eye's optical system are based on careful anatomical measurements and approximations. The model developed by Gullstrand (Fig 2-1, Table 2-1), a Swedish professor of ophthalmology, so closely approximated the human eye that he was awarded a Nobel Prize in 1911. Although very useful, this model is cumbersome for certain clinical calculations and can be simplified further.

Because the principal points of the cornea and lens are fairly close to each other, a single intermediate point can substitute for them. In a similar fashion, the nodal points of the cornea and lens can be combined into a single nodal point located 17.0 mm in front of the retina. Thus, we can treat the eye as if it were a single refracting element, an ideal spherical surface separating 2 media of different refractive indices: 1.000 for air and 1.333 for the eye (Fig 2-2). This concept is known as the *reduced schematic eye.*

Using this reduced schematic eye, we can calculate the retinal image size of an object in space (such as a Snellen letter). This calculation utilizes the simplified nodal point, through which light rays entering or leaving the eye pass undeviated. The geometric principle of similar triangles can be used for the calculation of retinal image size if the following information is given: (1) the actual height of a Snellen letter on the eye chart, (2) the

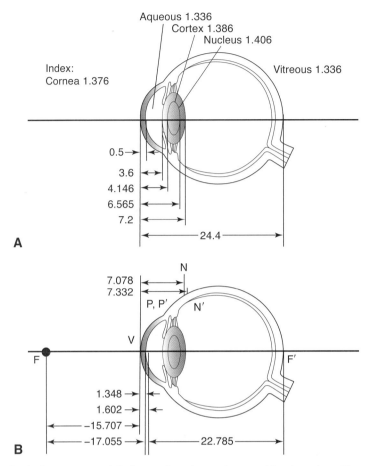

Figure 2-1 Optical constants of Gullstrand's schematic eye. All values in millimeters. **A,** Refractive indices of the media and positions of the refracting surfaces. **B,** Positions of the cardinal points, which are used for optical calculations. *(Illustration by C. H. Wooley.)*

distance from the eye chart to the eye, and (3) the distance from the nodal point to the retina. The formula for this calculation is as follows:

$$\frac{\text{Retinal Image Height}}{\text{Snellen Letter Height}} = \frac{\text{Nodal Point to Retina Distance}}{\text{Chart to Eye Distance}}$$

Although the distance from the eye chart to the nodal point should be measured, it is much easier to measure the distance to the surface of the cornea. The difference between these measurements is 5.6 mm, which is usually insignificant. For example, if the distance between the nodal point and the retina is 17.0 mm, the distance between the eye chart and the eye is 20 ft (6000 mm), and the height of a Snellen letter is 60 mm, then the resulting image size on the retina is 0.17 mm.

Katz M, Kruger PB. The human eye as an optical system. In: Tasman W, Jaeger EA, eds. *Duane's Clinical Ophthalmology* [CD-ROM]. Vol 1. Philadelphia: Lippincott Williams & Wilkins; 2006:chap 33.

Table 2-1 The Schematic Eye

	Accommodation Relaxed	Maximum Accommodation
Refractive index		
Cornea	1.376	1.376
Aqueous humor and vitreous body	1.336	1.336
Lens	1.386	1.386
Equivalent core lens	1.406	1.406
Position		
Anterior surface of cornea	0	0
Posterior surface of cornea	0.5	0.5
Anterior surface of lens	3.6	3.2
Anterior surface of equiv. core lens	4.146	3.8725
Posterior surface of equiv. core lens	6.565	6.5275
Posterior surface of lens	7.2	7.2
Radius of curvature		
Anterior surface of cornea	7.7	7.7
Posterior surface of cornea	6.8	6.8
Anterior surface of lens	10.0	5.33
Anterior surface of equiv. core lens	7.911	2.655
Posterior surface of equiv. core lens	−5.76	−2.655
Posterior surface of lens	−6.0	−5.33
Refracting power		
Anterior surface of cornea	48.83	48.83
Posterior surface of cornea	−5.88	−5.88
Anterior surface of lens	5.0	9.375
Core lens	5.985	14.96
Posterior surface of lens	8.33	9.375
Corneal system		
Refracting power	43.05	43.05
Position of first principal point	−0.0496	−0.0496
Position of second principal point	−0.0506	−0.0506
First focal length	−23.227	−23.227
Second focal length	31.031	31.031
Lens system		
Refracting power	19.11	33.06
Position of first principal point	5.678	5.145
Position of second principal point	5.808	5.255
Focal length	69.908	40.416
Complete optical system of eye		
Refracting power	58.64	70.57
Position of first principal point, P	1.348	1.772
Position of second principal point, P′	1.602	2.086
Position of first focal point, F	−15.707	−12.397
Position of second focal point, F′	24.387	21.016
First focal length	−17.055	−14.169
Second focal length	22.785	18.930
Position of first nodal point, N	7.078	NA
Position of second nodal point, N′	7.332	NA
Position of fovea centralis	24.0	24.0
Axial refraction	−1.0	−9.6

NA = not applicable.

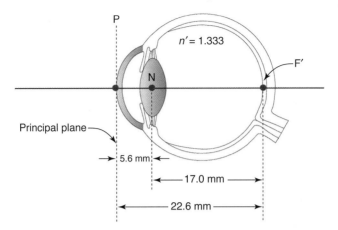

P

$n' = 1.333$

N

F'

Principal plane

5.6 mm

17.0 mm

22.6 mm

Figure 2-2 Dimensions of the reduced schematic eye, defined by the anterior corneal surface (P), the simplified nodal point of the eye (N), and the fovea (F'). The distance from the simplified nodal point to the fovea is 17.0 mm, and the distance from the anterior corneal surface to the nodal point is 5.6 mm. The refractive index for air is taken to be 1.000, and the simplified refractive index for the eye (n') is 1.333. The refractive power of this reduced schematic eye is 60.0 D, with its principal plane at the front surface of the cornea. *(Illustration by C. H. Wooley.)*

Important Axes of the Eye

Following are important definitions of terms used to describe the axes of the eye. The *principal line of vision* is the line passing through the fixation target, perpendicular to the corneal plane. The *pupillary axis* is the imaginary line perpendicular to the corneal surface and passing through the midpoint of the entrance pupil. The *visual axis* is the line connecting the fixation target and the fovea. The *optical axis* is the line that best approximates the line passing through the optical centers of the cornea, lens, and center of the fovea. Because the lens is usually decentered with respect to the cornea and the visual axis, no single line can precisely pass through each of these points. However, because the amount of decentration is small, the optical axis is considered the best approximation of this line.

The *angle alpha* (α) is the angle between the visual axis and the optical axis. This angle is considered positive when the visual axis in object space lies on the nasal side of the optical axis. The *angle kappa* (κ) is the angle between the pupillary axis and the visual axis (Fig 2-3).

Pupil Size and Its Effect on Visual Resolution

The size of the blur circle on the retina generally increases as the size of the pupil increases. If a pinhole aperture is placed immediately in front of an eye, it acts as an artificial pupil, and the size of the blur circle is reduced correspondingly (Fig 2-4; Clinical Problems 2-1).

The pinhole is used clinically to measure *pinhole visual acuity.* If visual acuity improves when measured through a pinhole aperture, a refractive error is usually present. The most useful pinhole diameter for general clinical purposes (refractive errors between

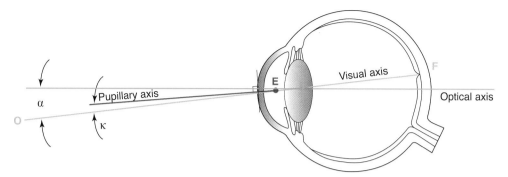

Figure 2-3 Angle kappa (κ). The pupillary axis *(red line)* is represented schematically as the line perpendicular to the corneal surface and passing through the midpoint of the entrance pupil (E). The visual axis *(green line)* is defined as the line connecting the fixation target (O) and the fovea (F). If all the optical elements of the human eye were in perfect alignment, these 2 lines would overlap. However, the fovea is normally displaced from its expected position. The angle between the pupillary axis and the visual axis is called *angle kappa* (κ) and is considered positive when the fovea is located temporally, as is the usual case. Conditions that cause temporal dragging of the retina, such as retinopathy of prematurity, can lead to a large positive angle kappa. Clinically, this will present as pseudoexotropia. A large positive angle kappa may also mask a small-angle esotropia, which can be detected by the cover-uncover test. Angle alpha (α) is the angle between the optical axis and the visual axis of the eye and is considered positive when the visual axis in object space lies on the nasal side of the optical axis, as is normally the case. *(Courtesy of Neal H. Atebara, MD. Redrawn by C. H. Wooley.)*

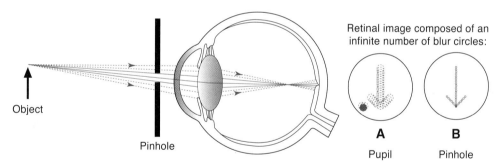

Figure 2-4 Light rays from each point on an object *(upright arrow)* form a blur circle on the retina of a myopic eye. The retinal image is the composite of all blur circles, the size of each being proportional to the diameter of the pupil **(A)** and the amount of defocus. If a pinhole is held in front of the eye, the size of each blur circle is decreased; as a result, the overall retinal image is sharpened **(B).** *(Courtesy of Neal H. Atebara, MD. Redrawn by C. H. Wooley.)*

−5.00 D and +5.00 D) is 1.2 mm. If the pinhole aperture is made smaller, the blurring effects of diffraction around the edges of the aperture overwhelm the image-sharpening effects of the small pupil. For refractive errors greater than 5.00 D, the clinician needs to use a lens that corrects most of the refractive error in addition to the pinhole.

After the best refractive correction has been determined, the pinhole can also be used with a dilated pupil. If visual acuity improves, optical irregularities such as corneal and lenticular light scattering or irregular astigmatism are likely to be present, given that the

> ### CLINICAL PROBLEMS 2-1
>
> *Why do persons with uncorrected myopia squint?*
> To obtain a pinhole effect (or rather a stenopeic slit effect). Better visual
> acuity results from smaller blur circles (or even smaller blur "slits").
>
> *Does pupil size affect the measured near point of accommodation?*
> Yes. With smaller pupil size, the eye's depth of focus increases, and ob-
> jects closer than the actual near point of the eye remain in better focus.
>
> *Why are patients less likely to need their glasses in bright light?*
> One reason is that the bright light causes the pupil to constrict, allowing
> the defocused image to be less blurred on the retina. Another reason is
> that bright light increases contrast.

pinhole serves to restrict light to a relatively normal area of the eye's optics. (This technique also can be used to identify optical causes of *monocular diplopia*.) If visual acuity
worsens, macular disease must be considered, as a diseased macula is often unable to
adapt to the reduced amount of light entering through the pinhole.

Because of the refractive effects of the cornea, the image of the pupil when viewed by
the clinician is about 13%–15% larger than the actual pupil; this enlarged image is called
the *entrance pupil.*

Visual Acuity

Clinicians often think of visual acuity primarily in terms of Snellen acuity, but visual perception is a far more complex process than is implied by this simple measuring system.
Indeed, there are a multitude of ways to measure visual function. The following are definitions of terms used in the measurement of visual function:

- The *minimum legible threshold* refers to the point at which a patient's visual ability
  cannot further distinguish progressively smaller letters or forms from one another;
  Snellen visual acuity is the most common method of determining this threshold.
- The *minimum visible threshold* is the minimum brightness of a target at which the
  patient can distinguish the target from the background.
- The *minimum separable threshold* refers to the smallest visual angle formed by the
  eye and 2 separate objects at which a patient can discriminate them individually.
- *Vernier acuity* is defined as the smallest detectable amount of misalignment of
  2 line segments.

Snellen visual acuity is measured with test letters (optotypes) constructed such that
each letter as a whole subtends an angle of *5 minutes of arc (arcmin),* whereas each stroke
of the letter subtends 1 arcmin. Letters of different sizes are designated by the distance
at which the letter subtends an angle of 5 arcmin (Fig 2-5). The Snellen chart is designed
to measure visual acuity in angular terms. However, the accepted convention does not

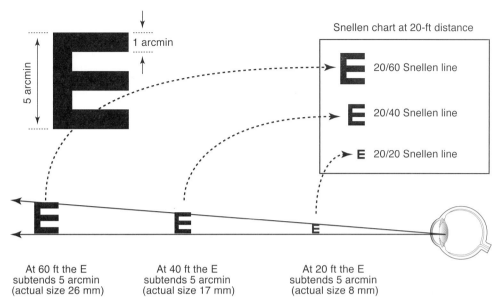

Figure 2-5 Snellen letters are constructed such that they subtend an angle of 5 arcmin when located at the distance specified by the denominator. For example, if a Snellen E is 26 mm in height, it subtends 5 arcmin at 60 ft. Correspondingly, a 26-mm letter occupies the 20/60 line of the Snellen chart at the standard testing distance of 20 ft. *(Courtesy of Neal H. Atebara, MD. Redrawn by C. H. Wooley.)*

specify visual acuity in angular measure; instead, it uses a notation in which the numerator is the *testing distance* (in feet or meters) and the denominator is the *distance at which a letter subtends the standard visual angle of 5 arcmin.* Thus, on the 20/20 line (6/6 in meters), the letters subtend an angle of 5 arcmin when viewed at 20 ft. In examination rooms with shorter distances than 20 ft (6 m), mirrors can be used to increase the viewing distance. On the 20/40 (6/12) line, the letters subtend an angle of 10 arcmin when viewed at 20 ft, or 5 arcmin when viewed at 40 ft. The "40" in the 20/40 letter (or the "12" in the 6/12 letter) refers to the viewing distance at which this letter subtends the "normal" visual angle of 5 arcmin. Table 2-2 lists conversions of visual acuity measurements for the various methods in use—the Snellen fraction, decimal notation (Visus), visual angle minute of arc, and *base-10 logarithm of the minimum angle of resolution* (logMAR). LogMAR is useful for determining the mean of Snellen visual acuity in a series.

Though widely accepted, the standard Snellen eye chart is not perfect. The letters on different Snellen lines are not related to one another by size in any geometric or logarithmic sense. For example, the increase in letter size from the 20/20 line to the 20/25 line differs from the increase from the 20/25 line to the 20/30 line. In addition, certain letters (such as C, D, O, and G) are inherently harder to recognize than others (such as A and J), partly because there are more letters of the alphabet with which they can be confused. For these reasons, alternative visual acuity charts have been developed and popularized in clinical trials (eg, the Early Treatment Diabetic Retinopathy Study [ETDRS] or Bailey-Lovie charts) (Fig 2-6). Computer-based acuity devices that display optotypes on

Table 2-2 Visual Acuity Conversion Chart

Snellen Fraction		4-Meter Standard	Decimal Notation (Visus)	Visual Angle Minute of Arc	LogMAR (Minimum Angle of Resolution)
Feet	Meters				
20/10	6/3	4/2	2.00	0.50	−0.30
20/15	6/4.5	4/3	1.33	0.75	−0.12
20/20	6/6	4/4	1.00	1.00	0.00
20/25	6/7.5	4/5	0.80	1.25	0.10
20/30	6/9	4/6	0.67	1.50	0.18
20/40	6/12	4/8	0.50	2.00	0.30
20/50	6/15	4/10	0.40	2.50	0.40
20/60	6/18	4/12	0.33	3.00	0.48
20/80	6/24	4/16	0.25	4.00	0.60
20/100	6/30	4/20	0.20	5.00	0.70
20/120	6/36	4/24	0.17	6.00	0.78
20/150	6/45	4/30	0.13	7.50	0.88
20/200	6/60	4/40	0.10	10.00	1.00
20/400	6/120	4/80	0.05	20.00	1.30

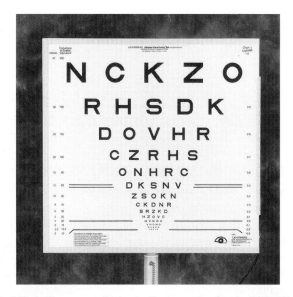

Figure 2-6 Modified Early Treatment Diabetic Retinopathy Study (ETDRS) visual acuity chart produced by the Lighthouse. The chart is intended for use at 20 ft (6 m) but can also be used at 10 ft (3 m) or 5 ft (1.5 m) with appropriate scaling. *(Courtesy of Kevin M. Miller, MD.)*

a monitor screen have also become popular because they allow presentation of a random assortment of optotypes and scrambling of letters, thereby eliminating problems associated with memorization by patients.

Westheimer G. Visual acuity. In: Kaufman PL, Alm A, eds. *Adler's Physiology of the Eye.* 10th ed. St Louis: Mosby; 2003.

Contrast Sensitivity and the Contrast Sensitivity Function

An underappreciated variable in measuring visual function is the degree of contrast between the optotype and its background. In general, the higher the contrast, the easier the optotype is to decipher. Good illumination makes it easier to read a book, for example, because the additional light creates a brighter background and therefore a higher contrast against the black letters on the page. If the brightness of an object (I_{min}) and the brightness of its background (I_{max}) are known, the following formula can be used to measure the degree of contrast between the object and its background:

$$\text{Contrast} = \frac{I_{max} - I_{min}}{I_{max} + I_{min}}$$

Thus, for letters printed with perfectly black ink (ie, 100% nonreflecting) on perfectly white paper (ie, 100% reflecting), the contrast would be 100%. Snellen visual acuity is commonly tested with targets, either illuminated or projected charts, that *approximate* 100% contrast. Therefore, when we measure Snellen visual acuity, we are measuring, at approximately 100% contrast, the smallest optotype that the visual system can resolve. In everyday life, however, 100% contrast is rarely encountered, and most visual tasks must be performed in lower-contrast conditions.

To take contrast sensitivity into account when measuring visual function, we can use the *modulation transfer function (MTF)*. Consider a target in which the light intensity varies from some peak value to zero in a sinusoidal fashion. The contrast is 100%, but instead of looking like a bar graph, it looks like a bar graph with softened edges. The number of light bands per unit length or per unit angle is called the *spatial frequency* and is closely related to Snellen acuity. For example, the 20/20 E optotype is composed of bands of light and dark, where each band is 1 arcmin. Thus, for a target at 100% contrast, 20/20 Snellen acuity corresponds roughly to 30 cycles per degree of resolution when expressed in spatial frequency notation. If we take sine wave gratings with various spatial frequencies and describe how the optical system alters the contrast of each of them, we have a set of information that constitutes the MTF.

In clinical practice, the ophthalmologist presents a patient with targets of various spatial frequencies and peak contrasts. A plot is then made of the minimum resolvable contrast target that can be seen for each spatial frequency. The minimum resolvable contrast is the *contrast threshold*. The reciprocal of the contrast threshold is defined as the *contrast sensitivity,* and the manner in which contrast sensitivity changes as a function of the spatial frequency of the targets is called the *contrast sensitivity function (CSF)* (Fig 2-7). A typical contrast sensitivity curve obtained with sinusoidal gratings is shown in Figure 2-8. Contrast sensitivity can also be tested with optotypes of variable contrast (such as the Pelli-Robson or Regan charts), which may be easier for patients to use. Which of these approaches is clinically more useful remains controversial.

It is important to perform contrast sensitivity testing with the best possible optical correction in place. In addition, luminance must be kept constant when CSF is tested, because mean luminance has an effect on the shape of the normal CSF. In low luminance, the low spatial frequency falloff disappears and the peak shifts toward the lower frequencies.

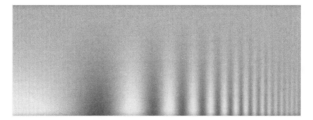

Figure 2-7 Contrast sensitivity grating. In this example, the contrast diminishes from bottom to top, and the spatial frequency of the pattern increases from left to right. The pattern appears to have a hump in the middle at the frequencies for which the human eye is most sensitive to contrasts. *(Courtesy of Brian Wandell, PhD.)*

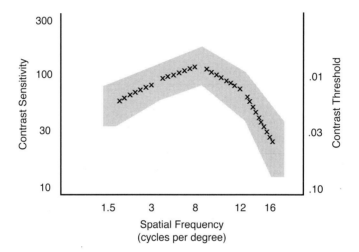

Figure 2-8 A typical contrast sensitivity curve is noted as x-x-x. The *shaded area* represents the range of normal values for 90% of the population. Expected deviations from normal due to specific diagnoses are noted in the text discussion. *(Developed by Arthur P. Ginsburg, PhD. Courtesy of Stereo Optical Company, Inc, Chicago.)*

In brighter light, there is little change in the shape of the normal CSF through a range of luminance for the higher spatial frequencies. Generally, contrast sensitivity is measured at normal room illumination, which is approximately 30–70 lux.

Contrast sensitivity is affected by various conditions of the eye, both physiologic and pathologic. Any corneal pathology that causes distortion or edema can affect contrast sensitivity. Lens changes, particularly incipient cataracts, may significantly decrease CSF, even with a normal Snellen visual acuity. Retinal pathology may affect contrast sensitivity more (as with retinitis pigmentosa or central serous retinopathy) or less (certain macular degenerations) than it does Snellen visual acuity. Glaucoma may produce a significant loss in the midrange. Optic neuritis may also be associated with a notch-type pattern loss. Amblyopia is associated with a generalized attenuation of the curve. Pupil size also has an effect on contrast sensitivity. With miotic pupils, diffraction reduces contrast sensitivity; with large pupils, optical aberrations may interfere with performance.

> Miller D. Glare and contrast sensitivity testing. In: Tasman W, Jaeger EA, eds. *Duane's Clinical Ophthalmology* [CD-ROM]. Vol 1. Philadelphia: Lippincott Williams & Wilkins; 2006:chap 35.

Refractive States of the Eyes

In considering the refractive state of the eye, we can use either of the following concepts:

1. The *focal point* concept: The location of the image formed by an object at optical infinity through a nonaccommodating eye determines the eye's refractive state. Objects focusing at points anterior or posterior to the retina form a blurred image on the retina, whereas objects that focus on the retina form a sharp image.
2. The *far point* concept: The far point is the point in space that is conjugate to the fovea of the nonaccommodating eye; that is, the far point is where the fovea would be imaged if the optics were reversed and the fovea became the object.

Emmetropia is the refractive state in which parallel rays of light from a distant object are brought to focus on the retina in the nonaccommodating eye (Fig 2-9A). The far point of the emmetropic eye is at infinity, and infinity is *conjugate* with the retina (Fig 2-9B). *Ametropia* refers to the absence of emmetropia and can be classified by presumptive etiology as *axial* or *refractive*. In *axial ametropia,* the eyeball is either unusually long *(myopia)* or short *(hyperopia)*. In *refractive ametropia,* the length of the eye is statistically normal, but the refractive power of the eye (cornea and/or lens) is abnormal, being either excessive (myopia) or deficient (hyperopia). *Aphakia* is an example of extreme refractive hyperopia unless the eye was highly myopic (>20.00 D) before lens removal. An ametropic eye requires either a diverging or a converging lens to image a distant object on the retina.

Ametropias may also be classified by the nature of the mismatch between the optical power and length of the eye. In myopia, the eye possesses too much optical power for its axial length, and (with accommodation relaxed) light rays from an object at infinity

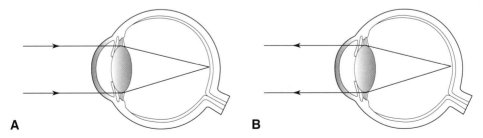

A **B**

Figure 2-9 Emmetropia with accommodation relaxed. **A,** Parallel light rays from infinity focus to a point on the retina. **B,** Similarly, light rays emanating from a point on the retina focus at the far point of the eye at optical infinity. *(Illustration by C. H. Wooley.)*

converge too soon and thus focus in front of the retina (Fig 2-10A). This results in a de-focused image on the retina; the far point of the eye is located in front of the eye, between the cornea and optical infinity (Fig 2-10B). In hyperopia, the eye does not possess enough optical power for its axial length, and (with accommodation relaxed) an object at infinity attempts to focus light behind the retina, again producing a defocused image on the retina (Fig 2-11A); the far point of the eye (actually a virtual point rather than a real point in space) is located behind the retina (Fig 2-11B).

Astigmatism (*a* = without, *stigmos* = point) is an optical condition of the eye in which light rays from an object do not focus to a single point because of variations in the curvature of the cornea or lens at different meridians. Instead, there is a set of 2 *focal lines*. Each astigmatic eye can be classified by the orientations and relative positions of these focal lines (Fig 2-12). If one of the focal lines lies in front of the retina and the other is on the retina, the condition is classified as *simple myopic astigmatism*. If both focal lines lie in front of the retina, the condition is classified as *compound myopic astigmatism*. If, in an unaccommodated state, one focal line lies behind the retina and the other is on the retina, the astigmatism is classified as *simple hyperopic astigmatism*. If both focal lines lie behind the retina, the astigmatism is classified as *compound hyperopic astigmatism*. If, in an unaccommodated state, one focal line lies in front of the retina and the other behind it, the condition is classified as *mixed astigmatism*.

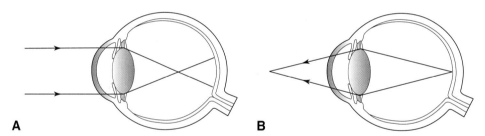

A　　　　　　　　　　　　　　　　**B**

Figure 2-10　Myopia with accommodation relaxed. **A,** Parallel light rays from infinity focus to a point anterior to the retina, forming a blurred image on the retina. **B,** Light rays emanating from a point on the retina focus to a far point in front of the eye, between optical infinity and the cornea. *(Illustration by C. H. Wooley.)*

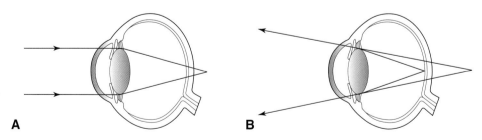

A　　　　　　　　　　　　　　　　**B**

Figure 2-11　Hyperopia with accommodation relaxed. **A,** Parallel light rays from infinity focus to a point posterior to the retina, forming a blurred image on the retina. **B,** Light rays emanating from a point on the retina are divergent as they exit the eye, appearing to have come from a virtual far point behind the eye. *(Illustration by C. H. Wooley.)*

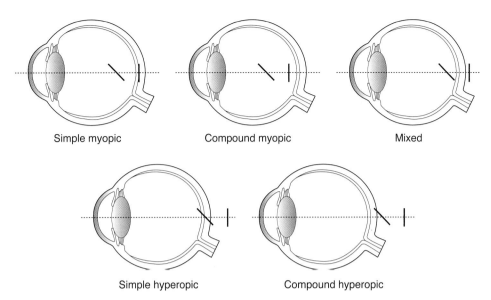

Figure 2-12 Types of astigmatism. The locations of the focal lines with respect to the retina define the type of astigmatism. The main difference between the types of astigmatism depicted in the illustration is the spherical equivalent refractive error. All of the astigmatisms depicted are with-the-rule astigmatisms—that is, they are corrected by using a plus cylinder with a vertical axis. If they were against-the-rule astigmatisms, the positions of the vertical and horizontal focal lines would be reversed.

If the principal corneal or lenticular meridians of astigmatism (or *axes,* which are 90° to the meridians) have constant orientation at every point across the pupil, and if the amount of astigmatism is the same at every point, the refractive condition is known as *regular astigmatism.* This condition is correctable by cylindrical spectacle lenses. Note that the axis of the cylindrical correction is perpendicular to the axis of the corneal or lenticular astigmatism. Regular astigmatism may itself be classified into *with-the-rule* or *against-the-rule astigmatism.* In *with-the-rule* astigmatism (the more common type in children), the vertical corneal meridian is steepest (resembling an American football lying on its side), and a correcting plus cylinder axis should be used at or near 90°. In *against-the-rule* astigmatism (the more common type in older adults), the horizontal meridian is steepest (resembling a football standing on its end), and a correcting plus cylinder axis should be used at or near 180°. The term *oblique astigmatism* is used to describe regular astigmatism in which the principal meridians do not lie at, or close to, 90° or 180° but instead lie near 45° or 135°.

In *irregular astigmatism,* the orientation of the principal meridians or the amount of astigmatism changes from point to point across the pupil. Although the principal meridians are 90° apart at every point, it may sometimes appear by retinoscopy or keratometry that the principal meridians of the cornea, as a whole, are not perpendicular to one another. All eyes have at least a small amount of irregular astigmatism, and instruments such as corneal topographers and wavefront aberrometers can be used to detect this condition clinically. These *higher-order* aberrations in the refractive properties of the cornea and lens have been characterized by Zernike polynomials, which are mathematical shapes that approximate various types of irregular astigmatism more closely than the simple "football" model. These aberrations include such shapes as spherical aberration, coma, and trefoil. See Chapter 6 of this book and BCSC Section 13, *Refractive Surgery*, for further discussion.

Binocular States of the Eyes

The spherical equivalent of a refractive state is defined as the algebraic sum of the spherical component and half of the astigmatic component. *Anisometropia* refers to any difference in the spherical equivalents between the 2 eyes. Uncorrected anisometropia in children may lead to amblyopia, especially if 1 eye is hyperopic. Although adults may be annoyed by uncorrected anisometropia, they may be intolerant of initial spectacle correction. Unequal image size, or *aniseikonia,* may occur, and the prismatic effect of the glasses will vary in different directions of gaze, inducing *anisophoria.* Anisophoria may be more bothersome than aniseikonia for patients with spectacle-corrected anisometropias.

Aniseikonia can also be due to a difference in the shape of the images formed in the 2 eyes. The most common cause is the differential magnification inherent in the spectacle correction of anisometropia. Even though aniseikonia is difficult to measure, anisometropic spectacle correction can be prescribed in such a manner as to reduce aniseikonia. Making the front surface power of a lens less positive can reduce magnification. Decreasing center thickness also reduces magnification. Decreasing vertex distance diminishes the magnifying effect of plus lenses as well as the minifying effect of minus lenses. These effects become increasingly noticeable as lens power increases. Contact lenses may provide a better solution than spectacles for most patients with anisometropia, particularly children, in whom fusion may be possible.

Unilateral aphakia is an extreme example of hyperopic anisometropia arising from refractive ametropia. In the adult patient, spectacle correction produces an intolerable aniseikonia of about 25%; contact lens correction produces aniseikonia of about 7%, which is usually tolerated. If necessary, the clinician may reduce aniseikonia still further by adjusting the powers of contact lenses and simultaneously worn spectacle lenses to provide the appropriate minifying or magnifying effect via the Galilean telescope principle. For further information on correcting aphakia, see Chapters 3, 4, and 5.

Accommodation and Presbyopia

Accommodation is the mechanism by which the eye changes refractive power by altering the shape of its crystalline lens. The mechanisms that achieve this alteration have been described by Helmholtz. The posterior focal point is moved forward in the eye during accommodation (Fig 2-13A). Correspondingly, the far point moves closer to the eye (Fig 2-13B). *Accommodative effort* occurs when the ciliary muscle contracts in response to parasympathetic stimulation, thus allowing the zonular fibers to relax. The

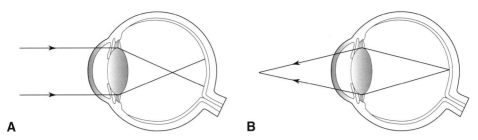

Figure 2-13 Emmetropia with accommodation stimulated. **A,** Parallel light rays now come to a point locus in front of the retina, forming a blurred image on the retina. **B,** Light rays emanating from a point on the retina focus to a near point in front of the eye, between optical infinity and the cornea. *(Illustration by C. H. Wooley.)*

outward-directed tension on the lens capsule is decreased, and the lens becomes more convex. *Accommodative response* results from the increase in lens convexity (primarily the anterior surface). It may be expressed as the *amplitude of accommodation* (in diopters) or as the *range of accommodation*, the distance between the far point of the eye and the nearest point at which the eye can maintain focus *(near point)*. It is evident that as the lens loses elasticity from the aging process, the accommodative response wanes (a condition called *presbyopia*), even though the amount of ciliary muscle contraction (or accommodative effort) is virtually unchanged. For an eye with presbyopia, the amplitude is a more useful measurement for calculating the power requirement of the additional spectacle lens. For appraising an individual's ability to perform a specific visual task, the range is more informative.

> Glasser A, Kaufman PL. The mechanism of accommodation in primates. *Ophthalmology.* 1999;106(5):863–872.

Epidemiology of Refractive Errors

An interplay among corneal power, lens power, anterior chamber depth, and axial length determines an individual's refractive status. All 4 elements change continuously as the eye grows. On average, babies are born with about 3.00 D of hyperopia. In the first few months of life, this hyperopia may increase slightly, but it then declines to an average of about 1.00 D of hyperopia by the end of the first year because of marked changes in corneal and lenticular powers, as well as axial length growth. By the end of the second year, the anterior segment attains adult proportions; however, the curvatures of the refracting surfaces continue to change measurably. One study found that average corneal power decreased 0.10–0.20 D and lens power decreased about 1.80 D between ages 3 years and 14 years.

From birth to age 6 years, the axial length of the eye grows by approximately 5 mm; thus, one might expect a high prevalence of myopia in children. However, most children's eyes are actually emmetropic, with only a 2% incidence of myopia at 6 years. This phenomenon is due to a still-undetermined mechanism called *emmetropization*. During this period of eye growth, a compensatory loss of 4.00 D of corneal power and 2.00 D of lens power keeps most eyes close to emmetropia. It appears that the immature human eye develops so as to reduce refractive errors.

American Academy of Ophthalmology. Refractive Management/Intervention Panel. Preferred Practice Pattern Guidelines. *Refractive Errors.* San Francisco: American Academy of Ophthalmology; 2002. Available at www.aao.org/ppp.

Lawrence MS, Azar DT. Myopia and models and mechanisms of refractive error control. *Ophthalmol Clin North Am.* 2002;15(1):127–133.

Prevent Blindness America; National Eye Institute. *Vision Problems in the U.S.: Prevalence of Adult Vision Impairment and Age-Related Eye Disease in America.* 5th ed. Chicago, IL: Prevent Blindness America; 2012.

Developmental Myopia

Myopia increases steadily with increasing age. In the United States, the prevalence of myopia has been estimated at 3% among children aged 5–7 years, 8% among those aged 8–10 years, 14% among those aged 11–12 years, and 25% among adolescents aged 12–17 years. In particular ethnic groups, a similar trend has been demonstrated, although the percentages in each age group may differ. Ethnic Chinese children have much higher rates of myopia at all ages. A national study in Taiwan found the prevalence was 12% among 6-year-olds and 84% among adolescents aged 16–18 years. Similar rates have been found in Singapore and Japan.

Different subsets of myopia have been characterized. *Juvenile-onset myopia,* defined as myopia with an onset between 7 years and 16 years of age, is due primarily to growth in axial length. Risk factors include *esophoria,* against-the-rule astigmatism, premature birth, family history, and intensive near work. In general, the earlier the onset of myopia is, the greater is the degree of progression. In the United States, the mean rate of childhood myopia progression is reported at about 0.50 D per year. In approximately 75% of teenagers, refractive errors stabilize at about age 15 or 16. In those whose errors do not stabilize, progression often continues into the 20s or 30s.

Adult-onset myopia begins at about 20 years of age, and extensive near work is a risk factor. A study of West Point cadets found myopia requiring corrective lenses in 46% at entrance, 54% after 1 year, and 65% after 2 years. The probability of myopic progression was related to the degree of initial refractive error. It is estimated that as many as 20%–40% of patients with low hyperopia or emmetropia who have extensive near-work requirements become myopic before age 25, compared with less than 10% of persons without such demands. Older Naval Academy recruits have a lower rate of myopia development than younger recruits over a 4-year curriculum (15% for 21-year-olds versus 77% for 18-year-olds). Some young adults are at risk for myopic progression even after a period of refractive stability. It has been theorized that persons who regularly perform considerable near work undergo a process similar to emmetropization for the customary close working distance, resulting in a myopic shift.

The etiologic factors concerning myopia are complex, involving both genetic and environmental factors. Regarding a genetic role, identical twins are more likely to have a similar degree of myopia than are fraternal twins, siblings, or parent and child. Identical twins separated at birth and having different work habits do not show significant differences in refractive error. Some forms of severe myopia suggest dominant, recessive, and even sex-linked inheritance patterns. However, studies of ethnic Chinese in Taiwan show an increase in the prevalence and severity of myopia over the span of 2 generations, a finding that implies that genetics alone are not entirely responsible for myopia. Some studies have reported that near work is not associated with a higher prevalence and progression of myopia, especially with respect to middle-distance activities such as tasks involving video displays. Higher educational achievement has been strongly associated with a higher prevalence of myopia. Poor nutrition has been implicated in the development of some refractive errors as well. Studies from Africa, for example, have found that children with malnutrition have an increased prevalence of high ametropia, astigmatism, and anisometropia.

Feldkämper M, Schaeffel F. Interactions of genes and environment in myopia. *Dev Ophthalmol.* 2003;37:34–49.

Fischer AJ, McGuire JJ, Schaeffel F, Stell WK. Light- and focus-dependent expression of the transcription factor ZENK in the chick retina. *Nat Neurosci.* 1999;2(8):706–712.

McCarty CA, Taylor HR. Myopia and vision 2020. *Am J Ophthalmol.* 2000;129(4):525–527.

Winawer J, Wallman J, Kee C. Differential responses of ocular length and choroidal thickness in chick eyes to brief periods of plus and minus lens-wear. *Invest Ophthalmol Vis Sci Suppl.* 1999;40:S963.

Developmental Hyperopia

Less is known about the epidemiology of hyperopia than that of myopia. There appears to be an increase in the prevalence of adult hyperopia with age that is separate from the development of nuclear sclerotic cataracts. Nuclear sclerosis is usually associated with a myopic shift. In Caucasians, the prevalence of hyperopia increases from about 20% among those in their 40s to about 60% among those in their 70s and 80s. In contrast to myopia, hyperopia has been associated with lower educational achievement.

Lee KE, Klein BE, Klein R. Changes in refractive error over a 5-year interval in the Beaver Dam Eye Study. *Invest Ophthalmol Vis Sci.* 1999;40(8):1645–1649.

Prevention of Refractive Errors

Over the years, many treatments have been proposed to prevent or slow the progression of myopia. Because accommodation is a postulated mechanism for the progression of myopia, optical correction through the use of bifocal or multifocal spectacles or the removal of distance spectacles when performing close work has been recommended to reduce the progression of myopia. Administration of atropine eyedrops also has long been proposed because it inhibits accommodation, which may exert forces on the eye that result in axial elongation. Use of a drug that lowers intraocular pressure has been suggested as an alternative pharmacologic intervention; this approach works presumably by reducing internal pressure on the eyewall. It has also been postulated that use of rigid contact lenses could slow the progression of myopia in children. Visual training purported to reduce myopia includes convergence exercises and those that incorporate changes in near–far focus. However, evidence reported in the peer-reviewed literature, including that from randomized clinical trials, is currently insufficient to support a recommendation for intervention using any of these proposed treatments.

The need to correct refractive errors depends on the patient's symptoms and visual needs. Patients with low refractive errors may not require correction, and small changes in refractive corrections in asymptomatic patients are not generally recommended. Correction options include spectacles, contact lenses, or surgery. Various occupational and recreational requirements, as well as personal preferences, affect the specific choices for any individual patient.

> Saw SM, Shih-Yen EC, Koh A, Tan D. Interventions to retard myopia progression in children: an evidence-based update. *Ophthalmology.* 2002;109(3):415–421.

Chapter Exercises

Questions

2.1. Using the reduced schematic eye and the concept of the nodal point, what is the retinal image height of an 18-mm 20/40 Snellen letter at a distance of 20 ft (6 m)?

    a. 0.5 mm

    b. 0.05 mm

    c. 1 mm

    d. 0.1 mm

    e. 0.01 mm

2.2. The angle subtended by the 20/40 Snellen letter at a distance of 20 ft (6 m) is approximately

    a. 1 arcmin

    b. 2 arcmin

    c. 5 arcmin

    d. 10 arcmin

    e. 40 arcmin

2.3. What is the relative size of target lights in a Goldmann perimeter (with a radius of 33 cm) relative to their corresponding retinal image?

    a. same

    b. 5 times larger

    c. 10 times larger

    d. 20 times larger

    e. 15 times larger

2.4. Which of the following statements is not true?

    a. In emmetropia with accommodation relaxed, parallel light rays from infinity focus to a point on the retina.

    b. In myopia with accommodation relaxed, parallel light rays from infinity focus to a point anterior to the retina, forming a blurred image on the retina.

    c. In myopia with accommodation relaxed, light rays emanating from a point on the retina focus to a far point in front of the eye between optical infinity and the cornea.

    d. In hyperopia with accommodation relaxed, parallel light rays from infinity focus on the far point posterior to the retina.

    e. In hyperopia with accommodation relaxed, light rays emanating from a point on the retina are divergent as they exit the eye, appearing to have come from a virtual far point behind the eye.

2.5. Which of the following statements is not true?

    a. If the principal meridians of astigmatism have constant orientation and the amount of astigmatism is the same at every point across the pupil, the refractive condition is known as regular astigmatism.

    b. With-the-rule astigmatism is more common in children.

    c. In with-the-rule astigmatism, the vertical meridian is steepest, and a correcting plus cylinder should be used at or near axis 90°.

    d. In against-the-rule astigmatism, the horizontal meridian is steepest, and a correcting minus cylinder should be used at or near axis 180°.

    e. Oblique astigmatism is the term used to describe regular astigmatism in which the principal meridians do not lie at, or close to, 90° and 180°.

2.6. A patient with myopic vision is wearing glasses that were prescribed incorrectly with an overminus of 1.00 D. When he wears them, his near point of accommodation is 20 cm. What is his amplitude of accommodation?

    a. none

    b. 1.00 D

    c. 5.00 D

    d. 6.00 D

    e. There is not enough information to solve this problem.

Answers

2.1. **b.** Utilizing the concepts of the nodal point and similar triangles, retinal image size is related to Snellen letter height (18 mm), the distance from the eye to the eye chart (6 m), and the distance from the nodal point to the retina (17 mm), as follows:

$$\frac{\text{Retinal Image Height}}{\text{Snellen Letter Height}} = \frac{\text{Retinal Image Distance From Nodal Point}}{\text{Snellen Letter Distance From Nodal Point}}$$

$$= \frac{17\,\text{mm}}{6000\,\text{mm}}$$

This implies

$$\text{Retinal Image Height} = \frac{18\,\text{mm} \times 17\,\text{mm}}{6000\,\text{mm}} = 0.05\,\text{mm}$$

2.2. **d.** Snellen letters are constructed such that they subtend an angle of 5 arcmin when located at the distance specified by the denominator (here, 40 ft). At a distance of 20 ft, the angle subtended by a 20/40 Snellen letter is twice that at 40 ft, or 10 arcmin.

2.3. **d.** The concept of the nodal point is applicable for the Goldmann perimeter, in which the target lights are located at 33 cm (330 mm) from the cornea. Because this distance is approximately 20 times greater than the 17-mm distance from the nodal point to the retina, the target lights in the perimeter are approximately 20 times larger than their corresponding retinal images.

2.4. **d.** In hyperopia with accommodation relaxed, parallel rays from infinity focus not on the far point but rather on another point that is also posterior to the retina.

2.5. **d.** In against-the-rule astigmatism (which is more common in older adults), the horizontal meridian is steepest and a corresponding plus cylinder is used at or near axis 180°. Moreover, the vertical meridian is flattest, which alternatively would be corrected with a minus cylinder at or near 90°.

2.6. **d.** We know the patient's amplitude of accommodation is 6.00 D because it takes 1.00 D of accommodation to focus to infinity and an additional 5.00 D of accommodation to focus to the false near point at 20 cm.

CHAPTER 3

Clinical Refraction

Objective Refraction Technique: Retinoscopy

Although autorefractors are easily accessible, retinoscopy remains an important skill and tool for the ophthalmologist to objectively determine the spherocylindrical refractive error of the eye. A *retinoscope* can also help the examiner detect optical aberrations, irregularities, and opacities, even through small pupils. Retinoscopy is especially useful for examinations of infants, children, and adults unable to cooperate.

Most retinoscopes in current use employ the streak projection system developed by Copeland. The illumination of the retinoscope is provided by a bulb with a straight filament that forms a streak in its projection. The light is reflected from a mirror that is either half silvered (Welch Allyn model) or totally silvered around a small circular aperture (Copeland instrument) (Fig 3-1). The filament light source can be moved in relation to a convex lens in the system. If the light is slightly divergent, it appears to come from a point behind the retinoscope, as if the light were reflected off a flat mirror (ie, a *plano mirror setting*) (Fig 3-2).

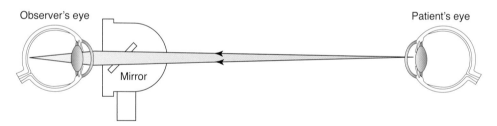

Figure 3-1   Observation system: light path from patient's pupil, through mirror, to observer's retina. *(Illustration by C. H. Wooley.)*

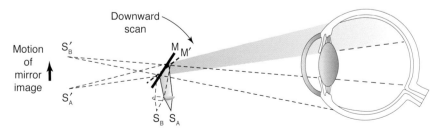

Figure 3-2   Illumination system: position of source (S) with plano mirror (M) effect.

Alternatively, when the distance between the convex lens and the filament is increased by moving the sleeve on the handle, convergent light is emitted. In this situation, the image of the filament appears between the examiner and the patient, as if the light were reflected off a concave mirror (Fig 3-3). Early retinoscopes actually used flat and concave mirrors to achieve these effects.

Retinoscopy is usually performed using the plano mirror setting. We restrict our discussion to the plano mirror effect; recall that in the concave mirror effect, the direction of motion is opposite that of the plano mirror effect. Not all retinoscopes employ the same sleeve position for the plano mirror setting. For example, the original Copeland retinoscope is in plano position with the sleeve up; the Welch Allyn instrument is in plano position with the sleeve down. The axis of the streak is rotated by rotating the sleeve.

Positioning and Alignment

Ordinarily, the examiner uses his or her right eye to perform retinoscopy on the patient's right eye, and the left eye for the patient's left eye. Doing so prevents the examiner's head from moving into the patient's line of sight and thus inadvertently stimulating accommodation. If the examiner looks directly through the optical centers of the trial lenses while performing retinoscopy, reflections from the lenses may interfere. In general, if the examiner is too far off-axis, unwanted spherical and cylindrical errors may occur. The optimal alignment is just off center, where the lens reflections can still be seen between the center of the pupil and the lateral edge of the lens.

Fixation and Fogging

Retinoscopy should be performed with the patient's accommodation relaxed. The patient should fixate at a distance on a nonaccommodative target. For example, the target may be a dim light at the end of the room or a large Snellen letter (20/200 or 20/400 size). Children typically require pharmacologic cycloplegia.

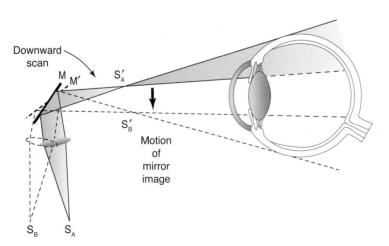

Figure 3-3 Illumination system: position of source with concave mirror effect.

The Retinal Reflex

The projected streak illuminates an area of the patient's retina, and this light returns to the examiner. By observing characteristics of this reflex, the examiner determines the refractive status of the eye. If the patient's eye is *emmetropic,* the light rays emerging from the patient's pupil are parallel to one another; if the eye is *myopic,* the rays are convergent (Fig 3-4); and if the eye is *hyperopic,* the rays are divergent. Through the peephole in the retinoscope, the emerging rays are seen as a red reflex in the patient's pupil. If the examiner (specifically, the peephole of the retinoscope) is at the patient's far point, all the light leaving the patient's pupil enters the peephole and illumination is uniform. However, if the far point of the patient's eye is not at the peephole of the retinoscope, only some of the rays emanating from the patient's pupil enter the peephole, and illumination of the pupil appears incomplete.

If the far point is between the examiner and the patient, the emerging rays will have focused and then diverged. The border between the dark and lighted portions of the pupil will move in a direction opposite to the motion (sweep) of the retinoscope streak (known as *against* movement) as it is moved across the patient's pupil. If the far point is behind the examiner, the light moves in the same direction as the sweep (known as *with* movement; Fig 3-5).

The condition in which the light fills the pupil and does not move is known as *neutrality* (Fig 3-6). The far point is moved with placement of a correcting lens in front of the patient's eye. At neutrality, if the examiner moves forward (in front of the far point),

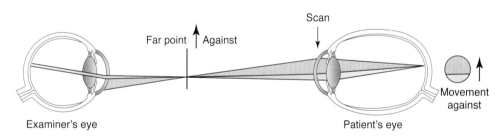

Figure 3-4   Observation system for myopia.

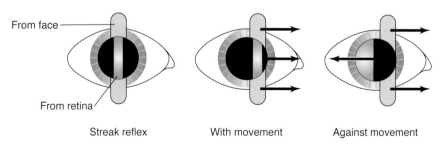

Figure 3-5   Retinal reflex movement. Note movement of the streak from face and from retina in *with* versus *against* movement. *(Illustration by C. H. Wooley.)*

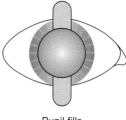

Figure 3-6 Neutrality reflex. Far point of the eye is conjugate with the peephole of the retinoscope. *(Illustration by C. H. Wooley.)*

Pupil fills

with movement is seen; if the examiner moves back and away from the far point, *against* movement is seen.

Characteristics of the reflex

The moving retinoscopic reflex has 3 main characteristics (Fig 3-7):

1. *Speed.* The reflex seen in the pupil moves slowest when the far point is distant from the examiner (peephole of the retinoscope). As the far point is moved toward the peephole, the speed of the reflex increases. In other words, large refractive errors have a slow-moving reflex, whereas small errors have a fast reflex.
2. *Brilliance.* The reflex is dull when the far point is distant from the examiner; it becomes brighter as neutrality is approached. *Against* reflexes are usually dimmer than *with* reflexes.
3. *Width.* When the far point is distant from the examiner, the streak is narrow. As the far point is moved closer to the examiner, the streak broadens and, at neutrality, fills the entire pupil. This situation applies only to *with* movement reflexes.

The Correcting Lens

When the examiner uses the appropriate correcting lenses (with either loose lenses or a *phoropter*), the retinoscopic reflex is neutralized. In other words, when the examiner brings the patient's far point to the peephole, the reflex fills the patient's entire pupil (Fig 3-8). The power of the correcting lens (or lenses) neutralizing the reflex helps determine the patient's refractive error.

The examiner determines the refractive error at the distance from which he or she is working. The dioptric equivalent of the *working distance* (ie, the inverse of the distance) must be subtracted from the power of the correcting lens to determine the actual refractive error of the patient's eye. Because a common working distance is 67 cm, many phoropters have a 1.50 D (1.00/0.67 m) "working-distance lens" for use during retinoscopy (however, this lens can produce bothersome reflexes).

Any working distance may be used. If the examiner prefers to move closer to the patient for a brighter reflex, the working-distance correction is adjusted accordingly. For example, suppose that an examiner obtains neutralization with a total of +4.00 D over the eye (gross retinoscopy) at a working distance of 67 cm. Subtracting 1.50 D for the working distance yields a refractive correction of +2.50 D.

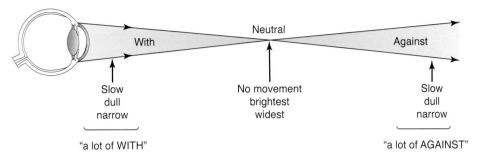

Figure 3-7 Characteristics of the moving retinal reflex on both sides of neutrality. The *vertical arrows* indicate the position of the retinoscope with regard to the point of neutrality. *(Illustration by C. H. Wooley.)*

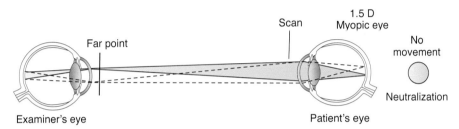

Figure 3-8 Observation system at neutralization.

Finding Neutrality

In *against* movement, the far point is between the examiner and the patient. Therefore, to bring the far point to the peephole of the retinoscope, a minus lens is placed in front of the patient's eye. Similarly, in the case of *with* movement, a plus lens is placed in front of the patient's eye. This procedure gives rise to the simple clinical rule: If *with* movement is observed, add plus power (or subtract minus power); if *against* movement is observed, add minus power (or subtract plus power) (Fig 3-9).

Because it is easier to work with the brighter, sharper *with* movement image, one should "overminus" the eye and obtain a *with* reflex; then reduce the minus power (or add plus power) until neutrality is reached. Be aware that the slow, dull reflexes of high-refractive errors may be confused with the neutrality reflex. Media opacities may also produce dull reflexes.

Retinoscopy of Regular Astigmatism

Most eyes have some regular astigmatism. In such cases, light is refracted differently by the 2 principal astigmatic meridians. Let us consider how the retinoscope works in greater detail and apply it to astigmatism.

Sweeping the retinoscope back and forth measures the power along only a single axis. Moving the retinoscope from side to side (with the streak oriented at 90°) measures the

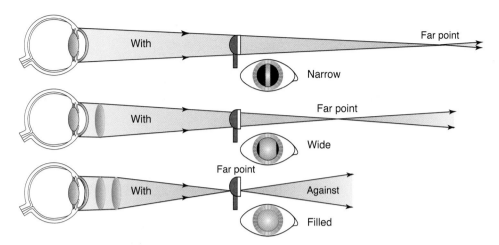

Figure 3-9 Approaching neutrality. Change in width of the reflex as neutrality is approached. Note that working distance remains constant, and the *far point* is pulled in with plus lenses. *(Illustration by C. H. Wooley.)*

optical power in the 180° meridian. Power in this meridian is provided by a cylinder at the 90° axis. The convenient result is that the streak of the retinoscope is aligned with the axis of the correcting cylinder being tested. In a patient with regular astigmatism, one seeks to neutralize 2 reflexes, 1 from each of the principal meridians.

Finding the cylinder axis

Before the powers in each of the principal meridians can be determined, the axes of the meridians must be determined. Four characteristics of the streak reflex aid in this determination:

1. *Break.* A break is observed when the streak is not oriented parallel to 1 of the principal meridians. The reflex streak in the pupil is not aligned with the streak projected on the iris and surface of the eye, and the line appears broken (Fig 3-10). The break disappears (ie, the line appears continuous) when the projected streak is rotated to the correct axis.
2. *Width.* The width of the reflex in the pupil varies as it is rotated around the correct axis. The reflex appears narrowest when the streak, or *intercept,* aligns with the axis (Fig 3-11).
3. *Intensity.* The intensity of the line is brighter when the streak is on the correct axis.
4. *Skew.* Skew (oblique motion of the streak reflex) may be used to refine the axis in small cylinders. If the retinoscope streak is off-axis, it moves in a slightly different direction from that of the pupillary reflex (Fig 3-12). The reflex and streak move in the same direction when the streak is aligned with 1 of the principal meridians.

When the streak is aligned at the correct axis, the sleeve may be lowered (Copeland instrument) or raised (Welch Allyn instrument) to narrow the streak, allowing the axis to be determined more easily (Fig 3-13).

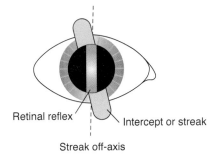

Figure 3-10 Break. The retinal reflex is discontinuous with the intercept when the streak is off the correct axis *(dashed lines)*. *(Illustration by C. H. Wooley.)*

Retinal reflex

Intercept or streak

Streak off-axis

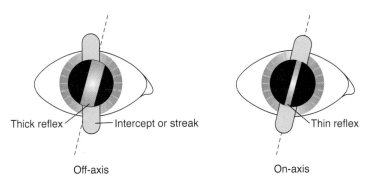

Thick reflex — Intercept or streak

Off-axis

Thin reflex

On-axis

Figure 3-11 Width, or thickness, of the retinal reflex. The examiner locates the axis where the reflex is thinnest *(dashed lines)*. *(Illustration by C. H. Wooley.)*

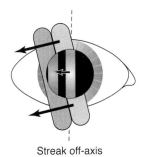

Figure 3-12 Skew. The *arrows* indicate that movements of the reflex *(single arrow)* and intercept *(2 arrows)* are not parallel. The reflex and intercept do not move in the same direction but are skewed when the streak is off-axis. *Dashed lines* indicate the on-axis line. *(Illustration by C. H. Wooley.)*

Streak off-axis

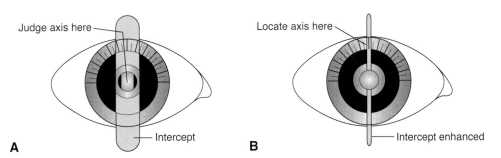

Judge axis here

Locate axis here

Intercept

Intercept enhanced

A

B

Figure 3-13 Locating axis on the protractor. **A,** First, determine the astigmatic axis. **B,** Second, adjust the sleeve to enhance the intercept until the filament is observed as a fine line pinpointing the axis. *(Illustration by C. H. Wooley.)*

This axis can be confirmed through a technique known as *straddling,* which is performed with the estimated correcting cylinder in place (Fig 3-14). The retinoscope streak is turned 45° off-axis in both directions, and if the axis is correct, the width of the reflex should be equal in both off-axis positions. If the axis is not correct, the widths are unequal in these 2 positions. The axis of the correcting plus-cylinder should be moved toward the narrower reflex and the straddling repeated until the widths are equal. This technique is often more accurate than subjective cross-cylinder axis refinement.

Finding the cylinder power

After the 2 principal meridians are identified, the previously explained spherical techniques are applied to each axis:

- *With 2 spheres.* Neutralize 1 axis with a spherical lens; then neutralize the axis 90° away. The difference between these readings is the cylinder power. For example, if the 90° axis is neutralized with a +1.50 sphere and the 180° axis is neutralized with a +2.25 sphere, the gross retinoscopy is +1.50 +0.75 × 180. The examiner's working distance (ie, +1.50) is subtracted from the sphere to obtain the final refractive correction: plano +0.75 × 180.
- *With a sphere and cylinder.* Neutralize 1 axis with a spherical lens. To enable the use of *with* reflexes, neutralize the *less plus* axis first. Then, with this spherical lens in place, neutralize the axis 90° away by adding a plus cylindrical lens. The spherocylindrical gross retinoscopy is read directly from the trial lens apparatus.

It is also possible to use 2 cylinders at right angles to each other for this gross retinoscopy.

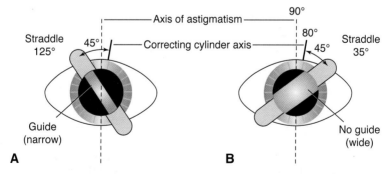

Figure 3-14 Straddling. The straddling meridians are 45° off the correcting cylinder axis, at roughly 35° and 125°. As the examiner moves back from the eye while comparing the meridians, the reflex at 125° remains narrow **(A)** at the same distance that the reflex at 35° has become wide **(B)**. This dissimilarity indicates an axis error; the narrow reflex **(A)** is the guide toward which the examiner must turn the correcting cylinder axis. *(Illustration by C. H. Wooley.)*

Aberrations of the Retinoscopic Reflex

With irregular astigmatism, almost any type of aberration may appear in the reflex. *Spherical aberrations* tend to increase the brightness at the center or periphery of the pupil, depending on whether they are positive or negative.

As neutrality is approached, 1 part of the reflex may be myopic, whereas the other may be hyperopic relative to the position of the retinoscope. This situation produces a *scissors reflex.* Causes of the scissors reflex include keratoconus, irregular corneal astigmatism, corneal or lenticular opacities, and spherical aberration.

All of these aberrant reflexes, in particular spherical aberration, are more noticeable in patients with large scotopic pupils. When a large pupil is observed during retinoscopy, the examiner should focus on neutralizing the central portion of the light reflex.

Table 3-1 provides a summary of the technique of retinoscopy using a plus-cylinder phoropter.

Corboy JM. *The Retinoscopy Book: An Introductory Manual for Eye Care Professionals.* 4th ed. Thorofare, NJ: Slack; 1995.

Wirtschafter JD, Schwartz GS. Retinoscopy. In: Tasman W, Jaeger EA, eds. *Duane's Clinical Ophthalmology* [CD-ROM]. Vol 1. Philadelphia: Lippincott Williams & Wilkins; 2006:chap 37.

Table 3-1 **Retinoscopy Summary (Using a Plus-Cylinder Phoropter)**

1. Set the phoropter to 0.00 D sphere and 0.00 D cylinder. Use cycloplegia if necessary. Otherwise, fog the eyes or use a nonaccommodative target.
2. Hold the sleeve of the retinoscope in the position that produces a divergent beam of light. (If the examiner can focus the linear filament of the retinoscope on a wall, the sleeve is in the wrong position.)
3. Sweep the streak of light (the intercept) across the pupil perpendicular to the long axis of the streak. Observe the pupillary light reflex. Sweep in several different meridians.
4. Add minus sphere until the retinoscopic reflex shows *with* movement in all meridians. Add some extra minus sphere if uncertain. If the reflexes are dim or indistinct, consider high refractive errors and make large changes in sphere (–3.00 D, –6.00 D, –9.00 D, and so on).
5. Continue examining multiple meridians while adding plus sphere until the retinoscopic reflex neutralizes in 1 meridian. (If all meridians neutralize simultaneously, the patient's refractive error is spherical; subtract the working distance to obtain the net retinoscopy.)
6. Rotate the streak 90° and position the axis of the correcting plus cylinder parallel to the streak. A sweep across this meridian reveals additional *with* movement. Add plus cylinder power with axis parallel to the streak until neutrality is achieved.
7. Refine the correcting cylinder axis by sweeping 45° to either side of it. Rotate the axis of the correcting plus cylinder a few degrees toward the "guide" line, the brighter and narrower reflex. Repeat until both reflexes are equal.
8. Refine the cylinder power by moving in closer to the patient to pick up *with* movement in all directions. Back away slowly, observing how the reflexes neutralize. Change sphere or cylinder power as appropriate to make all meridians neutralize simultaneously.
9. Subtract the dioptic equivalent of the working distance. For example, if the working distance is 67 cm, subtract 1.50 D (1.00/0.67).
10. Record the streak retinoscopy findings and, when possible, check the patient's visual acuity with the new prescription.

Subjective Refraction Techniques

In subjective refraction techniques, the examiner relies on the patient's responses to determine the refractive correction. If all refractive errors were spherical, subjective refraction would be easy. However, determining the astigmatic portion of the correction is more complex, and various subjective refraction techniques may be used. The Jackson cross cylinder is the most common instrument used in determining the astigmatic correction. However, we begin by discussing the astigmatic dial technique because it is easier to understand.

Astigmatic Dial Technique

An astigmatic dial is a test chart with radially arranged lines that may be used to determine the axes of astigmatism. A pencil of light from a point source is imaged by an astigmatic eye as a conoid of Sturm. The spokes of the astigmatic dial that are parallel to the principal meridians of the eye's astigmatism are imaged as sharp lines, which correspond to the focal lines of the conoid of Sturm.

Figure 3-15A shows an eye with compound hyperopic astigmatism and how it sees an astigmatic dial. The vertical line of the astigmatic dial is the blackest and sharpest because the vertical focal line of each conoid of Sturm is closer to the retina than the horizontal focal line is. By accommodating, however, the patient might pull both focal lines forward, far enough to make even the horizontal line of the astigmatic dial clear. To avoid accommodation, fogging is used. Sufficient plus sphere is placed before the eye to pull both focal lines into the vitreous, creating compound myopic astigmatism (Fig 3-15B).

Because accommodating with the eye fogged causes increased blurring of the lines, the patient relaxes accommodation. The focal line closest to the retina can then be identified with certainty as the horizontal line because it is now the blackest and sharpest line of the astigmatic dial. Note that the terms *blackest* and *sharpest* are more easily understood by patients and should be used in place of the word *clearest*.

After the examiner locates 1 of the principal meridians of the astigmatism, the conoid of Sturm can be collapsed by moving the anterior focal line back toward the posterior focal line. This task can be accomplished by adding a minus cylinder with an axis parallel to the anterior focal line. In Figure 3-15C, the vertical focal line has been moved back to the position of the horizontal focal line and collapsed to a point by the addition of a minus cylinder with an axis at 90°. Notice that the minus cylinder is placed with its axis *perpendicular* to the blackest meridian on the astigmatic dial. Also note that as the conoid of Sturm is collapsed, the focal lines disappear into a point focus.

All of the lines of the astigmatic dial now appear equally black but still are not in perfect focus, because the eye remains slightly fogged to control accommodation. At this point, a visual acuity chart is used; plus sphere is removed until the best visual acuity is obtained (Fig 3-15D).

In summary, the following steps are used in astigmatic dial refraction:

1. Obtain the best visual acuity using spheres only.
2. Fog the eye to approximately 20/50 by adding plus sphere.
3. Ask the patient to identify the blackest and sharpest line of the astigmatic dial.

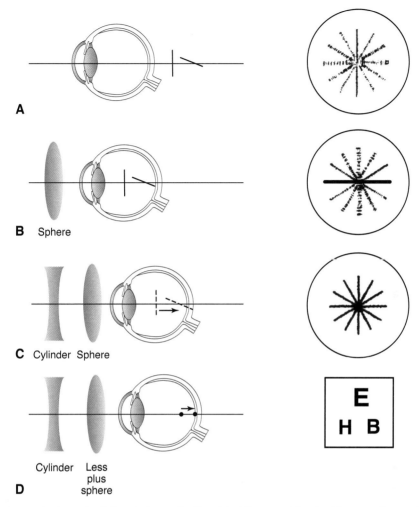

A

B Sphere

C Cylinder Sphere

D Cylinder   Less
plus
sphere

Figure 3-15 Astigmatic dial technique. **A,** Conoid of Sturm and retinal image of an astigmatic dial as viewed by an eye with compound hyperopic astigmatism. **B,** Fogging to produce compound myopic astigmatism. **C,** The conoid of Sturm is collapsed to a single point. **D,** Minus sphere is added (or plus sphere subtracted) to produce a sharp image, and a visual acuity chart is used for viewing.

4. Add minus cylinder with the axis perpendicular to the blackest and sharpest line until all lines appear equal. (If using a positive cylinder phoropter, add plus cylinder with the axis parallel to the blackest and sharpest line until all lines appear equal.)
5. Reduce plus sphere (or add minus) until the best visual acuity is obtained with the visual acuity chart.

Astigmatic dial refraction can also be performed with plus cylinder equipment, but this technique must be used in a way that simulates minus cylinder effect. All of the above steps remain the same except for step 4, which becomes "Add *plus* cylinder with the axis *parallel* to the blackest and sharpest line." As each 0.25 D of plus cylinder power is added, change the sphere simultaneously by 0.25 D in the minus direction. Doing so simulates minus cylinder effect exactly by moving the anterior focal line posteriorly without changing the position of the posterior focal line.

Michaels DD. *Visual Optics and Refraction: A Clinical Approach.* 3rd ed. St Louis: Mosby; 1985:319–322.

Stenopeic Slit Technique

The stenopeic slit is an opaque trial lens with an oblong slit whose width forms a pinhole with respect to vergence perpendicular to the slit (Fig 3-16). If an examiner is unable to decipher the astigmatism by performing the usual retinoscopy because of the subject eye's irregular astigmatism or unclear media, he or she may neutralize the refractive error with spherical lenses and the slit at various meridians to find a spherocylindrical correction. This correction can then be refined subjectively. This process is especially useful for patients with small pupils and lenticular or corneal opacities. If the subject can accommodate, fog and unfog using plus sphere to find the most plus power accepted. Then turn the slit until the subject says the image is sharpest. If, for example, –3.00 D sphere is best there, when the slit is oriented vertically, this finding indicates –3.00 D at 90° in a power cross. If the best sphere with the slit oriented horizontally is –5.00 D, then the result is –3.00 –2.00 × 90.

Cross-Cylinder Technique

The Jackson cross cylinder, in Edward Jackson's words, is probably "far more useful, and far more used" than any other lens in clinical refraction. Every ophthalmologist should be familiar with the principles involved in its use. Although the cross cylinder is usually used to *refine* the cylinder axis and power of a refraction that has already been obtained, it can also be used for the entire astigmatic refraction.

The first step in cross-cylinder refraction is adjusting the sphere to yield the best visual acuity with accommodation relaxed. Begin by placing the prescription the patient is wearing into a trial frame or phoropter. Fog the eye to be examined with plus sphere while the patient views a visual acuity chart; then decrease the fog until the best visual acuity is obtained. If astigmatism is present, decreasing the fog places the circle of least confusion on the retina, creating a mixed astigmatism. Then use test figures that are 1–2 lines larger than the patient's best visual acuity. At this point, introduce the cross cylinder, first for refinement of cylinder axis and then for refinement of cylinder power.

If no cylindrical correction is present initially, the cross cylinder may still be used, placed at 90° and 180°, to check for the presence of astigmatism. If a preferred flip position

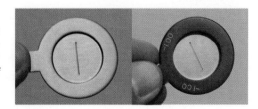

Figure 3-16 Stenopeic slit. The image on the right demonstrates the placement of a spherical lens in front of the stenopeic slit in order to determine the best visual acuity. *(Courtesy of Tommy Korn, MD.)*

is found, cylinder is added with the axis parallel to the respective plus or minus axis of the cross cylinder until the 2 flip choices are equal. If no preference is found with the cross-cylinder axes at 90° and 180°, then check the axes at 45° and 135° before assuming that no astigmatism is present. Once any cylinder power is found, axis and power should be refined in the usual manner.

Another method of determining the presence of astigmatism is to dial 0.50 D of cylinder into the phoropter (while preserving the spherical equivalent with a compensatory 0.25 D change in the sphere). Ask the patient to slowly rotate the cylinder axis once around using the knob on the phoropter. If doing so has no effect, there is no clinically significant astigmatism. If the patient finds a preferred position, it becomes the starting point for the cross-cylinder refinement.

Always refine cylinder axis before refining cylinder power. This sequence is necessary because the correct axis may be found in the presence of an incorrect power, but the full cylinder power is found only in the presence of the correct axis.

Refinement of cylinder axis involves the combination of cylinders at oblique axes. When the axis of the correcting cylinder is not aligned with that of the astigmatic eye's cylinder, the combined cylinders produce residual astigmatism with a meridian roughly 45° away from the principal meridians of the 2 cylinders. To refine the axis, position the principal meridians of the cross cylinder 45° away from those of the correcting cylinder (if using a handheld Jackson cross cylinder, the stem of the lens handle will be parallel to the axis of the correcting cylinder). Present the patient with alternative flip choices, and select the choice that is the blackest and sharpest to the patient. Then rotate the axis of the correcting cylinder toward the corresponding plus or minus axis of the cross cylinder (plus cylinder axis is rotated toward the plus cylinder axis of the cross cylinder, and minus cylinder axis is rotated toward the minus cylinder axis of the cross cylinder). Low-power cylinders are rotated in increments of 15°; high-power cylinders are rotated by smaller amounts, usually 5°. Repeat this procedure until the flip choices appear equal.

To refine cylinder power, align the cross-cylinder axes with the principal meridians of the correcting lens (Fig 3-17). The examiner should change cylinder power according to the patient's responses; the spherical equivalent of the refractive correction should remain constant to keep the circle of least confusion on the retina. Ensure that the correction

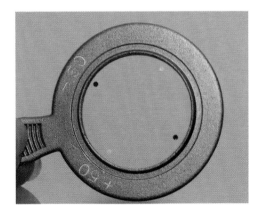

Figure 3-17 Jackson cross cylinder. *(Courtesy of Tommy Korn, MD.)*

remains constant by changing the sphere half as much and in the opposite direction as the cylinder power is changed. In other words, for every 0.50 D of cylinder power change, change the sphere by 0.25 D in the opposite direction. Periodically, the sphere power should be adjusted for the best visual acuity.

Continue to refine cylinder power until the patient reports that both flip choices appear equal. At that point, the 2 flip choices produce equal and opposite mixed astigmatism, blurring the visual acuity chart equally.

Remember to use the proper-power cross cylinder for the patient's visual acuity level. For example, a ±0.25 D cross cylinder is commonly used with visual acuity levels of 20/30 and better. A high-power cross cylinder (±0.50 D or ±1.00 D) allows a patient with poorer vision to recognize differences in the flip choices.

The patient may be confused with prior choices during cross-cylinder refinement. Giving different numbers to subsequent choices avoids this problem: "Which is better, 1 or 2, 3 or 4?" and so forth. If the patient persists in choosing either the first or second number, reverse the order of presentation to check for consistency.

Table 3-2 summarizes the cross-cylinder refraction technique.

Guyton DL. *Retinoscopy: Minus Cylinder Technique, 1986; Retinoscopy: Plus Cylinder Technique, 1986; Subjective Refraction: Cross-Cylinder Technique, 1987.* Reviewed for currency, 2007. Clinical Skills DVD Series [DVD]. San Francisco: American Academy of Ophthalmology.

Wunsh SE. The cross cylinder. In: Tasman W, Jaeger EA, eds. *Duane's Clinical Ophthalmology* [CD-ROM]. Vol 1. Philadelphia: Lippincott Williams & Wilkins; 2006:chap 38.

Refining the Sphere

After cylinder power and axis have been determined using either the astigmatic dial technique or the cross-cylinder method, the final step of determining monocular refraction is to refine the sphere. The endpoint in the refraction is the strongest plus sphere, or weakest minus sphere, that yields the best visual acuity. The following discussion briefly considers some of the methods used.

When the cross-cylinder technique has been used to determine the cylinder power and axis, the refractive error is presumed to a single point. Add plus sphere in +0.25 D increments

---

Table 3-2 Cross-Cylinder Refraction Summary

1. Adjust sphere to the most plus or least minus that gives the best visual acuity.
2. Use test figures that are 1 or 2 lines larger than the patient's best visual acuity.
3. If cylindrical correction is not already present, look for astigmatism by testing with the cross cylinder at axes 90° and 180°. If none is found there, test at 45° and 135°.
4. Refine axis first. Position the cross-cylinder axes 45° from the principal meridians of the correcting cylinder. Determine the preferred flip choice, and rotate the cylinder axis toward the corresponding axis of the cross cylinder. Repeat until the 2 flip choices appear equal.
5. Refine cylinder power. Align the cross-cylinder axes with the principal meridians of the correcting cylinder. Determine the preferred flip choice, and add or subtract cylinder power according to the preferred position of the cross cylinder. Compensate for the change in position of the circle of least confusion by adding half as much sphere in the opposite direction each time the cylinder power is changed.
6. Refine sphere, cylinder axis, and cylinder power until no further change is necessary.

until the patient reports decreased vision. If no additional plus sphere is accepted, add minus sphere in –0.25 D increments until the patient achieves the most optimal visual acuity.

Using accommodation, the patient can compensate for excess minus sphere. Therefore, it is important to use the least minus sphere necessary to reach the best visual acuity. In effect, accommodation creates a reverse Galilean telescope, whereby the eye generates more plus power as minus power is added to the trial lenses before the eye. As this minus power increases, the patient observes that the letters appear smaller and more distant.

The patient should be told what to look for. Before subtracting each 0.25 D increment, tell the patient that the letters may appear sharper and brighter or smaller and darker, and ask the patient to report any such change. Reduce the amount of plus sphere only if the patient can actually read more letters.

If the astigmatic dial technique has been used and the astigmatism is neutralized (ie, if all the lines on the astigmatic dial are equally sharp or equally blurred), the eye should still be fogged; additional plus sphere only increases the blur. Therefore, use minus sphere to reduce the sphere power until the best visual acuity is achieved. Again, the examiner should be careful not to add too much minus sphere.

To verify the spherical endpoint, the *duochrome test* (also known as the *red-green* or *bichrome test*) is used (Fig 3-18). A split red-green filter makes the background of the visual acuity chart appear vertically divided into a red half and a green half. Because of the chromatic aberration of the eye, the shorter (green) wavelengths are focused in front of the longer (red) wavelengths. The eye typically focuses near the midpoint of the spectrum, between the red and green wavelengths. With optimal spherical correction, the letters on the red and green halves of the chart appear equally sharp. The commercial filters used in the duochrome test produce a chromatic interval of approximately 0.50 D between the red and green wavelengths. When the image is clearly focused in white light, the eye is 0.25 D myopic for the green letters and 0.25 D hyperopic for the red letters.

Each eye is tested separately for the duochrome test, which is begun with the eye slightly fogged (by 0.50 D) to relax accommodation. The letters on the red side should appear sharper; the clinician should add minus sphere until the 2 sides appear the same. If the patient responds that the letters on the green side are sharper, the patient is over-minused, and more plus power should be added. Some clinicians use the RAM-GAP mnemonic—"*red add minus; green add plus*"—to recall how to use the duochrome test.

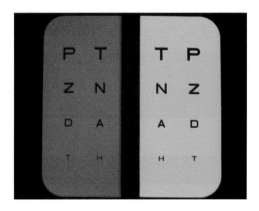

Figure 3-18 Duochrome test. *(Courtesy of Tommy Korn, MD.)*

Because this test is based on chromatic aberration and not on color discrimination, it is used even with color-blind patients (although it may be necessary to identify the sides of the chart as left and right rather than red and green). An eye with overactive accommodation may still require too much minus sphere in order to balance the red and green. Cycloplegia may be necessary. The duochrome test is not used with patients whose visual acuity is worse than 20/30 (6/9), because the 0.50 D difference between the 2 sides is too small to distinguish.

Binocular Balance

The final step of subjective refraction is to make certain that accommodation has been relaxed equally in both eyes. Several methods of binocular balance are commonly used. Most require that the corrected visual acuity be nearly equal in both eyes.

Fogging

When the endpoint refraction is fogged using a +2.00 D sphere before each eye, the visual acuity should be reduced to 20/200–20/100 (6/60–6/30). Place a –0.25 D sphere before first 1 eye and then the other, and rapidly alternate cover; the patient should then be able to identify the eye with the –0.25 D sphere before it as having the sharper image at the 20/100 (6/30) or 20/70 (6/20) level. If the eyes are not in balance, sphere should be added or subtracted in 0.25 increments until balance is achieved.

In addition to testing for binocular balance, the fogging method also provides information about appropriate sphere power. If either eye is overminused or underplussed, the patient should read farther down the chart—as far as 20/70 (6/20), 20/50 (6/15), or even 20/40 (6/12)—with the +2.00 D fogging spheres in place. In this case, the refraction endpoints should be reconsidered.

Prism dissociation

The most sensitive test of binocular balance is prism dissociation. For this test, the refractive endpoints are fogged with +1.00 D spheres, and vertical prisms of 4 or 5 prism diopters (Δ) are placed before 1 eye (Fig 3-19). Use of the prisms causes the patient to see 2 charts, 1 above the other. A single line, usually 20/40 (6/12), is isolated on the chart; the

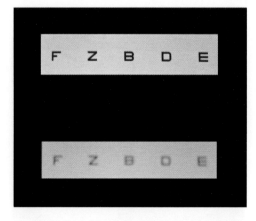

Figure 3-19 Binocular balancing by prism dissociation from patient perspective. *(Courtesy of Tommy Korn, MD.)*

patient sees 2 separate lines simultaneously, 1 for each eye. The patient can readily identify differences between the fogged images in the 2 eyes of as little as 0.25 D sphere. In practice, +0.25 D sphere is placed before 1 eye and then before the other. In each instance, if the eyes are balanced, the patient reports that the image corresponding to the eye with the additional +0.25 D sphere is blurrier. After a balance is established between the 2 eyes, remove the prism and reduce the fog binocularly until the best visual acuity is obtained.

Cycloplegic and Noncycloplegic Refraction

Ideally, refractive error is measured with accommodation relaxed. The amount of habitual accommodative tone varies from person to person, and even within an individual it varies at times and with age. Because determining this variable may not always be possible, cycloplegic drugs are sometimes used. The indication and appropriate dosage for a specific cycloplegic drug depend on the patient's age, accommodative amplitude, and refractive error.

A practical approach to obtaining satisfactory refraction is to perform a careful noncycloplegic (or manifest) refraction, ensuring relaxed accommodation with fogging or other nonpharmacologic techniques. If the results are inconsistent or variable, a cycloplegic refraction should be performed. If the findings of these 2 refractions are similar, the prescription may be based on the manifest refraction. If there is a disparity, a postcycloplegic evaluation may be necessary. Most children require cycloplegic refraction because of their high amplitude of accommodation. For more details on the cycloplegic drugs used in adults and children, please refer to the pharmacotherapeutics chapter in BCSC Section 2, *Fundamentals and Principles of Ophthalmology.*

Overrefraction

Phoropters may be used to refract the eyes of patients with highly ametropic vision. Variability in the vertex distance of the refraction (the distance from the back surface of the spectacle lens to the cornea) and other induced errors make prescribing directly from the phoropter findings unreliable.

Some of these problems can be avoided if highly ametropic eyes are refracted over the patients' current glasses (overrefraction). If the new lenses are prescribed with the same base curve as the current lenses and are fitted in the same frames, many potential difficulties can be circumvented, including vertex distance error and pantoscopic tilt error, as well as problems caused by marginal astigmatism and chromatic aberration. Overrefraction may be performed with loose lenses (using trial lens clips such as Halberg trial clips), with a standard phoropter in front of the patient's glasses, or with some automated refracting instruments.

If the patient is wearing spherical lenses, the new prescription is easy to calculate by combining the current spherical correction with the spherocylindrical overrefraction. If the current lenses are spherocylindrical and the cylinder axis of the overrefraction is not at 0° or 90° to the present correction, other methods previously discussed are used to determine the resultant refraction. Such lens combinations were often determined with a *lensmeter* used to read the resultant lens power through the combinations of the old glasses and the overrefraction correction. This procedure is awkward and prone to error because the lenses may rotate with respect to one another on transfer to the lensmeter. Manual calculation is possible but complicated. Programmable calculators can be used to perform the trigonometric combination of cylinders at oblique axes, but they may not be readily available in the clinic.

Overrefraction has other uses. For example, a patient wearing a soft toric contact lens may undergo overrefraction for the purpose of ordering new lenses. An overrefraction is especially useful for patients wearing rigid, gas-permeable, hard contact lenses for irregular corneal astigmatism or corneal transplants. Overrefraction can also be used in the retinoscopic examination of children.

Spectacle Correction of Ametropias

Ametropia is a refractive error; it is the absence of emmetropia. The most common method of correcting refractive error is through prescription of spectacle lenses.

Spherical Correcting Lenses and the Far Point Concept

The far point plane of the nonaccommodated eye is conjugate with the retina. For a simple lens, distant objects (those at optical infinity) come into sharp focus at the *secondary focal point* (F_2) of the lens. To correct the refractive error of an eye, a correcting lens must place the image it forms (or its F_2) at the eye's far point. The image at the far point plane becomes the object that is focused onto the retina. For example, in a myopic eye, the far point lies somewhere in front of the eye, between it and optical infinity. In this case, the correct *diverging lens* forms a virtual image of distant objects at its F_2, coincident with the far point of the eye (Fig 3-20).

The same principle holds for the correction of hyperopia (Fig 3-21). However, because the far point plane of a hyperopic eye is behind the retina, a *converging lens* must be chosen in the appropriate power to focus parallel rays of light to the far point plane.

The Importance of Vertex Distance

For any spherical correcting lens, the distance from the lens to its focal point is constant. Changing the position of the correcting lens relative to the eye also changes the relationship between the F_2 of the correcting lens and the far point plane of the eye. With

Figure 3-20 A diverging lens is used to correct myopia.

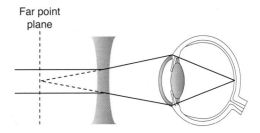

Far point
plane

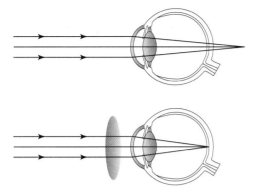

Figure 3-21 A converging lens is used to correct hyperopia.

high-power lenses, as used in the spectacle correction of aphakia or high myopia, a small change in the placement of the lens produces considerable blurring of vision unless the lens power is altered to compensate for the new lens position.

With refractive errors greater than ±5.00 D, the vertex distance must be accounted for in prescribing the power of the spectacle lens. A *distometer* (also called *vertexometer*) is used to measure the distance from the back surface of the spectacle lens to the cornea with the eyelid closed (Fig 3-22). Moving a correcting lens closer to the eye—whether the lens has plus or minus power—reduces its effective focusing power (the image moves posteriorly away from the fovea), whereas moving it farther from the eye increases its focusing power (the image moves anteriorly away from the fovea).

For example, in Figure 3-23, the +10.00 D lens placed 10 mm in front of the cornea provides sharp retinal imagery. Because the focal point of the correcting lens is identical to the far point plane of the eye and because this lens is placed 10 mm in front of the eye, the far point plane of the eye must be 90 mm behind the cornea. If the correcting lens is moved to a new position 20 mm in front of the eye and the far point plane of the eye is 90 mm, then the focal length of the new lens must be 110 mm, requiring a +9.10 D lens for correction. This example demonstrates the significance of vertex distance in spectacle correction of large refractive errors. Thus, the prescription must indicate not only the lens power but also the vertex distance at which the refraction was performed. The optician must recalculate the lens power as necessary for the actual vertex distance of the chosen spectacle–frame combination.

Cylindrical Correcting Lenses and the Far Point Concept

The far point principles used in the correction of hyperopia and myopia are also employed in the correction of astigmatism with spectacle lenses. However, in astigmatism, the required lens power must be determined separately for each of the 2 principal meridians.

Cylinders in spectacle lenses produce both monocular and binocular distortion. The primary cause is *meridional aniseikonia*—that is, unequal magnification of retinal images in the various meridians. Although aniseikonia may be corrected by iseikonic spectacles, such corrections may be complicated and expensive, and most practitioners prefer to prescribe cylinders according to their clinical judgment. Clinical experience also suggests

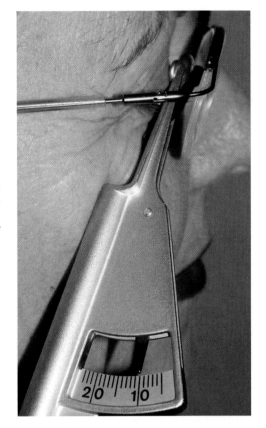

Figure 3-22 A vertexometer (distometer) is used to measure the vertex distance from the back surface of the spectacle lens to the cornea through a closed eyelid. *(Courtesy of Tommy Korn, MD.)*

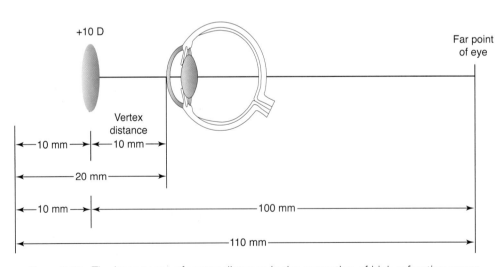

Figure 3-23 The importance of vertex distance in the correction of high refractive errors.

that adult patients vary in their ability to tolerate distortion, whereas young children always adapt to their cylindrical corrections.

The following guidelines may prove helpful in prescribing astigmatic spectacle corrections:

- For *children,* prescribe the full astigmatic correction at the correct axis.
- For *adults,* try the full correction initially. Give the patient a "walking-around" trial with trial frames before prescribing, if appropriate. Inform the patient about the need for adaptation. To reduce distortion, use minus cylinder lenses (most lenses dispensed today are minus cylinder) and minimize vertex distance.
- Because spatial distortion from astigmatic spectacles is a binocular phenomenon, occlude 1 eye to verify that spatial distortion is the cause of the patient's difficulty.
- If necessary, reduce distortion by rotating the axis of the cylinder toward 180° or 90° (or toward the old axis) and/or reduce the cylinder power. Adjust the sphere to maintain spherical equivalent, but rely on a final subjective check to obtain the most satisfactory visual result.
- If distortion cannot be reduced sufficiently, consider contact lenses or iseikonic corrections.

For a more detailed discussion of the problem of, and solutions for, spectacle correction of astigmatism, see Appendix 3.1 at the end of the chapter.

Prescribing for Children

The correction of ametropia in children presents several special and challenging problems. In adults, the correction of refractive errors has 1 measurable endpoint: the best-corrected visual acuity. Prescribing visual correction for children often has 2 goals: providing a focused retinal image and achieving the optimal balance between accommodation and convergence.

In some young patients, *subjective refraction* may be impossible or inappropriate, often because of the child's inability to cooperate with subjective refraction techniques. In addition, the optimal refraction in infants or small children (particularly those with esotropia) requires the *paralysis of accommodation* with complete cycloplegia. In such cases, objective techniques such as retinoscopy are the best way to determine the refractive correction. Moreover, the presence of *strabismus* may require modification of the normal prescribing guidelines.

Myopia

There are 2 types of childhood myopia: *congenital* (usually high) myopia and *developmental* myopia, which usually manifests itself between the ages of 7 and 10 years. Developmental myopia is less severe and easier to manage because the patients are older and refraction is less difficult. However, both forms of myopia are progressive; frequent refractions (every 6–12 months) and periodic prescription changes are necessary. The following are general guidelines for correction of significant childhood myopia:

- Cycloplegic refractions are mandatory. In infants, children with esotropia, and children with very high myopia (>10.00 D), atropine refraction may be necessary if tropicamide or cyclopentolate fails to paralyze accommodation in the office.
- In general, the full refractive error, including cylinder, should be corrected. Young children tolerate cylinder well.
- Some ophthalmologists undercorrect myopia, and others use bifocal lenses with or without atropine, on the basis of the theory that accommodation hastens or increases the development of myopia. This topic remains controversial among ophthalmologists.
- Intentional undercorrection of a child's myopic esotropia to decrease the angle of deviation is rarely tolerated.
- Intentional overcorrection of a myopic error (or undercorrection of a hyperopic error) may help control intermittent exodeviations. However, such overcorrection can cause additional accommodative stress.
- Parents should be educated about the natural progression of myopia and the need for frequent refractions and possible prescription changes.
- In older children, contact lenses may be desirable to avoid the problem of image minification that arises with high-minus lenses.

Hyperopia

The appropriate correction of childhood hyperopia is more complex than that of myopia for 2 reasons. First, children who are significantly hyperopic (>5.00 D) are more visually impaired than are their myopic counterparts, who can at least see clearly at near. Second, childhood hyperopia is more frequently associated with strabismus and abnormalities of the *accommodative convergence/accommodation (AC/A) ratio*. The following are general guidelines for correcting childhood hyperopia:

- Unless there is esodeviation or evidence of reduced vision, it is not necessary to correct low hyperopia. As with myopia, significant astigmatic errors should be fully corrected.
- When hyperopia and esotropia coexist, initial management includes full correction of the cycloplegic refractive error. Reductions in the amount of correction may be appropriate later, depending on the amount of esotropia and level of stereopsis with the full cycloplegic correction in place.
- In a school-aged child, the full refractive correction may cause blurring of distance vision because of the inability to relax accommodation fully. Reducing the amount of correction is sometimes necessary for the child to accept the glasses. A short course of cycloplegia may help a child accept the hyperopic correction.

Anisometropia

A child or infant with anisometropia is typically prescribed the full refractive difference between the 2 eyes, regardless of age, presence or amount of strabismus, or degree of anisometropia. Anisometropic amblyopia is frequently present and may require occlusion therapy. *Bilateral amblyopia* occasionally occurs when there is significant hyperopia, myopia, and/or astigmatism that occurs in both eyes.

Clinical Accommodative Problems

See Chapter 2 for a discussion of the terminology and mechanisms of accommodation.

Presbyopia

Presbyopia is the gradual loss of accommodative response resulting from reduced elasticity of the crystalline lens. Accommodative amplitude diminishes with age. It becomes a clinical problem when the remaining accommodative amplitude is insufficient for the patient to read and carry out near-vision tasks. Fortunately, appropriate convex lenses can compensate for the waning of accommodative power.

Symptoms of presbyopia usually begin to appear in patients after the age of 40 years. The age of onset depends on preexisting refractive error, depth of focus (pupil size), the patient's visual tasks, and other variables. Table 3-3 presents a simplified overview of age norms.

Accommodative Insufficiency

Accommodative insufficiency is the premature loss of accommodative amplitude. This problem may manifest itself by blurring of near visual objects (as in presbyopia) or by the

Table 3-3 Average Accommodative Amplitudes for Different Ages

Age	Average Accommodative Amplitude*
8	14.0 (±2 D)
12	13.0 (±2 D)
16	12.0 (±2 D)
20	11.0 (±2 D)
24	10.0 (±2 D)
28	9.0 (±2 D)
32	8.0 (±2 D)
36	7.0 (±2 D)
40	**6.0 (±2 D)**
44	4.5 (±1.5 D)
48	3.0 (±1.5 D)
52	2.5 (±1.5 D)
56	2.0 (±1.0 D)
60	1.5 (±1.0 D)
64	1.0 (±0.5 D)
68	0.5 (±0.5 D)

*Up to age 40, accommodation decreases by 1 D for each 4 years. After age 40, accommodation decreases more rapidly. From age 48 on, 0.5 D is lost every 4 years. Thus, one can recall the entire table by remembering the amplitudes at age 40 and age 48.

inability to sustain accommodative effort. The onset may be heralded by the appearance of asthenopic symptoms; the ultimate development is blurred near vision. Such "premature presbyopia" may signify concurrent or past debilitating illness, or it may be induced by medications such as tranquilizing drugs or the parasympatholytics used in treating some gastrointestinal disorders. In both cases, the condition may be reversible; however, permanent accommodative insufficiency may be associated with neurogenic disorders such as encephalitis or closed-head trauma. In some cases, the etiology may never be determined. These patients require additional reading plus power for near vision. The most common cause of premature presbyopia, however, is unrecognized hyperopia.

Accommodative Excess

Ciliary muscle spasm, often incorrectly termed spasm of accommodation, causes accommodative excess. A ciliary spasm has characteristic symptoms: headache, brow ache, variable blurring of distance vision, and an abnormally close near point. Ciliary spasm may be a manifestation of local disease such as iridocyclitis; it may be caused by medications such as the anticholinesterases used in the treatment of glaucoma; or it may be associated with uncorrected refractive errors, usually hyperopia but also astigmatism. In some patients, ciliary spasm exacerbates preexisting myopia. Postcycloplegic refraction often helps determine the patient's true refractive error in such cases.

Ciliary spasm may also occur after prolonged and intense periods of near work. *Spasm of the near reflex* is a characteristic clinical syndrome often observed in tense or anxious persons who present with (1) excess accommodation, (2) excess convergence, and (3) miosis.

Accommodative Convergence/Accommodation Ratio

Normally, accommodative effort is accompanied by a corresponding convergence effort (expressed in terms of meter angles). Thus, 1.00 D of accommodation is accompanied by a 1-m angle of convergence. For practical purposes, the AC/A ratio is ordinarily expressed in terms of prism diopters of deviation per diopter of accommodation. Using this type of expression, the normal AC/A ratio is 3:1–5:1.

The AC/A ratio is relatively constant in a given patient, but it should be noted that there is some variability among individuals. For example, a patient with an uncorrected 1.00 D of hyperopia may accommodate 1.00 D for clear distance vision without exercising a convergence effort. Conversely, a patient with uncorrected myopia must converge without accommodative effort to see clearly at the far point.

The AC/A ratio can be measured by varying the stimulus to accommodation in several ways. These methods are described in the following subsections.

Heterophoria method

The heterophoria method involves moving the fixation target. The heterophoria is measured at 6 m and again at 0.33 m.

$$AC/A = PD + \frac{\Delta n - \Delta d}{D}$$

where

> PD = interpupillary distance in centimeters
> Δn = near deviation in prism diopters
> Δd = distance deviation in prism diopters
> D = amount of accommodation in diopters

Sign convention:

> Esodeviations +
> Exodeviations –

Gradient method

The AC/A ratio can be measured in 1 of 2 ways with the gradient method. The first way is by *stimulating accommodation*. Measure the heterophoria with the target distance fixed at 6 m. Then remeasure the induced phoria after interposing a –1.00 D sphere in front of both eyes. The AC/A ratio is the difference between the 2 measurements.

The second way is by *relaxing accommodation*. With the target distance fixed at 0.33 m, measure the phoria before and after interposing +3.00 D spheres. The phoria difference divided by 3 is the AC/A ratio.

An abnormal AC/A ratio can place stress on the patient's fusional mechanisms at one distance or another, causing asthenopia or manifest strabismus. Abnormal AC/A ratios should be accounted for when prescribing corrective lenses.

> Parks MM. Vergences. In: Tasman W, Jaeger EA, eds. *Duane's Clinical Ophthalmology* [CD-ROM]. Vol 1. Philadelphia: Lippincott Williams & Wilkins; 2006:chap 7.

Effect of Spectacle and Contact Lens Correction on Accommodation and Convergence

Both accommodation and convergence requirements differ between contact lenses and spectacle lenses. The effects become more noticeable as the power of the correction increases.

Let us first consider accommodative requirements. Recall that because of vertex distance considerations, particularly with high-power corrections, the dioptric power of the distance correction in the spectacle plane is different from that in the contact lens plane: for a near object held at a constant distance, the amount that an eye needs to accommodate depends on the location of the refractive correction relative to the cornea. Patients with myopia must accommodate more for a given near object when wearing contact lenses than when wearing glasses. For example, patients in their early 40s with myopia who switch from single-vision glasses to contact lenses may suddenly experience presbyopic symptoms. The reverse is true with patients with hyperopia; spectacle correction requires more accommodation for a given near object than does contact lens correction. Patients with spectacle-corrected high myopia, when presbyopic, need only weak bifocal add power or none at all. For example, a patient with high myopia who wears –20.00 D glasses needs to accommodate only approximately 1.00 D to see an object at 33 cm.

Now let us consider convergence requirements and refractive correction. Because contact lenses move with the eyes and spectacles do not, different amounts of convergence are required for viewing near objects. Spectacle correction gives a myopic patient a base-in prism effect when converging and thus reduces the patient's requirement for convergence. (Fortunately, this reduction parallels the lessened requirement for accommodation.) In contrast, a patient with spectacle-corrected hyperopia encounters a base-out prism effect that increases the requirement for convergence. This effect is beneficial in the correction of residual esotropia at near in patients with hyperopia and accommodative esotropia. These effects may be the source of a patient's symptoms on switching between glasses and contact lenses. (See also Chapter 4.)

Prescribing Multifocal Lenses

A multifocal lens has 2 or more refractive elements. The power of each segment is prescribed separately.

Determining the Add Power of a Bifocal Lens

The information necessary to prescribe bifocal lenses includes (1) an accurate baseline refraction, (2) the accommodative amplitude, and (3) the patient's social or occupational activities that require near-vision correction (eg, reading, sewing, or computer use).

Measuring accommodative amplitude

Any of the following tests can provide useful information for determining the accommodative amplitude: (1) the near point of accommodation with accurate distance refractive correction in place, (2) the accommodative rule (eg, with a Prince rule), (3) the use of plus and minus spheres at near distance until the fixation target blurs. *Binocular amplitude of accommodation* is normally greater than the measurement for either eye alone by 0.50–1.00 D.

Near point of accommodation A practical method for measuring the near point of accommodation is to have the patient fixate on a near target (usually small print such as 5-point or Jaeger 2 type print) and move the test card toward the eye until the print blurs. If the eye is emmetropic (or rendered emmetropic by proper refractive correction), then the far point of the eye is at infinity and the near point can be converted into diopters of amplitude.

This method is subject to certain errors, including the apparent increased amplitude resulting from angular magnification of the letters as they approach the eye. In addition, if the eye is ametropic and not corrected for distance, the near point of accommodation cannot be converted into diopters of amplitude. In the following examples, each eye has 3 D of accommodative amplitude:

- A person with emmetropia would have a near point of 33 cm and a far point at optical infinity.
- A patient with an uncorrected 3.00 D of myopia would have a near point at 16.7 cm because at the far point of 33 cm, no accommodation is needed.
- A patient with an uncorrected 3.00 D of hyperopia would have a near point at infinity because all of the available accommodation is needed to overcome the hyperopia.

Accommodative rule Amplitude of accommodation can be measured with a device such as a Prince rule (Fig 3-24), which combines a reading card with a ruler calibrated in centimeters and diopters. Placing a +3.00 D lens before the emmetropic (or accurately corrected ametropic) eye places the far point of accommodation at 33 cm, and the near point is also brought closer by a corresponding 3.00 D. The amplitude is then determined by subtraction of the far point (in diopters) from the near point (in diopters).

Method of spheres Amplitude of accommodation may also be measured by having the patient fixate on a reading target at 40 cm. Accommodation is stimulated by the placement of successively stronger minus spheres before the eye until the print blurs; accommodation is then relaxed by the use of successively stronger plus lenses until blurring begins. The difference between the 2 lenses is a measure of accommodative amplitude. For example, if the patient accepts −3.00 D to blur (stimulus to accommodation) and +2.50 D to blur (relaxation of accommodation), the amplitude is 5.50 D.

Range of accommodation

Determining the range of accommodation, like measuring the amplitude of accommodation, is valuable in ensuring that the prescribed bifocal add power meets the patient's visual needs. The range of accommodation measures the useful range of clear vision when a given lens is employed. For this purpose, a measuring tape, meter stick, or accommodation rule may be used.

Selecting an add power

Determine the amount of accommodation required for the patient's near-vision tasks. For example, reading at 40 cm would require 2.50 D of accommodation. From the patient's measured accommodative amplitude, allow one-half to be held in reserve. This reserve allows for some comfortable movement should the patient move the reading material either closer or farther away from the optimal reading distance. For instance, if the patient has 2.00 D of accommodation, 1.00 D may be comfortably contributed by the patient. (Some patients may use more than one-half of their available accommodation with comfort.) Subtract the patient's available accommodation (1.00 D) from the total amount of accommodation required (2.50 D); the difference (1.50 D) is the approximate additional plus-lens power (add) needed.

Place a lens with this add power in front of the distance refractive correction, and measure the range of accommodation (near point to far point of accommodation in centimeters).

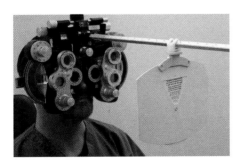

Figure 3-24 Prince rule. *(Courtesy of Tommy Korn, MD.)*

Does this range adequately meet the requirements of the patient's near-vision activities? If the accommodative range is too close, reduce the add power in increments of 0.25 D until the range is appropriate for the patient's requirement. Because binocular accommodative amplitude is usually 0.50–1.00 D greater than the monocular measurement, using the binocular measurement generally guards against prescribing an add power that is too high.

Types of Bifocal Lenses

Most bifocal lenses currently dispensed are 1-piece lenses that are made by generating the different refracting surfaces on a single lens blank (Fig 3-25). One-piece *round segment bifocal lenses* have their segment on the concave surface. One-piece *molded plastic bifocal lenses* are available in various shapes, including (1) round top with button on convex surface, (2) flat top with button on convex surface, and (3) Franklin (executive) style with split bifocal.

With *fused bifocal lenses,* the increased refracting power of the bifocal segment is produced by fusing a button of glass that has a higher refractive index than the basic crown glass lens into a countersink in the crown glass lens blank. With all such bifocal lenses, the add segment is fused into the convex surface of the lens; astigmatic corrections, when necessary, are ground on the concave surface.

Trifocal Lenses

A bifocal lens may not fully satisfy all the visual needs of an older patient with limited accommodation. Even when near and distant ranges are corrected appropriately, vision is not clear in the intermediate range, approximately at arm's length. This problem can be solved with trifocal spectacles, which incorporate a third segment of intermediate strength (typically one-half the power of the reading add) between the distance correction and the reading segment. The intermediate segment allows the patient to focus on objects beyond the reading distance but closer than 1 m. (See Clinical Example 3-1.)

Progressive Addition Lenses

Both bifocal and trifocal lenses have an abrupt change in power as the line of sight passes across the boundary between one portion of the lens and the next; image jump and diplopia can occur at the segment lines. Progressive addition lenses (PALs) avoid these difficulties by supplying power gradually as the line of sight is depressed toward the reading level. Unlike bifocal and trifocal lenses, PALs offer clear vision at all focal distances. Other advantages of PALs include lack of intermediate blur and absence of any visible segment lines.

The PAL form has 4 types of optical zones on the convex surface: a spherical distance zone, a reading zone, a transition zone (or "*corridor*"), and zones of peripheral distortion. The progressive change in lens power is generated on the convex surface of the lens by progressive aspheric changes in curvature from the top to the bottom of the lens. The concave surface is reserved for the sphere and cylinder of the patient's distance lens prescription.

However, there are certain drawbacks to PALs. Most notably, some degree of peripheral distortion is inherent in the design of all PALs. This peripheral aberration is caused by astigmatism resulting from the changing aspheric curves; these curves are most

Fused Bifocals

← Barium
crown glass
($n = 1.523$)

Flint glass button
($n = 1.654$)

Round top

Usual segment diameter 22 mm
(from 13.22 mm)

Flat top

Segment diameter
20 22 25 28 35 45 mm

Curved top

Ribbon segments

This fused bifocal is designed to permit
distance vision viewing below the segment.

One-Piece Bifocals

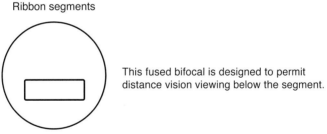

Split lens (or "Benjamin Franklin") **bifocal**.
Correction for astigmatism is ground
on the **concave** surface.

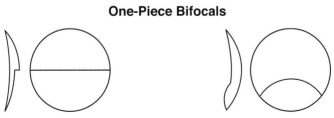

Ultex-type bifocals in segment diameters.

Ultex A   38 mm
Ultex AL   38 mm (up to 33 mm high)

Astigmatism correction is ground on
the **convex** surface.

Figure 3-25   Bifocal lens styles. n = index of refraction.

CLINICAL EXAMPLE 3-1

Consider a patient with 1.00 D of available accommodation. He wears a bifocal lens with a +2.00 add. His accommodative range for each part of the spectacle lens is

Distance segment: Infinity to 100 cm
Bifocal segment: 50–33 cm

He now has a blurred zone between 50 and 100 cm. An intermediate segment, in this case +1.00 D (half the power of the reading segment), would provide sharp vision from 50 cm (using all of his available accommodation plus the +1.00 D add) to 100 cm (using the add only). This trifocal lens combination therefore provides the following ranges:

Distance segment: Infinity to 100 cm
Intermediate segment: 100–50 cm
Near segment: 50–33 cm

pronounced in the lower inner and outer quadrants of the lens. These distortions produce a "swimming" sensation with head movement.

The vertical meridian joining the distance and reading optical centers is free of surface astigmatism and provides the optimal visual acuity. To either side of this distortion-free vertical meridian, induced astigmatism and a concomitant degradation of visual acuity occur. If the lens is designed such that the peripheral distortions are spread out over a relatively wide portion of the lens, there is a concomitant decrease in the distortion-free principal zones. This effect is the basis of *soft-design PALs* (Fig 3-26). Conversely, a wider distortion-free zone for distance and reading means a more intense lateral deformity. This effect is the basis of hard-design PALs. If the transition corridor is lengthened, the distortions are less pronounced, but problems arise because of the greater vertical separation between the distance optical center and the reading zone. Therefore, each PAL design represents a series of compromises. Some manufacturers prefer less distortion at the expense of less useful aberration-free distance and near visual acuity; others opt for maximum acuity over a wider usable area, with smaller but more pronounced lateral distortion zones.

PALs are readily available from −8.00 to +7.50 D spheres and up to 4.00 D cylinders; the available add powers are from +1.50 to +3.50 D. Some vendors also make custom lenses with parameters outside these limits. Prism can be incorporated into PALs.

The best candidates for PALs are patients with early presbyopia who have not previously worn bifocal lenses, patients who do not require wide near-vision fields, and highly motivated patients. Patients who change from conventional multifocal lenses to PALs should be advised that distortion will be present and that adaptation will be necessary. Small-frame PALs can reduce the usable reading zone to a small area at the bottom edge of the lens. Also, the differential magnification through the progressive zone can make computer screens appear trapezoidal. Progressive designs are also available for indoor use, with large zones devoted to computer monitor and reading distances (eg, 23 inches and 16 inches from the eye).

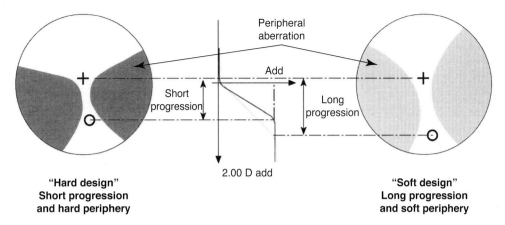

Figure 3-26 Comparison of hard-design and soft-design *progressive addition lenses (PALs)*. These illustrations compare the power progression and peripheral aberration of these 2 PAL designs. *(From Wisnicki HJ. Bifocals, trifocals, and progressive-addition lenses. Focal Points: Clinical Modules for Ophthalmologists. San Francisco: American Academy of Ophthalmology; 1999, module 6.)*

The Prentice Rule and Bifocal Lens Design

There are special considerations when prescribing lenses for patients with significant anisometropias.

Prismatic effects of lenses

All lenses act as prisms when one looks through the lens at any point other than the optical center. The amount of the induced prismatic effect depends on the power of the lens and the distance from the optical center. Specifically, the amount of prismatic effect (measured in prism diopters) is equal to the distance (in centimeters) from the optical center multiplied by the lens power (in diopters). This equation is known as the *Prentice rule:*

$$\Delta = hD$$

where

Δ = prismatic effect (in prism diopters)
h = distance from the optical center (in centimeters)
D = lens power (in diopters)

Image displacement

When reading at near through a point below the optical center, a patient wearing spectacle lenses of unequal power may notice vertical double vision. With a bifocal segment, the gaze is usually directed 8–10 mm below and 1.5–3.0 mm nasal to the distance optical center of the distance lens (in the following examples, we assume the usual 8 mm down and 2 mm nasal). As long as the bifocal segments are of the same power and type, the prismatic displacement is determined by the power of the distance lens alone.

If the lens powers are the same for the 2 eyes, the displacement of each is the same (Figs 3-27, 3-28). However, if the patient's vision is anisometropic, a phoria is induced by

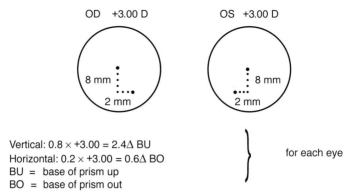

Vertical: 0.8 × +3.00 = 2.4Δ BU
Horizontal: 0.2 × +3.00 = 0.6Δ BO
BU = base of prism up
BO = base of prism out

} for each eye

Figure 3-27 Prismatic effect of bifocal lenses in isometropic hyperopia.

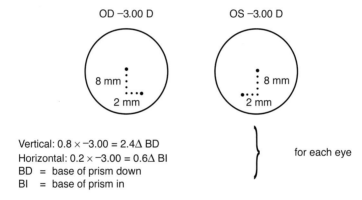

Vertical: 0.8 × −3.00 = 2.4Δ BD
Horizontal: 0.2 × −3.00 = 0.6Δ BI
BD = base of prism down
BI = base of prism in

} for each eye

Figure 3-28 Prismatic effect of bifocal lenses in isometropic myopia.

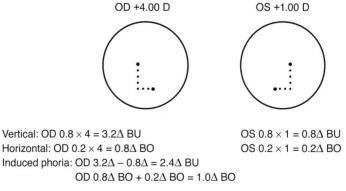

Vertical: OD 0.8 × 4 = 3.2Δ BU   OS 0.8 × 1 = 0.8Δ BU
Horizontal: OD 0.2 × 4 = 0.8Δ BO   OS 0.2 × 1 = 0.2Δ BO
Induced phoria: OD 3.2Δ − 0.8Δ = 2.4Δ BU
            OD 0.8Δ BO + 0.2Δ BO = 1.0Δ BO

Figure 3-29 Prismatic effect of bifocal lenses in anisometropic hyperopia.

OD +2.00   OS −2.00

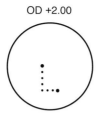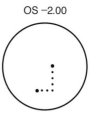

Vertical: OD 0.8 × +2 = 1.6Δ BU   OS 0.8 × −2 = 1.6Δ BD
Horizontal: OD 0.2 × +2 = 0.4Δ BO   OS 0.2 × −2 = 0.4Δ BI
Induced phoria: OD 1.6Δ + 1.6Δ = 3.2Δ BU
              OD 0.4Δ BO − OS 0.4Δ BI = 0
              (no horizontal induced phoria)

Figure 3-30 Prismatic effect of bifocal lenses in antimetropia.

the unequal prismatic displacement of the 2 lenses (Figs 3-29, 3-30). The amount of *vertical phoria* is determined by subtracting the smaller prismatic displacement from the larger if both lenses are myopic or hyperopic (see Fig 3-29) or by adding the 2 lenses if the patient is hyperopic in 1 eye and myopic in the other (see Fig 3-30).

For determination of the induced *horizontal phoria,* the induced prisms are added if both eyes are hyperopic or if both eyes are myopic. If 1 eye is hyperopic and the other is myopic, the smaller amount of prismatic displacement is subtracted from the larger (see Fig 3-30). Image displacement is minimized when round-top segment bifocal lenses are used with plus lenses and flat-top segment bifocal lenses are used with minus lenses (Fig 3-31).

Image jump

The usual position of the top of a bifocal segment is 5 mm below the optical center of the distance lens. As the eyes are directed downward through a lens, the prismatic displacement of the image increases (downward in plus lenses, upward in minus lenses). When the eyes encounter the top of a bifocal segment, they meet a new plus lens with a different optical center, and the object appears to jump upward unless the optical center of the add is at the very top of the segment (Fig 3-32). Executive-style segments have their optical centers at the top of the segment. The optical center of a typical flat-top segment is located 3 mm below the top of the segment. The closer the optical center of the segment approaches the top edge of the segment, the less the image jump is. Thus, flat-top segments produce less image jump than do round-top segments because the latter have much lower optical centers.

Patients with myopia who wear round-top bifocal lenses would be more bothered by image jump than would patients with hyperopia because the jump occurs in the direction of image displacement. Thus, it is good practice to avoid prescribing round-top bifocal segments to patients with myopia.

With plus lenses:

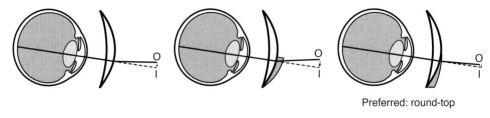

Preferred: round-top

With minus lenses:

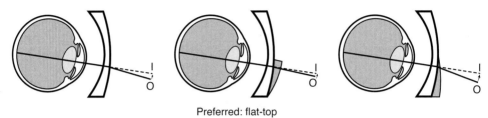

Preferred: flat-top

Figure 3-31 Image displacement through bifocal segments. *(From Wisnicki HJ. Bifocals, trifocals, and progressive-addition lenses. Focal Points: Clinical Modules for Ophthalmologists. San Francisco: American Academy of Ophthalmology; 1999, module 6. Reprinted with permission from Guyton DL. Ophthalmic Optics and Clinical Refraction. Baltimore: Prism Press; 1998. Redrawn by C. H. Wooley.)*

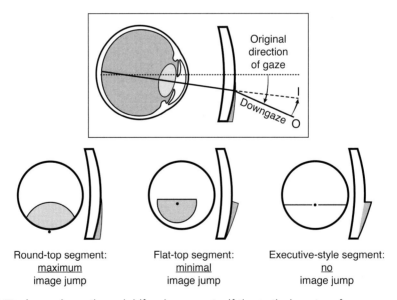

Round-top segment:
<u>maximum</u>
image jump

Flat-top segment:
<u>minimal</u>
image jump

Executive-style segment:
<u>no</u>
image jump

Figure 3-32 Image jump through bifocal segments. If the optical center of a segment is at its top, no image jump occurs. *(From Wisnicki HJ. Bifocals, trifocals, and progressive-addition lenses. Focal Points: Clinical Modules for Ophthalmologists. San Francisco: American Academy of Ophthalmology; 1999, module 6. Reprinted with permission from Guyton DL. Ophthalmic Optics and Clinical Refraction. Baltimore: Prism Press; 1998. Redrawn by C. H. Wooley.)*

Compensating for induced anisophoria

When anisometropia is corrected with spectacle lenses, unequal prism is introduced in all secondary positions of gaze. This prism may be the source of symptoms, even diplopia. *Symptomatic anisophoria* occurs especially when a patient with early presbyopia uses his or her first pair of bifocal lenses or when the anisometropia is of recent and/or sudden origin, as occurs after retinal detachment surgery, with gradual asymmetric progression of cataracts, or after unilateral intraocular lens implantation. The patient usually adapts to horizontal imbalance by increasing head rotation but may have symptoms when looking down, in the reading position. Recall that horizontal vergence amplitudes are large compared with vertical fusional amplitudes, which are typically less than 2Δ. We can calculate the amount of induced phoria by using the Prentice rule (Fig 3-33).

At the reading point, 8 mm below distance optical center:

OD	4.00×0.80	=	3.20Δ BU
OS	1.00×0.80	=	0.80Δ BU
Net difference			2.40Δ BU

In this example, there is an induced right hyperdeviation of 2.40Δ. Conforming to the usual practice in the management of heterophorias, approximately two-thirds to three-fourths of the vertical phoria should be corrected—in this case, 1.75Δ. This correction may be accomplished in several ways.

Press-on prisms With press-on prisms, 2.00Δ of base down (BD) may be added to the right segment in the preceding example or 2.00Δ of base up (BU) to the left segment.

Slab-off The most satisfactory method of compensating for the induced vertical phoria in anisometropia is the technique of bicentric grinding, known as *slab-off* (Fig 3-34). In this

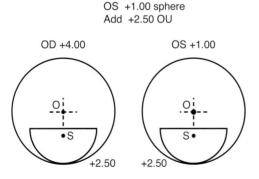

Rx: OD +4.00 sphere
    OS +1.00 sphere
    Add +2.50 OU

OD +4.00   OS +1.00

Figure 3-33 Calculation of induced anisophoria.

O = optical center, distance
S = optical center of segment
R (= S): Reading position 8 mm below distance
        optical center

Figure 3-34 Bicentric grinding (slab-off). **A,** Lens form with a dummy lens cemented to the front surface. **B,** Both surfaces of the lens are reground with the same curvatures but removing base-up prism from the top segment of the front surface and removing base-down prism from the entire rear surface. **C,** The effect is a lens from which base-down prism has been removed from the lower segment only.

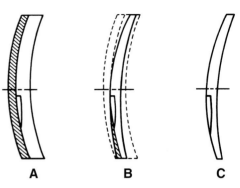

A   B   C

method, 2 optical centers are created in the lens that has the greater minus (or less plus) power, thereby counteracting the base-down effect of the greater minus lens in the reading position. It is convenient to think of the slab-off process as creating *base-up prism* over the reading area of the lens.

Bicentric grinding is used for single-vision lenses as well as for multifocal lenses. By increasing the distance between the 2 optical centers, this method achieves as much as 4.00Δ of prism compensation at the reading position.

Reverse slab-off Prism correction in the reading position is achieved not only by removing *base-down prism* from the lower part of the more minus lens (slabbing off) but also by adding base-down prism to the lower half of the more plus lens. This technique is known as *reverse slab-off.*

Historically, it was easy to remove material from a standard lens. Currently, because plastic lenses are fabricated by molding, it is more convenient to add material to create a base-down prism in the lower half of what will be the more plus lens. Because plastic lenses account for most lenses dispensed, reverse slab-off is the most common method of correcting anisometropically induced anisophoria.

When the clinician is ordering a lens that requires prism correction for an anisophoria in downgaze, it is often appropriate to leave the choice of slab-off versus reverse slab-off to the optician by including a statement in the prescription, such as, "Slab-off right lens 3.00Δ (or reverse slab-off left lens)." In either case, the prescribed prism should be measured in the reading position, not calculated, because the patient may have partially adapted to the anisophoria.

Dissimilar segments In anisometropic bifocal lens prescriptions, vertical prism compensation can also be achieved by the use of dissimilar bifocal segments with their optical centers at 2 different heights. The segment with the lower optical center should be placed in front of the more hyperopic (or less myopic) eye to provide base-down prism. (This method contrasts with the bicentric grinding method, which produces base-up prism and is therefore employed on the lesser plus or greater minus lens.)

In the example in Figure 3-35, a 22-mm round segment is used for the right eye, and the top of its segment is at the usual 5 mm below the distance optical center. For the left eye, a 22-mm flat-top segment is used, again with the top of the segment 5 mm below the optical center.

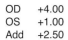

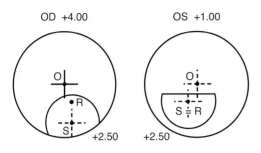

Figure 3-35 Dissimilar segments used to compensate for anisophoria in anisometropic bifocal prescriptions.

O = optical center, distance
S = optical center of segment
R (= S): Reading position 8 mm below distance
        optical center

Because the optical center of the flat-top segment is 3 mm below the top of the segment, it is at the patient's reading position and that segment will introduce no prismatic effect. However, for the right eye, the optical center of the round segment is 8 mm below the patient's reading position; according to the Prentice rule, this 2.50 D segment will produce $2.50 \times 0.8 = 2.00\Delta$ base-down prism.

Single-vision reading glasses with lowered optical centers Partial compensation for the induced vertical phoria at the reading position can be obtained with single-vision reading glasses when the optical centers are placed 3–4 mm below the pupillary centers in primary gaze. The patient's gaze will be directed much closer to the optical centers of the lenses when reading.

Contact lenses Contact lenses can be prescribed for patients with significant anisometropia that causes a symptomatic anisophoria in downgaze. Reading glasses can be worn over the contacts if the patient's vision is presbyopic.

Refractive surgery Corneal refractive surgery may be an option for some patients with symptomatic anisometropia or anisophoria.

Occupation and Bifocal Segment

The *dioptric power* of a segment depends on the patient's accommodative reserve and the working distance required for a specific job. Such focal length determinations are a characteristic not of the job but of the individual patient's adaptation to that job. If the patient is allowed to use half of his or her available accommodation (which must be measured), the remainder of the dioptric requirement will be met by the bifocal add. For example, if the job entails proofreading at 40 cm, the dioptric requirement for that focal length is 2.50 D. If the patient's accommodative amplitude is 2.00 D, and half of that (1.00 D) is used for the job, the balance of 1.50 D becomes the necessary bifocal add. It is essential that the accommodative range (near point to far point) be measured and that it be adequate for the job tasks.

Lens design

The most important characteristic of the bifocal segment is the *segment height* in relation to the patient's pupillary center. The lenses will be unsuitable if the segment is placed too high or too low for the specific occupational need.

Segment width is substantially less important. The popular impression that very large bifocal lenses mean better reading capability is not supported by projection measurements. At a 40-cm reading distance, a 25-mm flat-top segment provides a horizontal reading field of 50–55 cm.

At a 40-cm distance, an individual habitually uses face rotation to increase his or her fixation field when it exceeds 45 cm (30° of arc); therefore, a 25-mm-wide segment is more than adequate for all but a few special occupations, such as a graphic artist or an architectural drafter using a drawing board. Furthermore, with a 35-mm segment producing a horizontal field 75 cm wide, the focal length at the extremes of the fixation field would be 55 cm, not 40 cm! Therefore, the split bifocal is useful not because it is a wider bifocal lens but because of its monocentric construction.

The *shape* of the segment must also be considered. For example, round-top segments (Kryptok, Ultex type) require the user to look far enough down in the segment to employ his or her maximum horizontal dimension. In addition, these segments exaggerate image jump, especially in myopic corrections.

Segment decentration To avoid inducing a base-out prism effect when the bifocal lens–wearing patient converges for near-vision tasks, the reading segment is generally decentered inward. This design is especially important in aphakic spectacles. Consider the following points for proper decentration:

- *Working distance.* Because the convergence requirement increases as the focal length decreases, additional inward decentration of the bifocal segment is required.
- *Interpupillary distance.* The wider the interpupillary distance, the greater the convergence requirement and, correspondingly, the need for inward decentration of the segments.
- *Lens power.* If the distance lens is a high-plus lens, it will create a greater base-out prism effect (ie, induced exophoria) as the viewer converges. Additional inward decentration of the segments may be helpful. The reverse is true for high-minus lenses.
- *Existing heterophoria.* As with lens-induced phorias, the presence of an existing exophoria suggests that increasing the inward decentration would be effective. An esophoria calls for the opposite approach.

Prescribing Special Lenses

Aphakic Lenses

The problems of correcting aphakia with high-plus spectacle lenses are well known and were described eloquently by Alan C. Woods. They include

- magnification of approximately 20%–35%
- altered depth perception resulting from the magnification

- pincushion distortion; for example, doors appear to bow inward
- difficulty with hand–eye coordination
- ring scotoma generated by prismatic effects at the edge of the lens (causing the "jack-in-the-box" phenomenon)
- extreme sensitivity of the lenses to minor misadjustment in vertex distance, pantoscopic tilt, and height
- in monocular aphakia, loss of useful binocular vision because of differential magnification

In addition, aphakic spectacles create cosmetic problems. The patient's eyes appear magnified and, if viewed obliquely, may seem displaced because of prismatic effects. The high-power lenticular lens is itself unattractive, given its "fried-egg" appearance (Fig 3-36).

For all these reasons, intraocular lenses and aphakic contact lenses now account for nearly all aphakic corrections. Nevertheless, spectacle correction of aphakia is sometimes appropriate, as in bilateral infantile pediatric aphakia.

Refracting technique

Because of the sensitivity of aphakic glasses to vertex distance and pantoscopic tilt, it is nearly impossible to refract an aphakic eye reliably by using a phoropter. The vertex distance and the pantoscopic tilt are not well controlled, nor are they necessarily close to the values for the final spectacles. Rather than a phoropter, trial frames or lens clips are used.

The trial frame allows the refractionist to control vertex distance and pantoscopic tilt. It should be adjusted for minimal vertex distance and for the same pantoscopic tilt planned for the actual spectacles (approximately 5°–7°, not the larger values that are appropriate for conventional glasses).

Another good technique is to refract with clip-on trial lens holders placed over the patient's existing aphakic glasses (overrefraction). Take care that the center of the clip coincides with the optical center of the existing lens. Even if the present lens contains a cylinder at an axis different from what is needed, it is possible to calculate the resultant spherocylindrical correction with an electronic calculator, by hand, or with measurement of the combination in a lensmeter.

Guyton DL. *Retinoscopy: Minus Cylinder Technique, 1986; Retinoscopy: Plus Cylinder Technique, 1986; Subjective Refraction: Cross-Cylinder Technique, 1987.* Reviewed for currency, 2007. Clinical Skills DVD Series [DVD]. San Francisco: American Academy of Ophthalmology.

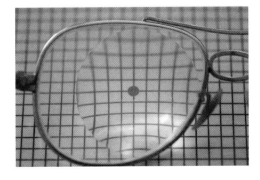

Figure 3-36 Aphakic lens with magnification and pincushion distortion. *(Courtesy of Tommy Korn, MD.)*

Absorptive Lenses

In certain high-illumination situations, sunglasses allow for better visual function in a number of ways.

Improvement of contrast sensitivity

On a bright, sunny day, irradiance from the sun ranges from 10,000–30,000 foot-lamberts. These high light levels tend to saturate the retina and therefore decrease finer levels of contrast sensitivity. The major function of dark (gray, green, or brown) sunglasses is to allow the retina to remain at its normal level of contrast sensitivity. Most dark sunglasses absorb 70%–80% of the incident light of all wavelengths.

Improvement of dark adaptation

A full day at the beach or on the ski slopes on a sunny day (without dark sunglasses) can impair dark adaptation for more than 2 days. Thus, dark sunglasses are recommended for prolonged periods in bright sun.

Reduction of glare sensitivity

Various types of sunglasses can reduce glare sensitivity. Because light reflected off a horizontal surface is polarized in the horizontal plane, properly oriented *polarized lenses* reduce the intensity of glare from road surfaces, glass windows, metal surfaces, and lake and river surfaces. *Graded-density sunglasses* are deeply tinted at the top and gradually become lighter toward the lens center. They are effective in removing glare from sources above the line of sight, such as the sun. Wide-temple sunglasses work by reducing glare from temporal light sources.

Use of photochromic lenses

When short-wavelength light (300–400+ nm) interacts with photochromic lenses, the lenses darken by means of a chemical reaction that converts silver ions to elemental silver. This process is similar to the reaction that occurs when photographic film is exposed to light. Unlike that in photographic film, however, the chemical reaction in photochromic lenses is reversible. Current photochromic lenses incorporate complex organic compounds in which UV light changes the molecules into different configuration states (ie, *cis* to *trans*); this process darkens the lenses (Fig 3-37). Photochromic lenses can darken enough to absorb approximately 80% of the incident light; when the amount of illumination falls, they can lighten to absorb only a small part of the incident light. Note that these lenses take some time to darken and, in particular, take longer to lighten than to darken. This discrepancy can be problematic in patients who move frequently between outdoor and indoor environments. Because automobile glass and the window glass in many residences and commercial buildings absorb light in the UV spectrum, most photochromics do not darken inside cars or buildings. In colder weather, patients should also be warned that these lenses darken more than usual, especially during a cloudy day. Nevertheless, photochromic lenses are excellent UV absorbers.

Ultraviolet-absorbing lenses

The spectrum of UV light is divided into 3 types: UVA contains wavelengths of 400–320 nm, UVB contains wavelengths of 320–290 nm, and UVC contains wavelengths below

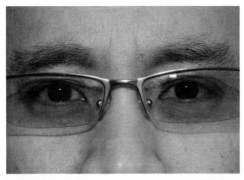

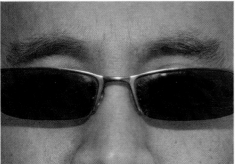

Figure 3-37 Photochromic lenses. *(Courtesy of Tommy Korn, MD.)*

290 nm. The ozone layer of the atmosphere absorbs almost all UVC coming from the sun. Most exposure to UVC is from manufactured sources, including welding arcs, germicidal lamps, and excimer lasers. Of the total solar radiation falling on the earth, approximately 5% is UV light, of which 90% is UVA and 10% UVB.

The amount of UV light striking the earth varies with season (greatest in the summer), latitude (greatest near the equator), time of day (greatest at noon), and elevation (greatest at high elevation). UV light can also strike the eye by reflection. Fresh snow reflects between 60% and 80% of incident light; sand (beach, desert) reflects approximately 15% of incident light; and water reflects approximately 5% of incident light.

Laboratory experiments have shown that UV light damages living tissue in 2 ways. First, chemicals such as proteins, enzymes, nucleic acids, and cell-membrane components absorb UV light. When they do so, their molecular bonds (primarily the double bonds) may become disrupted. Second, these essential biochemicals may become disrupted by the action of free radicals (such as the superoxide radical). Free radicals can often be produced by UV light in the presence of oxygen and a photosensitizing pigment. For a fuller discussion of free radicals, see BCSC Section 2, *Fundamentals and Principles of Ophthalmology*.

Because it may take many years for UV light to damage eye tissue, a tight linkage between cause and effect is difficult to prove. Therefore, proof that UV light damages the eye comes primarily from acute animal experiments and epidemiologic studies covering large numbers of patients.

The available data on the effects of exposure to UV light have suggested a benefit to protecting patients from UV light after cataract surgery. Some surgeons routinely prescribe UV-absorbing glasses after surgery. Intraocular lenses incorporating UV-absorbing chromophores are now the norm. For further information regarding the effects of UV radiation on various ocular structures, see BCSC Section 8, *External Disease and Cornea;* and Section 12, *Retina and Vitreous.*

Almost all dark sunglasses absorb most incident UV light. The same is true for certain coated clear-glass lenses and clear plastic lenses made of CR-39 or polycarbonate. One suggestion has been that certain sunglasses (primarily light blue ones) may cause light damage to the eye. Proponents of this theory contended that the pupil dilates behind dark glasses and that if the sunglasses do not then absorb significant amounts of UV light, they will actually allow more UV light to enter the eye than if no sunglasses were worn. In fact, dark sunglasses reduce light levels striking the eye on a bright, sunny day to the range of 2000–6000 foot-lamberts. Such levels are approximately 10 times higher than those of an average lighted room. At such light levels, the pupil is significantly constricted. Thus, contrary to the preceding argument, dark sunglasses used on a bright day allow pupillary dilation of only a fraction of a millimeter and do not lead to light injury of the eye.

Special Lens Materials

It is important for the ophthalmologist to be aware of the variety of spectacle lens materials available. Four major properties are commonly discussed in relation to lens materials:

1. *Index of refraction.* As the refractive index increases, the thickness of the lens can be decreased to obtain the same optical power.
2. *Specific gravity.* As the specific gravity of a material decreases, the lens weight can be reduced.
3. *Abbe number (value).* This value indicates the degree of chromatic aberration or distortion that occurs because of the dispersion of light, primarily with off-axis viewing. Materials with a higher Abbe number exhibit less chromatic aberration and thus allow for higher optical quality.
4. *Impact resistance.* All lenses dispensed in the United States must meet impact-resistance requirements defined by the US Food and Drug Administration (FDA) (in 21CFR801.410), except in special cases wherein the physician or optometrist communicates in writing that such lenses would not fulfill the visual requirements of the particular patient. Lenses used for occupational and educational personal eye protection must also meet the impact-resistance requirements defined in the American National Standards Institute (ANSI) high-velocity impact standard (Z87.1). Lenses prescribed for children and active adults should also meet the ANSI Z87.1 standard, unless the patient is duly warned that he or she is not getting the most impact-resistant lenses available.

Standard glass

Glass lenses provide superior optics and are scratch resistant but also have several limitations, including low impact resistance, increased thickness, and heavy weight. Once the standard in the industry, glass lenses are less frequently used in current practice; many patients select plastic lenses. Without special treatment, glass lenses may be easily shattered.

Chemical or thermal *tempering* increases the shatter resistance of glass, but if it is scratched or worked on with any tool after tempering, the shatter resistance is lost. Farmers appreciate photoreactive glass for its scratch resistance and easy care. Welders and grinders are better off with plastic, as small hot particles can become embedded in glass. Persons with myopia who desire thin glasses may choose high-index glass. The highest-index versions cannot be tempered and require that waivers be signed by patients who accept the danger of their breakage. High-index glass does not block UV light unless a coating is applied. (Characteristics of standard glass lenses are as follows: index of refraction, 1.52; Abbe number, 59; specific gravity, 2.54; impact resistance, pass FDA 21CFR801.410 if thick enough and chemically or heat treated.)

Standard plastic

Because of its high optical quality and light weight, standard plastic (also known as hard resin or CR-39) is the most commonly used lens material and is inexpensive. Standard plastic lenses are almost 50% lighter than glass lenses owing to the lower specific gravity of their material. They block 80% of UV light without treatment, can be tinted easily if desired, and can be coated to resist scratching and to provide further UV-light blocking. The index of refraction is not high, so the lenses are not thin. CR-39 lenses do not have the shatter resistance of polycarbonate or Trivex. (Characteristics of standard plastic lenses are as follows: index of refraction, 1.49; Abbe number, 58; specific gravity, 1.32; impact resistance, pass FDA 21CFR801.410.)

Polycarbonate

Introduced in the 1970s for ophthalmic lens use, the high-index plastic material polycarbonate has a low specific gravity and a higher refractive index, which allow for a light, thin lens. Polycarbonate is also durable and meets the high-velocity impact standard (ANSI Z87.1). One disadvantage of this material is the high degree of chromatic aberration, as indicated by its low Abbe number (30). Thus, color fringing can be an annoyance, particularly in strong prescriptions. Another disadvantage is that polycarbonate is the most easily scratched plastic, so a scratch-resistant coating is required. Also, if polycarbonate is cut too thin, it can flex on impact and pop out of the frame. (Characteristics of polycarbonate lenses are as follows: index of refraction, 1.58; Abbe number, 30; specific gravity, 1.20; impact resistance, pass FDA 21CFR801.410 and ANSI Z87.1.)

Trivex

Introduced in 2001, Trivex is a highly impact-resistant, low-density material that delivers strong optical performance and provides clear vision because of its high Abbe number. Its impact resistance is close to that of polycarbonate, and it blocks all UV light. Its index of refraction is not high, however, so the lenses are not thin. Trivex is the lightest lens material currently available and meets the high-velocity impact standard (ANSI Z87.1). Trivex material allows a comparably thin lens for the ±3.00 D prescription range. A scratch-resistant coating is required. (Characteristics of Trivex lenses are as follows: index of refraction, 1.53; Abbe number, 45; specific gravity, 1.11; impact resistance, pass FDA 21CFR801.410 and ANSI Z87.1.)

High-index materials

A lens with a refractive index of 1.60 or higher is referred to as a *high-index lens.* High-index materials can be either glass or plastic and are most often used for higher-power prescriptions to create thin, cosmetically attractive lenses. The weight, optical clarity, and impact resistance of high-index lenses vary depending on the specific material used and the refractive index; in general, as the index of refraction increases, the weight of the material increases and the optical clarity (Abbe number) decreases. None of the high-index materials passes the ANSI Z87.1 standard for impact resistance. Plastic high-index materials require a scratch-resistant coating.

> Strauss L. Spectacle lens materials, coatings, tints, and designs. *Focal Points: Clinical Modules for Ophthalmologists.* San Francisco: American Academy of Ophthalmology; 2005, module 11.

Therapeutic Use of Prisms

Small horizontal and vertical deviations can be corrected conveniently in spectacle lenses by the addition of prisms.

Horizontal heterophorias

Asthenopic symptoms may develop in patients (usually adults) if fusion is disrupted by inadequate vergence amplitudes; if fusion cannot be maintained, diplopia results. Thus, in patients with an exophoria at near, symptoms develop when the convergence reserve is inadequate for the task. Some patients can compensate for this fusional inadequacy through the improvement of fusional amplitudes. Younger patients may be able to do so through orthoptic exercises, which are sometimes used in conjunction with prisms that further stimulate their fusional capability (base-out prisms to enhance convergence reserve).

Symptoms may arise in some patients because of abnormally high accommodative convergence. Thus, an esophoria at near may be improved by full hyperopic correction for distance and/or by the use of bifocal lenses to decrease accommodative demand. In adult patients, orthoptic training and maximum refractive correction may be inadequate, and prisms or surgery may be necessary to restore binocularity.

Prisms are especially useful if a patient experiences an abrupt onset of symptoms secondary to a basic heterophoria or heterotropia. The prisms may be needed only temporarily, and the minimum amount of prism correction necessary to reestablish and maintain binocularity should be used.

Vertical heterophorias

Vertical fusional amplitudes are small (<2.00Δ). Thus, if a vertical muscle imbalance is sufficient to cause asthenopic symptoms or diplopia, it should be compensated for by the incorporation of prisms into the refractive correction. Once again, the minimum amount of prism needed to eliminate symptoms should be prescribed. In a noncomitant vertical heterophoria, the prism should be sufficient to correct the imbalance in primary gaze. With combined vertical and horizontal muscle imbalance, correcting only the vertical deviation may help improve control of the horizontal deviation as well. If the horizontal deviation is not adequately corrected, an oblique Fresnel prism may be helpful. A brief period of clinical heterophoria testing may be insufficient to unmask a latent muscle imbalance. Often, after prisms have been worn for a time, the phoria appears to increase, and the prism correction must be correspondingly increased.

Methods of prism correction

The potential effect of prisms should be evaluated by having the patient test the indicated prism in trial frames or trial lens clips over the current refractive correction. Temporary prisms in the form of clip-on lenses or Fresnel press-on prisms can be used to evaluate and alter the final prism requirement. The Fresnel prisms have several advantages: (1) they are lighter in weight (1 mm thick) and more acceptable cosmetically because they are affixed to the concave surface of the spectacle lens, and (2) they allow much larger prism corrections (up to 40.0Δ). With higher prism powers, however, it is not uncommon to observe a decrease in the visual acuity of the corrected eye. Patients may also observe chromatic fringes.

Prisms can be incorporated into spectacle lenses within the limits of cost, appearance, weight, and the technical skill of the optician. Prisms should be incorporated into the spectacle lens prescription only after an adequate trial of temporary prisms has established that the correction is appropriate and the deviation is stable.

Prism correction may also be achieved by decentering the optical center of the lens relative to the visual axis, although a substantial prism effect by means of this method is possible only with higher-power lenses. Aspheric lens designs are not suitable for decentration. (See earlier discussion of lens decentration and the Prentice rule.) Bifocal segments may be decentered *in* more than the customary amount to give a modest additional base-in effect to help patients with convergence insufficiency.

Chapter Exercises

Questions

3.1. Which of the following represents a Jackson cross cylinder?
   a. −2.00 +4.00 × 180
   b. −1.00 +3.00 × 90
   c. +2.00 +3.00 × 180
   d. +1.00 −1.00 × 90

3.2. When performing cycloplegic retinoscopy on an anxious 7-year-old boy, you notice that the central reflex shows *with* movement while the peripheral reflex shows *against* movement. What is the most likely cause?
   a. keratoconus
   b. congenital cataract
   c. spherical aberration
   d. insufficient time for maximum cycloplegia

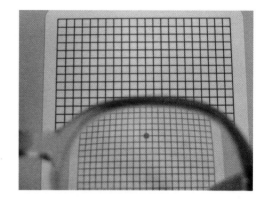

Figure 3-38 *(Courtesy of Tommy Korn, MD.)*

3.3. What type of distortion is shown in Figure 3-38?
   a. pincushion distortion
   b. barrel distortion
   c. image jump
   d. image displacement
3.4. A patient with +9.00 D spectacle lenses (vertex distance is 12 mm) requires a new spectacle frame because of recent nasal surgery. The vertex distance of the new frame is required to be 22 mm to avoid any nasal discomfort. What power is required for the new spectacles?
   a. +7.25 D
   b. +8.25 D
   c. +9.25 D
   d. +10.25 D
3.5. On the basis of the type of spectacle lenses shown in Figure 3-39, what is the patient's probable occupation?
   a. retired investment banker or stockbroker
   b. professional senior golfer
   c. airline pilot
   d. jewelry or watch-repair technician

Figure 3-39 *(Courtesy of Tommy Korn, MD.)*

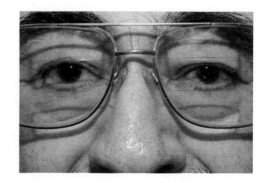

3.6. The Abbe number is a measure of
   a. spherical aberration
   b. chromatic aberration
   c. image displacement in plus lenses
   d. curvature of spectacle lenses

3.7. Your refraction determines that a −8.00 D lens in a trial frame with a vertex distance of 10 mm from the patient's cornea provides 20/15 visual acuity. What is the minus-power lens needed if the patient requires a vertex distance of 14 mm to use her favorite existing spectacle frame?
   a. −7.25 D
   b. −8.25 D
   c. −9.25 D
   d. −10.25 D

3.8. The primary reason that patients with presbyopia cannot tolerate significant anisometropia in bifocal lenses is
   a. asthenopia
   b. inability of the lens to accommodate and correct any hyperopic error
   c. reduced vertical fusion amplitude
   d. spherical aberration

3.9. In bifocal lens design, image jump may be minimized by
   a. placing the optical center of the segment as close as possible to the top of the segment
   b. placing the top of the segment as close as possible to the distance optical center
   c. using a smaller bifocal segment
   d. using a blended bifocal segment that has no visible line of separation
   e. lowering the bifocal segment by 3 mm

3.10. An angle of 45° corresponds to how many prism diopters (Δ)?
   a. 45.0Δ
   b. 22.5Δ
   c. 90.0Δ
   d. 100.0Δ

3.11. When bifocal lenses are prescribed for a patient with myopia,
   a. the practitioner should leave the choice of the segment type to the optician
   b. a round-top segment is preferred because of its thin upper edge, which causes less prismatic effect
   c. a flat-top segment is preferred because it lessens image jump
   d. the 1-piece shape is indicated for adds greater than +2.00 D
   e. a split bifocal should be used because patients with myopia do not accept bifocal lenses easily

Answers

3.1. **a.** The Jackson cross cylinder is a lens made of 2 cylinders of equal but opposite magnitude placed at 90° relative to each other; the spherical equivalent of the resulting lens is zero (see Fig 3-17). High-power Jackson cross cylinders are especially useful in refining the refraction in low vision patients.

3.2. **c.** Spherical aberration occurs in patients with large or dilated pupils. This aberration is caused when light rays are refracted as they travel through a widely dilated pupil and strike the peripheral crystalline lens. The periphery of the human lens is more curved than the center, so the incoming light rays show increased refraction compared with the light rays that strike the central lens. In retinoscopy, this can result in the appearance of different central and peripheral reflexes. Thus, it is always important to concentrate on the central light reflex when performing retinoscopy.

3.3. **b.** Figure 3-38 depicts a high-minus spectacle lens where there is minification of the image. Note the barrel-shaped distortion of the Amsler grid as viewed through the lens.

3.4. **b.** The far point of a +9.00 D lens is 111 mm (1/9 m) behind the lens. However, for the old lens to focus the image on the retina, it must be held by the frame 12 mm in front of the cornea. Thus, the far point of the patient's hyperopia is located 99 mm (111 mm – 12 mm) behind the cornea. If the new frame is to be located 22 mm in front of the cornea, it should be placed 121 mm (99 mm + 22 mm) in front of the far point of the patient's hyperopia. The power required for this new lens, therefore, is 1/0.121 m = +8.26 D. Because spectacle lenses come in 0.25 D steps, the answer is +8.25 D.

3.5. **c.** Figure 3-39 depicts an occupational multifocal lens known as a *double D*. This type of lens has the additive near power at the top and bottom of the spectacle lens; the distance power is in the middle. This design is especially useful for airline pilots, who must frequently look up at cockpit instrument panels that are in close proximity to one another and look down at printed flight material.

3.6. **b.** The Abbe number is a measure of chromatic aberration. The lower the Abbe number, the higher the amount of chromatic aberration present in the lens material. Spectacle lenses with a low Abbe number often require antireflective coating to minimize chromatic aberration that arises particularly when bright indoor light reflects off the lenses.

3.7. **b.** The far point of a –8.00 D lens is 125 mm (1/8 m) and is located in front of the lens. A patient's myopic refractive error is corrected with a –8.00 D trial lens when the lens is placed 10 mm in front of the cornea (Fig 3-40). If the lens is moved to 14 mm in front of the cornea with her existing frame, the far point remains the same distance from the original –8.00 D lens. The location of the existing frame from the far point is 135 mm – 14 mm = 121 mm. The power of the lens must then be 1/0.121 m = –8.26 D. Because spectacle lenses come in 0.25 D increments, the answer is –8.25 D.

3.8. **c.** When a patient has anisometropia, which may arise after cataract surgery, for example, a large vertical prismatic effect is induced in the bifocal add. When the patient suddenly looks through the top of the bifocal segment, image jump occurs because of vertical prismatic effects through the spectacle lenses. Image jump is a problem because the human brain has a very limited capacity to fuse 2 images that are separated vertically, as in the case of a bifocal lens with anisometropia.

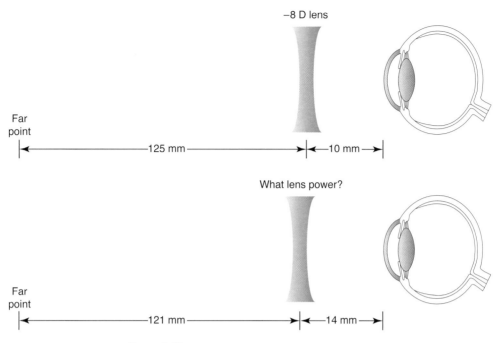

Figure 3-40 *(Illustration developed by Tommy Korn, MD.)*

3.9. **a.** As the eyes look down to read through the add segment, there is an abrupt upward image jump at the top edge of the segment. This jump is due to the prismatic effect of the plus lens (the add segment). On the basis of the Prentice rule, the amount of jump depends on the power of the segment and on the distance from the top of the segment to the optical center of the segment.

3.10. **d.** As a rule of thumb, the number of prism diopters is approximately twice the angle in degrees. However, this equation works only for small angles (<20°). An angle of 45° means that at 1 m, a beam is deviated by 1 m (100 cm). Thus, 45° corresponds to 100.0Δ. An angle of 90° corresponds to infinity in prism diopters.

3.11. **c.** In general, patients perceive image jump as a greater problem than image displacement. Flat-top segments minimize image jump because the optical center is near the top. In patients with myopia, flat-top segments also reduce prism displacement because the base-down effect of the distance portion is reduced by the base-up effect of the segment.

Appendix 3.1

Common Guidelines for Prescribing Cylinders for Spectacle Correction

[The material in this appendix is modified from Guyton DL. Prescribing cylinders: the problem of distortion. *Surv Ophthalmol.* 1977;22(3):177–188. Copyright © 1977, Survey of Ophthalmology]

Commonly taught guidelines for spectacle correction are the following:

1. Children accept the full astigmatic correction.
2. If an adult cannot tolerate the full astigmatic correction, rotate the cylinder axis toward 90° or 180° and/or reduce the cylinder power to decrease distortion. When reducing the cylinder power, keep the spherical equivalent constant by making the appropriate adjustment of sphere.
3. With older patients, beware of changing the cylinder axis.

The problem: distortion

Why have such guidelines been developed? Why can some patients not tolerate the full astigmatic correction in the first place? One text on clinical refraction states that full correction of a high astigmatic error may initially result in considerable blurring of vision. Another teaching is that with the full astigmatic correction the image is too sharp—the patient is not used to seeing so clearly. Statements such as these are not only misleading; they are incorrect.

The reason for intolerance of astigmatic spectacle corrections is distortion caused by meridional magnification. Unequal magnification of the retinal image in the various meridians produces monocular distortion manifested by tilting lines or altered shapes of objects (Fig 3-41). But monocular distortion by itself is rarely a problem; the effect is too small. Maximum tilting of vertical lines (declination error) in the retinal image occurs when the correcting cylinder axis is at 45° or 135°, but even under these conditions each diopter of correcting cylinder power produces only approximately 0.4° of tilt.

The clinically significant problem occurs only under binocular conditions. Minor degrees of monocular distortion can produce major alterations in binocular spatial perception. Consider, for example, a patient with symmetrical oblique astigmatism wearing a +1.00 diopter cylinder, axis 135° before the right eye, and a +1.00 diopter cylinder, axis 45° before the left eye. If the patient looks at a vertical rod 3 m away, the retinal images of the rod will be tilted toward each other at the top (declination error) by approximately 0.4° each, a barely perceptible amount under monocular conditions. But under

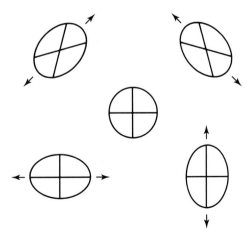

Figure 3-41 Monocular distortion caused by meridional magnification. If the retinal image is magnified more in one direction than the other (as indicated by the *arrows*), vertical lines may become slanted, horizontal lines may become tilted, and objects may appear taller or shorter.

binocular conditions, the vertical rod will theoretically appear tilted toward the patient (inclination) by approximately 35°! Such large errors in stereoscopic spatial localization are clearly intolerable, seemingly out of proportion to the amount of monocular distortion that produces them. Oblique distortion in 1 or both eyes causes more distressing binocular symptoms than does vertical or horizontal distortion, and movement accentuates the symptoms.

Fortunately, errors in stereoscopic spatial localization are usually compensated for in most patients by experiential factors: perspective clues, the known size and shape of familiar objects, the knowledge of what is level and what is perpendicular, etc. The possibility of permanent adaptation to binocular distortion is discussed later, but the fact remains that some patients cannot or will not tolerate binocular spatial distortion, and herein lies our problem.

We have no effective means of treating binocular spatial distortion except by altering or eliminating the monocular distortion that produces it. Complete understanding of the causes and management of monocular distortion is difficult, involving several areas of physiological optics that the average practitioner would prefer to avoid: blur theory, spectacle lens design, obliquely crossed cylinders, and theory of the Jackson cross cylinder. However, with a few key facts from each of these areas, we can quickly gain a working understanding of astigmatic spectacle corrections.

Sources of monocular distortion

As illustrated in Figure 3-41, monocular distortion is caused by meridional magnification. We can identify 2 basic sources of meridional magnification, 1 involving the design of the spectacle lens and the other involving the location of the spectacle lens with respect to the entrance pupil of the eye.

Shape factor of the spectacle lens All spectacle lenses having curved front surfaces produce a magnification inherent to the lens itself. The more convex the front surface and the thicker the lens, the greater this *shape factor* magnification. If the front surface of the lens is spherical, the shape factor magnification will be the same in all meridians, producing only an overall size change in the retinal image. However, if the front surface of the lens is cylindrical or toric, the shape factor magnification will vary from 1 meridian to another, producing distortion of the retinal image. Again, this occurs only with lenses in which the cylinder ground is on the front surface, the so-called *plus cylinder form* or anterior toric spectacle lens. Lenses in which the cylinder ground is on the back surface (minus cylinder lenses, posterior toric lenses, *iseikonic* lenses) do not produce differential meridional magnification due to the shape factor, because the front surface power is the same in all meridians. The lens clock may be used to check the front and back curves.

Meridional magnification arising from the shape factor of plus cylinder spectacle lenses is rarely more than 1% to 2%. Many patients can perceive this difference, however, and for this reason and others, since the mid-1960s, minus cylinder spectacle lenses have become the preferred form for routine dispensing.

Distance of the spectacle lens from the entrance pupil More important than the shape factor of the spectacle lens in producing distortion is the location of the spectacle lens relative to the entrance pupil of the eye. We consider both the conventional method and the general method of analyzing the magnification produced.

The conventional analysis: a special case

The conventional method of calculating the total magnification produced by a spectacle lens is to multiply the shape factor magnification by the *power factor* magnification. The power factor magnification is a function of the dioptric power of the correcting lens and the distance of the correcting lens from the *seat of ametropia*. For example, consider a +4.00 D cylindrical lens placed at a vertex distance of 12 mm from an eye with simple hyperopic astigmatism. Assume that the eye's astigmatism arises in the cornea and that the +4.00 D cylindrical lens fully corrects the astigmatic error. This lens will produce a power factor magnification of 0% in the axis meridian and 5% in the meridian perpendicular to the axis meridian, for a differential meridional magnification of 5%. Figure 3-42 shows the (differential) meridional magnification to be expected for this lens as a function of vertex distance. The shorter the vertex distance is, the less will be the meridional magnification, an important point to remember when trying to minimize distortion.

The conventional analysis is valid only when the spectacle lens actually *corrects* the corneal astigmatism. What sort of meridional magnification and resulting distortion can we expect with *uncorrected* astigmatism, or with astigmatism that is only partially, or inappropriately, corrected?

The general case: blurred retinal images

To investigate the general nature of meridional magnification, we must consider what happens in the case of blurred retinal images. The size of a blurred retinal image is defined as the distance between the centers of those blur circles which represent the extremities of the object.[1] Each blur circle is formed by a bundle of rays limited by the entrance pupil of the eye; the chief ray of the bundle passes toward the center of the entrance pupil and forms the center of the blur circle on the retina. Therefore, the chief rays from the extremities of the object determine the size of the retinal image, and because the chief rays pass toward the center of the entrance pupil, the angle subtended by the object *at the entrance pupil* is proportional to the size of the retinal image.[2]

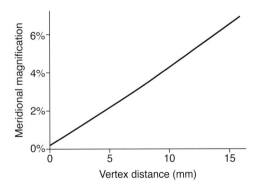

Figure 3-42 Meridional magnification as a function of vertex distance for a +4.00 D cylindrical spectacle lens.

Illustrating the location effect of cylindrical lenses

Figure 3-43 illustrates the general case of distortion of the retinal image produced by a cylindrical lens placed before a nonastigmatic eye. In Figure 3-43, rays *ef* and *gh* represent the chief rays from the vertical extremities of the object. These chief rays cross at the center of the entrance pupil and continue on to form the vertical extremities of the retinal image.[3] No distortion of the retinal image is present in Figure 3-43A.

In Figure 3-43B, a cylindrical lens is placed before the eye in the usual spectacle plane with its axis *xy* oriented in the 45° meridian. Chief rays *ijk* and *lmn* pass through the cylindrical lens at points away from the axis *xy* and are therefore bent by the lens. Chief ray *ijk* undergoes a small prismatic deviation down and to the patient's left, while chief ray *lmn* undergoes a small prismatic deviation up and to the patient's right. The chief rays continue on through the center of the entrance pupil to the retina, but the ray segments *jk* and *mn* lie in a tilted plane because of the prismatic deviations that occurred in opposite horizontal directions at the cylindrical lens. (Note that ray segments *i* and *I* do not lie in the same common plane as the segments *jk* and *mn,* and neither do they follow the same paths as ray segments *e* and *g* in Figure 3-43A.) Because ray segments *jk* and *mn* lie in a tilted plane, the vertical arrow in the retinal image of Figure 3-43B is tilted. In fact, the entire retinal image in Figure 3-43B is distorted. In the case of this retinal image as a whole, we may speak of the distortion as arising from meridional magnification caused by the cylindrical lens—a meridional magnification in the direction of the double arrows (at corners), perpendicular to axis *xy* of the cylindrical lens.

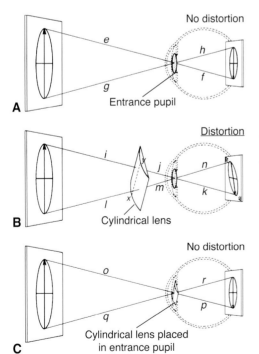

A

B

C

Figure 3-43 The relationship between the position of a cylindrical lens relative to the entrance pupil of a nonastigmatic eye and the distortion of the retinal image produced. **A,** No distortion in the absence of the cylindrical lens. **B,** Distortion produced by the cylindrical lens located in the usual spectacle plane. **C,** No distortion when the cylindrical lens is placed hypothetically in the entrance pupil of the eye.

In Figure 3-43C, the cylindrical lens has been moved toward the eye until it is located hypothetically within the entrance pupil. Chief rays *op* and *qr* pass to the center of the entrance pupil, where they now pass *undeviated* through the cylindrical lens because they strike the lens along its axis. Chief rays *op* and *qr* continue on to the retina and may be seen to be identical with rays *ef* and *gh* of Figure 3-43A, causing no distortion of the retinal image.

Summary of the general case

To summarize the lesson learned from Figure 3-43, astigmatic refracting surfaces located away from the entrance pupil of the eye cause meridional magnification and distortion of the retinal image. The direction of meridional magnification is determined by the axis orientation of the astigmatic refracting surface, and the amount of meridional magnification increases not only with the power of the astigmatic refracting surface but also with increased distance of the astigmatic refracting surface from the entrance pupil of the eye.[4]

Distortion with uncorrected and inappropriately corrected astigmatism

We can now predict what sort of meridional magnification and resultant distortion to expect in the case of uncorrected astigmatism or inappropriately corrected astigmatism. In uncorrected astigmatism, the astigmatic refracting surfaces are those of the cornea or lens. Because these surfaces are located near the entrance pupil, meridional magnification and distortion will be minimal. The meridional magnification produced by uncorrected corneal astigmatism is approximately 0.3% per diopter of astigmatism, which is a rather small amount.

The situation with inappropriately corrected astigmatism is much the same as the situation with properly corrected astigmatism. Whenever an astigmatic spectacle lens is placed before an eye, whether it is the correct lens or not, significant meridional magnification is likely to occur because of the relatively remote location of the spectacle lens from the entrance pupil. Even though the eye may be astigmatic, the effect of astigmatic surfaces located near the entrance pupil is so small that the direction and amount of meridional magnification are determined, not by the astigmatism of the eye itself, but primarily by the axis and power of the astigmatic spectacle lens—whatever the axis and power may be, correct or not.

Minimizing monocular distortion

Specifying minus cylinder (posterior toric) spectacle lenses The small amount of meridional magnification caused by plus cylinder (anterior toric) spectacle lenses is avoided simply by specifying minus cylinder lenses in the prescriptions. In practice, this distinction is rarely necessary because minus cylinder lenses have become the preferred form for routine dispensing. Most dispensers will choose the minus cylinder form automatically and reserve the plus cylinder form only for duplication of an old pair of plus cylinder lenses.

Minimizing vertex distance As previously discussed, meridional magnification decreases as the correcting spectacle lens is placed closer and closer to the eye (see Fig 3-42). There is often little room for manipulation of vertex distance with common styles of frames, but when distortion is anticipated, we can at least avoid the so-called fashionable glasses that sit at the end of the patient's nose.

With contact lenses, the vertex distance is reduced to zero and distortion is practically eliminated. Contact lenses should always be considered an alternative to spectacle correction if the patient remains unsatisfied with other attempts to reduce distortion. In fact, contact lenses may be the only means available (other than iseikonic corrections) to reduce distortion while maintaining clear imagery, given that further attempts to reduce distortion by manipulating the spectacle lens correction, as discussed in the next section, involve a certain sacrifice in the sharpness of the retinal image.

Altering the astigmatic correction: rotating the cylinder axis Clinical experience suggests that new astigmatic spectacle corrections in adults are better tolerated if the axis of the cylinder is at 90° or 180° rather than in an oblique meridian. In fact, it has long been taught that oblique axes should be rotated toward 90° or 180°, if visual acuity does not suffer too much, to avoid problems from oblique distortion. This makes sense because the *direction* of meridional magnification is determined principally by the axis orientation of the correcting cylinder, whether or not the axis is correct, and vertical or horizontal aniseikonia is known to be more tolerable than oblique aniseikonia.

There have been recurrent arguments in the literature regarding why spectacle cylinder axes should not be rotated away from the correct position, but these arguments are based primarily on the misconception that the axis and power of the *residual* astigmatism determine the direction and amount of distortion. Rather, it is the axis and power of the spectacle lens itself, correct or not, that principally determine the direction and amount of distortion. With this concept understood, and on the basis of clinical experience, we may thus state that the *direction* of distortion may be made more tolerable, if necessary, by rotating the cylinder axis toward 90° or 180°.

There is another situation in which the cylinder axis should sometimes be rotated away from the correct position. An older patient may have *adapted* to an incorrect axis position in his or her previous spectacles, and may not tolerate the change in direction of distortion produced by rotating the cylinder axis to the correct position. The nature of such adaptation is discussed elsewhere, but there is no question that it occurs and can cause problems. In this case, the cylinder axis should be rotated toward the position of the *old* cylinder axis, even if the old cylinder axis is oblique. This maneuver does not *reduce* distortion but does change the *direction* of distortion back toward the position of adaptation.

Altering the astigmatic correction: reducing the cylinder power The other method that is commonly used to lessen distortion is reduction of the power of the correcting cylinder. This method makes sense, for we have seen that the *amount* of meridional magnification is largely determined by the power of the correcting cylinder—the less the cylinder power, the less the meridional magnification.

Altering the astigmatic correction: residual astigmatism Whenever the cylinder power is reduced from its correct value, or the cylinder axis is rotated away from its correct position, residual astigmatism appears. The residual astigmatism does not produce distortion, but it does produce blur of the retinal image, limiting the amount that the cylinder power may be reduced or the amount that the cylinder axis may be rotated away from its correct position. If we must minimize distortion, we must be careful at the same time not to create excessive blur from residual astigmatism.

It is the *amount* of residual astigmatism that produces the blur, not the axis[5] of the residual astigmatism. It is easy to judge the amount of residual astigmatism when reducing the cylinder power of a spectacle correction, for the residual astigmatism is simply equal to the amount the cylinder power is reduced. It is more difficult, however, to judge the amount of residual astigmatism induced by rotating the cylinder axis away from the correct position. The resulting residual astigmatism may always be calculated using the rules for combination of obliquely crossed cylinders, but this calculation requires considerable mental gymnastics. Residual astigmatism may be minimized with the Jackson cross-cylinder test for cylinder power. The spherical equivalent concept will guide the adjustment of the sphere. The guidelines for prescribing cylinders for spectacle correction are summarized below.

Revised guidelines for prescribing cylinders for spectacle correction

1. In *children,* give the full astigmatic correction.
2. In *adults,* try the full astigmatic correction first. Give warning and encouragement. If problems are anticipated, try a walking-around trial with trial frames before prescribing.
3. To minimize distortion, use minus cylinder lenses and minimize vertex distances.
4. Spatial distortion from astigmatic spectacle corrections is a *binocular* phenomenon. Occlude 1 eye to verify that this is indeed the cause of the patient's complaints.
5. If necessary, reduce distortion still further by rotating the cylinder axis toward 180° or 90° (or toward the *old* axis) and/or by reducing the cylinder power. Balance the resulting blur with the remaining distortion, using careful adjustment of cylinder power and sphere. Residual astigmatism at *any* position of the cylinder axis may be minimized with the Jackson cross-cylinder test for cylinder power. Adjust the sphere using the spherical equivalent concept as a guide, but rely on a final subjective check to obtain best visual acuity.
6. If distortion cannot be reduced sufficiently by altering the astigmatic spectacle correction, consider contact lenses (which cause no appreciable distortion) or iseikonic corrections.

Special cases occasionally arise. If a patient's sense of spatial distortion seems out of proportion to his or her astigmatic correction, consider the possibility of spherical aniseikonia as the cause of his symptoms, and prescribe accordingly.

If patients with moderate to high astigmatism have no complaints about distance spectacle correction but have difficulty reading at near, remember that changes in the astigmatic axes of the eyes (from cyclorotations) and changes in the effectivity of astigmatic corrections may cause problems at near. Such patients may require separate reading glasses.

Finally, patients who desire spectacles only for part-time wear may not be able to adapt to distortion during short periods of wear. In such cases, the astigmatic correction should be altered to reduce distortion according to the principles outlined above.

The revised set of guidelines for prescribing cylinders is now complete. With a rational basis for these guidelines, we should be able to place our confidence in them and prescribe cylinders more from knowledge and less from empirical rumors.

For a complete list of references, see the original article: Guyton DL. Prescribing cylinders: The problem of distortion. *Surv Ophthalmol.* 1977;22(3):177–188.

Appendix Notes

1. In the case of astigmatism, the blur patches on the retina may be ellipses or lines instead of blur circles, and the size of the blurred retinal image may appear somewhat altered by the effect of the *shape* of the blur patches on the outline of the image. This effect, however, only affects the *outline* of the retinal image and does not cause the type of monocular distortion (tilting of lines, etc.) that concerns us here.

2. The size of the retinal image is usually computed as proportional to the angle subtended by the object at the first nodal point of the eye (which is approximately 4 mm posterior to the center of the entrance pupil), but this is true only for sharp retinal images. The nodal point cannot be used to compute the size of blurred retinal images.

3. Chief rays such as those in Figure 3-43, although they initially pass *toward* the center of the entrance pupil, are actually refracted by the cornea, pass through the center of the *real* pupil, and are further refracted by the crystalline lens before continuing on to the retina. However, each pair of chief rays, such as *ef* and *gh* or *jk* and *mn,* because of the axial symmetry of the ocular media, remain in the same plane as one another other as they pass through the eye's optics. Therefore, although the retinal images in Figure 3-43 are not exactly the proper size because of the simplified representation of the chief rays, the presence or absence of distortion is accurately represented.

4. An alternate way to analyze the effect of a cylindrical lens is to consider the lens an integral part of the eye's optical system and calculate the position of the entrance pupil for the system as a whole in each principal meridian. The pairs of chief rays in the 2 principal meridians would then cross the optical axis at different points, producing the same differential meridional magnification as obtained with the present analysis.

5. The axis of residual astigmatism is of no consequence in the consideration of blur, except perhaps as it may affect the reading of letters that have predominantly vertical strokes. If the axis of the residual astigmatism is vertical or horizontal, and if the patient is able to clear the vertical strokes of the letters by accommodating, his or her reading ability may be somewhat better than would otherwise be predicted.

CHAPTER 4

Contact Lenses

Introduction

The first documented use of contact lenses occurred in the 1880s. Those lenses were large and made of glass, and they extended to the sclera. Corneal lenses were introduced in the 1940s and were made of a plastic called *polymethylmethacrylate (PMMA)*. Soft hydrogel lenses were introduced in the United States in the 1950s and led to the widespread use of contact lenses. Current estimates are that 51% of US adults use some kind of vision correction; of those, 25% use contact lenses. Therefore, more than 30 million Americans use contact lenses. While the vast majority of contact lens wearers are younger than 50 years, contact lenses also have important uses in older patients, such as for the correction of aphakia. The large number of contact lens users means that all ophthalmologists will interact with this group of patients—for fitting, follow-up care, and/or the treatment of complications. Some knowledge of contact lenses is thus essential for all practitioners.

Contact Lens Glossary

It is important for ophthalmologists to know the vocabulary related to contact lenses. The 3 most important terms are base curve, diameter, and power (Fig 4-1):

Base curve　The curvature of the central posterior surface of the lens, which is adjacent to the cornea; it is measured by its radius of curvature (mm) or may be converted to diopters (D) by taking the reciprocal of the radius.

Diameter (chord diameter)　The width of the contact lens, which typically varies with the lens material; the diameter of soft contact lenses, for example, ranges from 13 mm to 15 mm, whereas that of rigid gas-permeable (RGP) lenses ranges from 9 mm to 10 mm.

Power　Determined by lens shape and calculated indirectly by Snell's law: $D = [n_2 - n_1]/r$; for measurement of the posterior vertex power (as with spectacles), the lens (convex surface facing the observer) can be placed on a lensmeter.

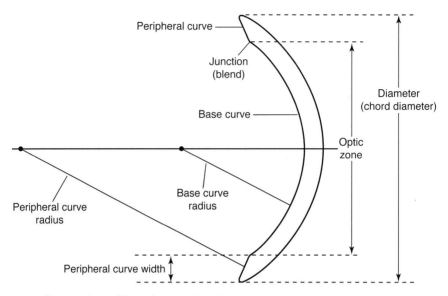

Figure 4-1 Contact lens. Note the relationship among the parts. *(Modified with permission from Stein HA, Freeman MI, Stein RM. CLAO Residents Contact Lens Curriculum Manual. New Orleans: Contact Lens Association of Ophthalmologists; 1996. Redrawn by Christine Gralapp.)*

The following terms are also important to know:

Apical zone   The steep part of the cornea, generally including its geometric center; usually 3–4 mm in diameter.

Corneal apex   The steepest part of the cornea.

Dk   The oxygen permeability of a lens material, where D is the diffusion coefficient for oxygen movement in the material and k is the solubility constant of oxygen in the material.

Dk/L   A term describing the oxygen transmissibility of the lens; depends on the lens material and the central thickness (L).

Edge lift   Description of the peripheral lens and its position in relation to the underlying cornea; adequate edge lift (as documented during fluorescein evaluation by a ring of fluorescein appearing under the lens periphery) prevents edges from digging into the flatter corneal periphery.

Fluorescein pattern   The color intensity of fluorescein dye in the tear lens beneath a rigid contact lens. Areas of contact appear black; green reflects clearance between the lens and the cornea.

K reading   Keratometry reading; determined by a manual or automated keratometer.

Lenticular contact lens   A lens with a central optical zone and a nonoptical peripheral zone known as the carrier; designed to improve lens comfort.

Optic zone   The area of the front surface of the contact lens that has the refractive power of the lens.

Peripheral curves   Secondary curves just outside the base curve at the edge of a contact lens. They are typically flatter than the base curve to approximate the normal flattening of the peripheral cornea. Typically, junctions between posterior curves (base curve and peripheral curve, for example) are smoothed or "blended" to enhance lens comfort.

Polymethylmethacrylate (PMMA)   The first plastic used in the manufacture of contact lenses.

Radiuscope   A device that measures radius of curvature, such as the base curve of an RGP lens. Flatter surfaces have larger radii of curvature, and steeper surfaces have smaller radii of curvature.

Sagittal depth or vault   A term describing the depth (or vault) of a lens; measuring the distance between the center of the posterior surface (or the center of the base curve) to the plane connecting the edges of the lens determines sagittal depth. In general, if the diameter is held constant, the sagittal depth decreases as the base curve increases. Although sagittal depth is critical for determining good fit, designation of the base curve for a particular lens type typically ensures the appropriate sagittal depth.

Tear lens   The optical lens formed by the tear-film layer between the posterior surface of a contact lens and the anterior surface of the cornea. In general, with soft lenses, the tear lens has plano power; with rigid lenses, the power varies, depending on the shape of the lens and the cornea.

Wetting angle   The wettability of a lens surface. A low wetting angle means water will spread over the surface, increasing surface wettability, whereas a high wetting angle means that water will bead up, decreasing surface wettability. A lower wetting angle (greater wettability) generally translates into greater lens comfort and better lens optics.

Clinically Important Features of Contact Lens Optics

Contact lenses and conventional lenses have 4 parameters in common: posterior surface curvature *(base curve)*, anterior surface curvature *(power curve)*, *diameter*, and *power* (see Fig 4-1). However, unlike for spectacle lenses, the shape of contact lenses' posterior surface is designed primarily to have certain fitting relationships with the anterior surface of the eye.

The refractive performance of contact lenses differs from that of spectacle lenses for 2 primary reasons: (1) contact lenses have a shorter vertex distance and (2) tears, rather than air, form the interface between the contact lens and the cornea. Unique optical considerations that are related to contact lenses include field of vision, image size, accommodation, convergence demand, the tear lens, correction of astigmatism, and correction of presbyopia. Each type of contact lens has unique optical considerations (Table 4-1).

Field of Vision

Spectacle frames reduce the field of vision by approximately 20°. Owing to their proximity to the entrance pupils and lack of frames, contact lenses provide a larger field of corrected

Table 4-1 Optical Considerations of Contact Lenses

Type of Lens	Indications	Optical Characteristics
Soft spherical	Myopia or hyperopia with no or small amount of astigmatism	No correction of corneal astigmatism
Soft toric	Myopia, hyperopia, mild to moderate amount of regular astigmatism	Lens must maintain toric axis position through mechanisms such as prism ballast, thin areas. May be used to correct corneal and lenticular astigmatism
Soft bifocal alternating vision	Presbyopia, regular refractive errors	The lens translates up on the cornea during downgaze by the lower lid. The inferior periphery of the lens contains the near prescription
Soft bifocal simultaneous vision	Presbyopia, regular refractive errors	Concentric rings, diffractive, or aspheric design gives simultaneous focus of distance and near objects
RGP spherical	Myopia, hyperopia, regular and irregular astigmatism	Corrects corneal but not lenticular astigmatism
RGP posterior toric	Has a posterior toric surface to match the cornea; especially effective to treat against-the-rule astigmatism	The toric surface is used for fitting purposes
RGP bitoric	Anterior toric surface may be used to compensate for the optical effects of a posterior toric surface or for correction of residual astigmatism	If the anterior toric surface is used to correct for residual astigmatism, the lens must maintain axis alignment through prism ballast or truncation
RGP bifocal alternating or simultaneous	May be used with regular and irregular corneas	Similar to soft bifocal lenses
Hybrid	Keratoconus, postkeratoplasty; other irregular corneas	Combines the comfort and fitting properties of soft contact lenses with the ability of rigid lenses to correct irregular corneas
Scleral	Keratoconus, postkeratoplasty; other irregular corneas. Also useful in creating a therapeutic environment in ocular surface disease such as Stevens-Johnson syndrome and graft-vs-host disease	The lens creates a stable optical surface when corneal contact lenses cannot be successfully fitted

RGP = rigid gas-permeable.

vision and avoid much of the peripheral distortion, such as spherical aberration, created by high-power spectacle lenses.

Image Size

Retinal image size is influenced by the vertex distance and power of corrective lenses. Contact lenses have shorter vertex distances than do spectacles, so image size changes less with contact lenses than with spectacles.

Anisometropia and image size

Axial ametropia is predominant in eyes with higher (non–surgically induced) refractive errors. Theoretically, the anisometropic aniseikonia of such eyes is minimized when the corrective lens is placed in the eyes' anterior focal plane (see discussion of Knapp's law in Chapter 1), which is, on average, approximately 15.7 mm anterior to the corneal vertex. In axial myopia, moving the corrective lens posterior to the eye's focal plane (closer to the cornea) increases the size of the retinal image compared with that of an emmetropic eye. The reverse is true in axial hyperopia. In practice, however, using contact lenses to correct the refractive error of the eyes is usually best for managing anisometropia because aniso-phoria generated by induced prism in off-axis viewing of spectacle lenses is eliminated. In addition, the greater separation between the elements in the stretched retinas of larger myopic eyes may explain the less-than-perceived magnification observed with contact lenses. Surgically induced anisometropia (resulting from, for example, cataract or refrac-tive surgery) without an axial component is usually managed best through use of contact lenses or additional surgery; in either method, the images will be closer in size than if spectacles are used.

Monocular aphakia and aniseikonia

Minimizing aniseikonia in monocular aphakia improves the functional level of binocular vision. An optical model of surgical aphakia can be represented by inserting a neutralizing (minus-power) lens in the location of the crystalline lens and correcting the resulting ametro-pia with a forward-placed plus-power lens. Doing so effectively creates a Galilean telescope within the optical system of the eye. Accordingly, magnification is reduced as the effective plus-power corrective lens (corrected for vertex distance) is moved closer to the neutralizing minus-power lens (the former site of the crystalline lens). This model illustrates why contact lens correction of aphakia creates significantly less magnification than does a spectacle lens correction; a posterior chamber intraocular lens creates the least magnification of all.

Although the ametropia of an aphakic eye is predominantly refractive, it can also have a significant preexisting axial component. For example, the coexistence of axial myopia would further increase the magnification of a contact lens–corrected aphakic eye (com-pared with the image size of the spectacle-corrected fellow phakic myopic eye). Even if the image size of the fellow myopic eye were to be increased by fitting this eye with a contact lens, the residual aniseikonia might still exceed the limits of fusion and cause diplopia (Clinical Example 4-1). Divergent strabismus can develop in aphakic adult eyes (and eso-tropia may develop in children) if fusion is interrupted for a significant period. If diplo-pia does not resolve within several weeks, excessive aniseikonia should be suspected and

> ## CLINICAL EXAMPLE 4-1
>
> *Fitting a unilateral aphakic eye causes diplopia that persists in the presence of prisms that superimpose the 2 images. The refractive error of the fellow eye is –5.00 D, and the image of the aphakic eye is described as being larger than that of the fellow myopic eye. How can the diplopia be resolved?*
>
> The goal is to reduce the aniseikonia of the 2 eyes by magnifying the image size of the phakic eye and/or reducing the image size of the contact lens–corrected aphakic eye. To achieve the former, correct the myopic phakic eye with a contact lens to increase its image size. If doing so is inadequate, overcorrect the contact lens by 5.00 D and prescribe a spectacle lens of –5.00 D for that eye, thereby introducing a reverse Galilean telescope into the optical system of the eye. (If, however, the phakic eye were hyperopic, its image size would be increased by correcting its refractive error with a spectacle lens rather than a contact lens.)

confirmed by demonstration of the patient's inability to fuse images superimposed with the aid of prisms. Such patients are usually aware that the retinal image in the aphakic eye is larger than that in the fellow phakic eye.

When the fellow phakic eye is significantly myopic, correcting it with a contact lens increases its image size and often reduces the aniseikonia sufficiently to resolve the diplopia. If excessive aniseikonia persists, the clinician should aim to further reduce the image size of the contact lens–corrected aphakic eye. Overcorrecting the aphakic contact lens and neutralizing the resulting induced myopia with a forward-placed spectacle lens of appropriate minus power can achieve the additional reduction in image size. In effect, this process introduces a reverse Galilean telescope into the optical system of that eye. Empirically, increasing the power of the distance aphakic contact lens by +3 D and prescribing a –3 D spectacle lens for that eye usually suffice. Alternatively, if it is impractical to fit the fellow myopic eye with a contact lens, the clinician may elect to add plus power to the aphakic contact lens by an amount equal to the spherical equivalent of the refractive error of the fellow eye, in effect equalizing the myopia of the 2 eyes. The resulting decrease in the residual aniseikonia usually improves fusional potential and facilitates the recovery of fusion even of significant aniseikonic exotropia over several weeks. However, the resolution of aphakic esotropia or cyclotropia is less certain.

In contrast with axial myopia, coexisting axial hyperopia reduces the magnification of a contact lens–corrected aphakic eye. Residual aniseikonia can be further mitigated by correction of the fellow hyperopic eye with a spectacle lens (rather than a contact lens) to maximize image size.

Infantile aphakia

Management of aphakia in infants and young children represents a challenge because of the possibility of amblyopia and permanent vision loss. Contact lens wear may be ineffective in children because of poor patient adherence; therefore, intraocular lens implants may be a better option. Aphakia may be corrected in infants with contact lenses or lens implants. The optimal method in this group of patients is not yet known. The rapid change in axial length and corneal power during infancy (see Chapter 2) may make the selection of implant power difficult. Aggressive management of both optical correction and amblyopia treatment is necessary to achieve an optimal outcome in such young patients.

Autrata R, Rehurek J, Vodicková K. Visual results after primary intraocular lens implantation or contact lens correction for aphakia in the first year of age. *Ophthalmologica*. 2005; 219(2):72–79.

Infant Aphakia Treatment Group; Lambert SR, Buckley EG, et al. The infant aphakia treatment study: design and clinical measures at enrollment. *Arch Ophthalmol*. 2010;128(1):21–27.

Accommodation

Accommodation is defined as the difference in vergence at the first principal point of the eye (1.35 mm behind the cornea) between rays originating at infinity and those originating at a near point. This disparity creates different accommodative demands for spectacle and contact lenses. Compared with spectacles, contact lenses increase the accommodative requirements of myopic eyes and decrease those of hyperopic eyes in proportion to the size of the refractive error. The difference between the accommodative efficiency of spectacle lenses and that of contact lenses results from the effect of these 2 modalities on the vergence of light rays as they pass through the respective lenses. Contact lens correction requires an accommodative effort equal to that of emmetropic eyes. In other words, contact lenses eliminate the *accommodative advantage* enjoyed by those with spectacle-corrected myopia and the *disadvantage* experienced by those with spectacle-corrected hyperopia. The accommodative advantage observed in patients with spectacle-corrected myopia is consistent with the clinical observation that patients with spectacle-corrected high myopia can read through their distance correction at older ages than can patients with emmetropia. The opposite is true of patients with spectacle-corrected hyperopia (Clinical Example 4-2).

CLINICAL EXAMPLE 4-2

What is the accommodative demand of a –7 D myopic eye corrected with a spectacle lens compared with a contact lens? A 7 D hyperopic eye? Assume a vertex distance of 15 mm and a near-object distance of 33.3 cm.

The myopic refractive error of the first eye is –7 D at a vertex distance of 15 mm, and the object distance is 33.3 cm. The vergence of rays originating at infinity and exiting the spectacle lens is –7 D. Due to the vertex distance, the vergence of these rays at the front surface of the cornea (which is approximately the location of the first principal point) is –6.3 D. Use the focal point of the –7 D spectacle lens, 1/7 = 0.143 m, plus the vertex distance of 0.015 m (0.158 m) to find the vergence at the corneal surface: 1/0.158 m = –6.3 D (Fig 4-2A).

(Continued)

(continued)

The vergence of rays originating at a distance of 33.3 cm after exiting the spectacle lens is –10 D (Fig 4-2B). The vergence is calculated by using the vergence of the light after it leaves the spectacle lens: –3 + (–7) = –10. Due to the vertex distance, the vergence of these rays at the front surface of the cornea (which is approximately the location of the first principal point) is –8.7 D. Use the focal point of the vergence after the light travels through the lens, –10 D, 1/10 = 0.1 m, plus the vertex distance of 0.015 m (0.115 m) to find the vergence at the corneal surface: 1/0.115 m = –8.7 D).

Accommodation is the difference between the vergence at the first principal point between rays originating at infinity and the vergence of rays originating at a distance of 33.3 cm. In this case, the accommodation is 2.4 D: –6.3 – (–8.7) = 2.4. In contrast, the accommodation required with a contact lens correction is approximately 3 D (Fig 4-2C, D). Therefore, this myopic eye would need 0.6 D more accommodation to focus an object at 33.3 cm when wearing a contact lens compared with correction with a spectacle lens. Similarly, the accommodative demands of an eye corrected with a +7 D spectacle lens would be 3.5 D compared with approximately 3 D for a contact lens (Table 4-2).

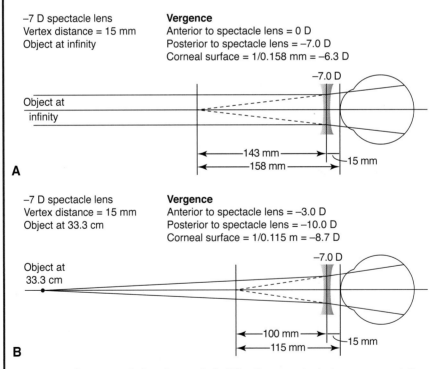

-7 D spectacle lens
Vertex distance = 15 mm
Object at infinity

Vergence
Anterior to spectacle lens = 0 D
Posterior to spectacle lens = –7.0 D
Corneal surface = 1/0.158 mm = –6.3 D

–7.0 D

Object at infinity

―143 mm―
―158 mm―
–15 mm

A

-7 D spectacle lens
Vertex distance = 15 mm
Object at 33.3 cm

Vergence
Anterior to spectacle lens = –3.0 D
Posterior to spectacle lens = –10.0 D
Corneal surface = 1/0.115 m = –8.7 D

–7.0 D

Object at 33.3 cm

―100 mm―
―115 mm―
–15 mm

B

Figure 4-2 Accommodative demand. **A,** Effective spectacle lens power at the corneal surface. **B,** Accommodative demand with a –7.0 D spectacle lens.

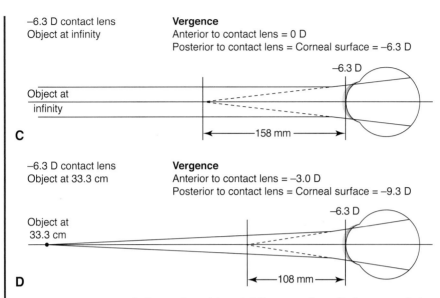

Figure 4-2 *(continued)* **C,** Correction with a –6.3 D contact lens. **D,** Accommodative demand with a –6.3 D contact lens. *(Illustrations developed by Thomas F. Mauger, MD.)*

Table 4-2 Accommodation Through Spectacles and Contact Lenses

	–7.0 D Spectacle Lens		–6.3 D Contact Lens*	
Object at:	Infinity	33.3 cm	Infinity	33.3 cm
Vergence *(D)* at anterior spectacle lens surface	0	–3.0		
Power of lens	–7.0	–7.0	–6.3	–6.3
Vergence at posterior spectacle lens surface	–7.0	–10.0		
Vergence at corneal surface with 15 mm vertex distance	–6.3	–8.7	–6.3	–9.3
Accommodative demand		–6.3 – (–8.7) = **2.4 D**		–6.3 – (–9.3) = **3.0 D**

	+7.0 D Spectacle Lens		+7.8 D Contact Lens†	
Object at:	Infinity	33.3 cm	Infinity	33.3 cm
Vergence *(D)* at anterior spectacle lens surface	0	–3.0		
Power of lens	+7.0	+7.0	+7.8	+7.8
Vergence at posterior spectacle lens surface	+7.0	+4.0		
Vergence at corneal surface with 15-mm vertex distance	+7.8	+4.3	+7.8	+4.8
Accommodative demand		+7.8 – (+4.3) = **3.5 D**		+7.8 – (+4.8) = **3.0 D**

*The effective power of a –7.0 D spectacle lens with a vertex distance of 15 mm is –6.3 D.
†The effective power of a +7.0 D spectacle lens with a vertex distance of 15 mm is +7.8 D.

Convergence Demands

Depending on their power, spectacle lenses (optically centered for distance) and contact lenses require different convergences. Myopic spectacle lenses induce *base-in prisms* for near objects. This benefit is eliminated with contact lenses. Conversely, hyperopic spectacles increase the convergence demands by inducing *base-out prisms.* In this case, contact lenses provide a benefit by eliminating the incremental convergence requirement.

In summary, correction of myopia with contact lenses, as opposed to spectacle lenses, increases both accommodative and convergence demands of focusing near objects proportional to the size of the refractive error. The reverse is true in hyperopia (Fig 4-3).

Tear Lens

The presence of fluid, rather than air, between a contact lens and the corneal surface is responsible for another major difference between the optical performance of contact lenses and that of spectacle lenses. The tear layer between a contact lens and the corneal surface is an optical lens in its own right. As with all lenses, the power of this *tear,* or *fluid,* lens is determined by the curvatures of the anterior surface (formed by the back surface of the contact lens) and the posterior surface (formed by the front surface of the cornea).

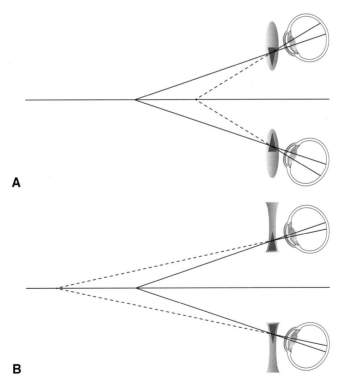

A

B

Figure 4-3 Effect of spectacle lenses on convergence demands. **A,** Lenses for correction of hyperopia create induced base-out prism with convergence, which increases the convergence demand. **B,** Lenses for correction of myopia create induced base-in prism, which decreases the convergence demand. *(Illustrations developed by Thomas F. Mauger, MD.)*

Because flexible (soft) contact lenses conform to the shape of the cornea and the curvatures of the anterior and posterior surfaces of the intervening tear layer are identical, the power of their tear lenses is always *plano.* This statement is not generally true of rigid contact lenses: the shape of the posterior surface (which defines the anterior surface of the tear lens) can differ from the shape of the underlying cornea (which forms the posterior surface of the tear lens). Under these circumstances, the tear layer introduces power that is added to the eye's optical system.

The power of the tear lens is approximately 0.25 D for every 0.05-mm radius-of-curvature difference between the base curve of the contact lens and the central curvature of the cornea *(K),* and this power becomes somewhat greater for corneas steeper than 7.00 mm. Tear lenses created by rigid contact lenses with base curves that are steeper than *K* (ie, have a smaller radius of curvature) have plus power, whereas tear lenses formed by base curves that are flatter than *K* (ie, have a larger radius of curvature) have minus power (Fig 4-4). Therefore, the power of a rigid contact lens must account for both the eye's refractive error and the power introduced by the tear lens. An easy way of remembering this is to use the rules *steeper add minus (SAM)* and *flatter add plus (FAP)* (Clinical Example 4-3).

Because the refractive index of the tear lens (1.336) is almost identical to that of a cornea (1.3765), the anterior surface of the tear lens virtually masks the optical effect of the corneal surface. If the back surface of a contact lens is spherical, then the anterior surface of the tear lens is also spherical, regardless of the corneal topography. In other words, the tear layer created by a spherical rigid contact lens neutralizes more than 90% of regular and irregular corneal astigmatism. This principle simplifies the calculation of the tear lens power on astigmatic corneas: because the powers of the steeper corneal meridians are effectively neutralized, they can be ignored, and only the flattest meridians need to be considered. The refractive error along the flattest meridian is represented by the spherical component of refractive errors expressed in *minus cylinder form.* For this reason,

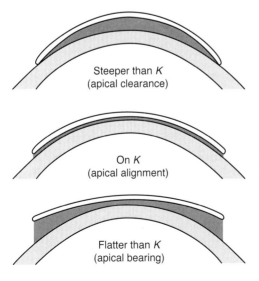

Figure 4-4 A rigid contact lens creates a tear (or fluid) lens whose power is determined by the difference between the curvature of the cornea *(K)* and that of the base curve of the contact lens. *(Courtesy of Perry Rosenthal, MD. Redrawn by Christine Gralapp.)*

> ## CLINICAL EXAMPLE 4-3
>
> *The refractive error of an eye is –3.00 D, the K measurement is 7.80 mm (43.25 D), and the base curve chosen for the rigid contact lens is 7.95 mm (42.50 D). What is the anticipated power of the contact lens?*
>
> The power of the resulting tear lens is –0.75 D. This power would correct –0.75 D of the refractive error. Therefore, the remaining refractive error that the contact lens is required to correct is –2.25 D (recall the FAP rule: flatter add plus). Conversely, if the refractive error were +3.00 D (hyperopia), then the necessary contact lens power would be +3.75 D to correct the refractive error and the –0.75 D tear lens (Fig 4-5).

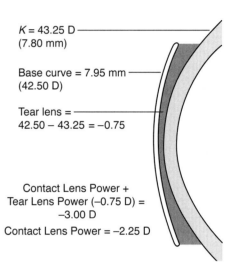

$K = 43.25$ D
(7.80 mm)

Base curve = 7.95 mm
(42.50 D)

Tear lens =
$42.50 - 43.25 = -0.75$

Contact Lens Power +
Tear Lens Power (–0.75 D) =
–3.00 D
Contact Lens Power = –2.25 D

Figure 4-5 Determining the power of a contact lens using the FAP-SAM rules. *(Illustration developed by Thomas F. Mauger, MD.)*

clinicians should use only the minus cylinder format when dealing with contact lenses (Clinical Example 4-4).

Correcting Astigmatism

Because rigid (and toric soft) contact lenses neutralize astigmatism at the corneal surface, the meridional aniseikonia created by the 2 different powers incorporated within each spectacle lens is avoided. For this reason, contact lens–wearing patients with significant corneal astigmatism often experience an annoying change in spatial orientation when they switch to spectacles. However, refractive astigmatism is the sum of *corneal* and *lenticular astigmatism*. Lenticular astigmatism, if present, is not corrected by spherical contact lenses. Because lenticular astigmatism usually has an against-the-rule orientation (vertical axis minus cylinder), it persists as residual astigmatism when the corneal astigmatism component is neutralized by rigid contact lenses. This finding is more

CLINICAL EXAMPLE 4-4

The refractive correction is −3.50 +1.75 × 90, and the K measurements along the 2 principal meridians are 7.80 mm horizontal (43.25 D at 180°) and 7.50 mm vertical (45.00 D at 90°). The contact lens base curve is 7.50 mm. What is the anticipated power of the contact lens?

The refractive correction along the flattest corneal meridian (7.80 mm) is −1.75 D (convert the refractive error to minus cylinder form), and the lens has been fitted steeper than flat *K*, creating a tear lens of +1.75 D. Thus, a corresponding amount of minus power must be added (recall the SAM rule: steeper add minus), giving a corrective power of −3.50 D in that meridian.

The refractive correction along the steepest meridian (7.50 mm) is −3.50 D. The lens is fitted "on *K*"; therefore, no tear lens power is created. The corrective power for this meridian is also −3.50 D.

Accordingly, the power of the contact lens should be −3.50 D (Fig 4-6).

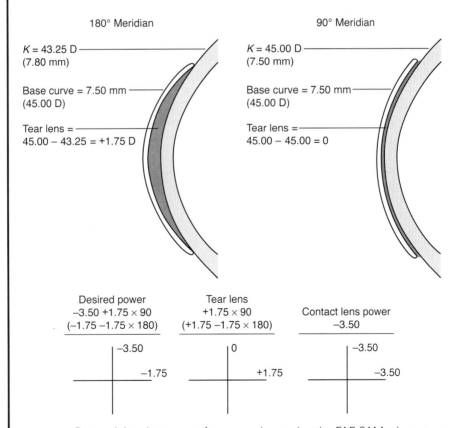

Figure 4-6   Determining the power of a contact lens using the FAP-SAM rules. *(Illustrations developed by Thomas F. Mauger, MD.)*

common among older patients and often explains why their hard contact lenses fail to provide the anticipated vision correction. These cases can be identified via spherocylinder refraction over the contact lens. However, against-the-rule lenticular astigmatism is probably present when against-the-rule refractive astigmatism (adjusted to reflect the power at the corneal surface) exceeds the keratometric corneal astigmatism. Such eyes may have less residual astigmatism when the refractive error is corrected with soft rather than rigid spherical contact lenses if the corneal astigmatism is compensating for lenticular astigmatism.

For example, consider a patient whose refraction is –3.50 –0.50 × 180 and K measurements of the affected eye are 42.5 D (7.94 mm) horizontal and 44.0 D (7.67 mm) vertical. Would a soft or rigid contact lens provide better vision (ie, less residual astigmatism)? The disparity between the corneal astigmatism of 1.50 D and the refractive astigmatism of 0.50 D reveals 1.00 D of against-the-rule lenticular astigmatism that neutralizes a similar amount of with-the-rule corneal astigmatism. Neutralizing the corneal component of the refractive astigmatism with a rigid contact lens exposes the lenticular residual astigmatism. Therefore, a spherical soft contact lens would provide better vision because the residual astigmatism is 1.00 D for a rigid contact lens.

Correcting Presbyopia

Correcting presbyopia with contact lenses can be done in several different ways:

- reading glasses over contact lenses
- alternating vision contact lenses (segmented or annular)
- simultaneous vision contact lenses (aspheric [multifocal] or diffractive)
- monovision

From an optical point of view, the use of reading glasses or alternating vision contact lenses is similar to standard spectacle correction for presbyopia. Simultaneous vision contact lenses direct light from 2 points in space—one near, one far—to the retina, resulting in a loss of contrast. Distant targets are "washed out" by light coming in through the near segment(s), and near objects are "washed out" by light coming in through the distance segment(s). Monovision allows one eye to have better distance vision and the other to have better near vision, but this arrangement interferes with binocular function, and the patient then has reduced stereopsis. For these reasons, it is important to fully explain the options to contact lens wearers with presbyopia. As previously demonstrated, it is important to explain to a new contact lens wearer with presbyopia and myopia that he or she may need near correction or one of the other aforementioned options when presbyopic correction with the spectacles had not previously been required. The contact lens correction of presbyopia is discussed in greater detail in the section Contact Lenses for Presbyopia.

Kastl PR, ed. *Contact Lenses: The CLAO Guide to Basic Science and Clinical Practice.* 4 vols. Dubuque, IA: Kendall-Hunt; 1995.

Contact Lens Materials and Manufacturing

Various materials have been used to make contact lenses. The choice of material can affect contact lens parameters such as wettability, oxygen permeability, and deposits on the lens. In addition, material choice affects the flexibility and comfort of the lens and the stability and quality of vision. Manufacturing techniques primarily address the ability to make reproducible lenses in a cost-effective manner.

Materials

Contact lens materials can be described in terms of flexibility (hard, rigid gas-permeable [RGP], soft, or hybrid). The first popular corneal contact lenses were made of PMMA, a plastic that is durable but not oxygen permeable. Gas-permeable materials are rigid but usually more flexible than PMMA. RGP lenses allow some oxygen permeability *(Dk);* this factor may vary from *Dk* 15 to more than *Dk* 100. This feature has allowed some RGP lenses to be approved for overnight or extended wear. Currently, most RGP lenses are made of silicone acrylate. This material provides the hardness needed for sharp vision, which is associated with PMMA lenses, and the oxygen permeability associated with silicone. Despite advances, wettability still poses a challenge (Fig 4-7).

The newest lenses are made of *fluoropolymer,* which provides greater oxygen permeability than does PMMA. Disadvantages of fluoropolymer lenses are rigidity and discomfort.

The gas permeability of a material is related to (1) the size of the intermolecular voids that allow the transmission of gas molecules, and (2) the gas solubility of the material. Silicon monomers are the most commonly used materials because their characteristic bulky molecular structure creates a more open polymer architecture. The addition of fluorine increases the gas solubility of polymers and somewhat counteracts the tendency of silicon to bind hydrophobic debris (such as lipid-containing mucus) to the contact lens surface.

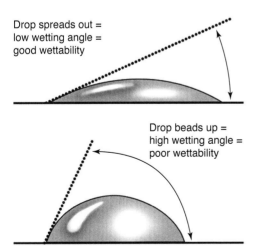

Drop spreads out =
low wetting angle =
good wettability

Drop beads up =
high wetting angle =
poor wettability

Figure 4-7 The wettability of a lens surface determines whether a wetting angle will be low (greater wettability, greater comfort) or high (less wettability, less comfort). *(Modified with permission from Stein HA, Freeman MI, Stein RM. CLAO Residents Contact Lens Curriculum Manual. New Orleans: Contact Lens Association of Ophthalmologists; 1996. Redrawn by Christine Gralapp.)*

In general, polymers that incorporate more silicon offer greater gas permeability at the expense of surface biocompatibility.

Soft contact lenses are typically made of a soft hydrogel polymer, *hydroxyethylmethacrylate*. The surface characteristics of hydrogels can change instantaneously, depending on their external environment. When hydrogel lenses are exposed to water, their hydrophilic elements are attracted to (and their hydrophobic components are repelled from) the surface, which becomes more wettable. However, drying of the surface repels the hydrophilic elements inward, making the lens surfaces less wettable. The hydrophobic surface elements have a strong affinity for nonpolar lipid tear components through forces known as *hydrophobic interactions*. Such interactions further reduce surface wettability, accelerate evaporative drying, and compromise the clinical properties of soft lenses.

The oxygen and carbon dioxide permeability of traditional hydrogel polymers is directly related to their water content. Because tear exchange under soft lenses is minimal, corneal respiration depends almost entirely on the transmission of oxygen and carbon dioxide through the polymer matrix. Although the oxygen permeability of hydrogel polymers increases with water content, so does their tendency to dehydrate. To maintain the integrity of the tear compartment and avoid corneal epithelial desiccation in dry environments, these lenses are made thicker, thereby limiting their oxygen transmissibility.

High-oxygen-permeability, low-water-content silicone hydrogels are used for extended wear. The oxygen transmission of these lenses is a function of their silicon (rather than water) content and is sufficient to meet the oxygen needs of most patients' corneas during sleep. The surfaces of these lenses require special coatings to mask their hydrophobic properties. Other clinically important properties of contact lens hydrogels include light transmission, modulus (resistance to flexure), rate of recovery from deformation, elasticity, tear resistance, dimensional sensitivity to pH and the osmolality of the soaking solution and tears, chemical stability, deposit resistance, and surface water-binding properties.

Manufacturing

Several methods are used to manufacture contact lenses. Some contact lenses are *spin-cast*, a technique popularized with the first soft contact lenses. In spin-casting, the liquid plastic polymer is placed in a mold that is spun on a centrifuge; the shape of the mold and the rate of spin determine the final shape of the contact lens. Soft contact lenses can also be made on a lathe, starting with a hard, dry plastic button; this method is similar to the way that RGP lenses are made. Once the soft lens lathe process is complete, the lens is hydrated in saline solution to create the characteristic softness. Lathes may be either manually operated or automated. In either case, manufacturers can create very complex, variable shapes that provide correction for many different types of refractive error; lenses can even be customized to meet individual needs.

Following the introduction of disposable contact lenses—and thus the need to manufacture large quantities of lenses—cast molding was developed. In this technique, different metal dies, or molds, are used for specific refractive corrections. Liquid polymer is injected into the mold and then polymerized to create a soft contact lens of the desired dimensions. This process is completely automated from start to finish, enabling cost-effective production of large quantities of lenses.

Scleral contact lenses have very large diameters and touch the sclera 2–4 mm beyond the limbus. They have been available for years, but because they were originally made of PMMA—and thus were oxygen impermeable—the lenses were not comfortable. With the use of newer RGP materials, interest in these lenses has resurfaced, especially for patients with abnormal corneas. Scleral contact lenses are made from a mold taken of the anterior surface of the eye; the mold is made of an alginate mix, which hardens in the shape of the ocular surface. This alginate mold is then used to make a plaster mold, which, in turn, is used to make the actual scleral lens.

Patient Examination and Contact Lens Selection

As in all patient care, a complete history and eye examination are needed to rule out serious ocular problems such as glaucoma and macular degeneration.

Patient Examination

A clinician needs specific information to select a contact lens for a particular patient. This information includes the patient's daily activities (desk work, driving, and so on) and reason for using contact lenses (eg, full-time vision, sports only, social events only, changing eye color, avoiding use of reading glasses). If a patient is already a contact lens user, the fitter must also find out the following: the number of years the patient has worn contact lenses, the current type of lens worn, the wear schedule, and the care system used. In addition, the fitter must determine whether the patient currently has or previously had any problems with lens use.

Factors that may suggest an increased risk of complications with contact lens use include diabetes mellitus, especially if uncontrolled; immunosuppression; long-term use of topical medications such as corticosteroids; and environmental exposure to dust, vapors, or chemicals. Other relative contraindications to contact lens use include an inability to handle and/or care for contact lenses; monocularity; abnormal eyelid function, such as with Bell palsy; severe dry eye; and corneal neovascularization. The primary indications for contact lenses in a patient with preexisting corneal disease are therapeutic or bandage lenses and a rigid contact lens for the correction of irregular astigmatism.

Key areas to observe during slit-lamp examination include the eyelids (to rule out blepharitis or mechanical lid abnormalities such as trichiasis, ectropion, and entropion), the tear film, and the ocular surface (to rule out dry eye). Eyelid movement and blink should also be observed. The cornea and conjunctiva should be evaluated carefully for signs of ocular surface disease, allergy, scarring, symblepharon, or other signs of conjunctival scarring diseases, such as ocular cicatricial pemphigoid (mucous membrane pemphigoid). Through refraction and keratometry, the ophthalmologist can determine whether there is significant corneal, lenticular, or irregular astigmatism. The identification of irregular astigmatism may suggest other pathologies, such as keratoconus, that would require further evaluation.

Contact Lens Selection

The selection of a contact lens for an individual patient and eye is a complex process. Optical, biological, mechanical, and social considerations are among the factors that enter into this process (see Table 4-1).

Soft contact lenses are currently the most frequently prescribed and worn lenses in the United States. They can be classified according to various characteristics. Given this variety, selection of the appropriate lens for each patient may be difficult. Typically, an experienced fitter knows the characteristics of several lenses that cover the needs of most patients.

The main advantages of soft contact lenses are their shorter period of adaptation and their high level of comfort (Table 4-3). They are available with many parameters so that all regular refractive errors are covered. Furthermore, the ease of fitting soft lenses makes them the first choice of many practitioners.

The decision about a replacement schedule may be made on a cost basis. Conventional lenses (changed every 6–12 months) are often the least expensive, but disposable lenses and conventional lenses that are replaced more frequently are typically associated with less irritation, such as red eyes, and more consistent quality of vision. Daily disposable lenses require the least amount of care, so less expense is involved for lens-care solutions. Disposable lenses are generally more expensive than reusable contact lenses, but they offer advantages to patients who are either unable or unwilling to properly care for and disinfect contact lenses. They are also helpful in patients who have unacceptable reactions to lens-care solutions or protein deposits on contact lenses.

Daily wear (DW) is the most favored wear pattern in the United States. Extended wear (EW)—that is, leaving the lens in during sleep—is less popular, primarily because of reports from the 1980s of the increased incidence of keratitis with EW lenses. However, improved materials that have far greater oxygen permeability (Dk = 60 to 140) have been approved for EW; use of these materials may decrease the risk of infection compared with the risk associated with earlier materials (although it is difficult to document the incidence because serious infections are rare with all lenses currently in use). Patients who want EW

Table 4-3 Comparative Advantages of Soft and Rigid Gas-Permeable Contact Lenses

Soft Contact Lenses	RGP Contact Lenses
Immediate comfort	Clear and sharp quality of vision
Shorter adaptation period	Correction of small and large amounts of astigmatism, as well as irregular astigmatism
Flexible wear schedule	
Less sensitivity to environmental foreign bodies, dust	Ease of handling
	Acceptable for patients with dry eye, ocular surface disease, and similar disorders
Variety of lens types (eg, disposable lenses, lenses replaced frequently)	Stability and durability
Ability to change eye color	Ease of care

lenses should understand the risks and benefits of this modality. Specifically, patients are at increased risk of bacterial keratitis and other ocular infections (see BCSC Section 8, *External Disease and Cornea.*). Risk factors for EW complications include a previous history of eye infections, lens use while swimming, and any exposure to smoke. To avoid complications associated with EW lenses, the clinician should make sure that the lenses fit properly, that they feel comfortable to the patient, that the patient's vision is good, and most importantly, that the patient is informed of and will adhere to care instructions. Patients should understand the need for careful contact lens care and replacement, as well as the signs and symptoms of eye problems that require the attention of a physician.

Rigid contact lenses continue to be used today, but only by a small percentage (<20%) of lens wearers in the United States. The original hard contact lenses, made of PMMA, are rarely used now because of their oxygen impermeability. Currently, commonly used RGP materials include fluorinated silicone acrylate with oxygen permeability ranging from the 20s to more than 250 and are manufactured with many parameters. Modern RGP lenses are approved for DW—some even for extended, overnight wear. Because of the manufacturing costs and the many parameters available, RGP lenses are not usually offered in disposable packs, but yearly replacement is recommended. The main advantages of RGP lenses are the quality of vision they offer and the ease with which they correct astigmatism (see Table 4-3). The main disadvantages are initial discomfort, a longer period of adaptation, and greater difficulty in fitting. Because of the added time and skill involved in RGP lens fitting, not every contact lens practitioner chooses to offer these lenses.

Schein OD, Glynn RJ, Poggio EC, Seddon JM, Kenyon KR. The relative risk of ulcerative keratitis among users of daily-wear and extended-wear soft contact lenses. A case-control study. Microbial Keratitis Study Group. *N Engl J Med.* 1989;321(12):773–778.

Contact Lens Fitting

The goals of lens fitting include patient satisfaction (good vision that does not fluctuate with blinking or eye movement) and good fit (the lens is centered and moves slightly with each blink). The details of what constitutes a good fit vary between soft and RGP lenses and involve the "art" of contact lens fitting. For example, a patient who wants contact lenses only for skiing or tennis should probably be fitted with soft contact lenses because of the rapid adaptation that is possible with these lenses. However, a patient with 3 D of astigmatism would probably have the best vision with RGP contact lenses (see Table 4-3).

Soft Contact Lenses

Soft contact lenses are comfortable primarily because the material is soft and the diameter is large, extending beyond the cornea to the sclera. Most manufacturers make a specific style of lens that varies in only 1 parameter, such as a lens that comes in 3 base curves, with all other parameters being the same. The first lens is fit empirically; often, the lens chosen is one that the manufacturer reports "will fit 80% of patients." Then, on the basis of the patient's comfort and vision and a slit-lamp evaluation of the fit, the lens may be changed for another base curve and then reevaluated.

A good soft contact lens fit is often described as having a "3-point touch," which means that the lens touches the surface of the eye at the corneal apex and at the limbus on either side of the cornea (in cross section, the lens would touch the limbus at 2 places). To find a light 3-point touch, one may need to choose a lens with a different *sagittal depth*. Changing the lens diameter and/or changing the base curve can alter the sagittal depth of a lens. If the base curve is kept constant, as the diameter is increased, the sagittal depth increases and the lens fits more tightly; that is, there is less lens movement. If the diameter is kept constant and the base curve is decreased, the sagittal depth increases, and again, the fit is tightened (Table 4-4).

In evaluating the soft lens fit, the clinician should observe the lens movement and centration. In a good fit, the lens will move approximately 0.5–1.0 mm with upward gaze or blink, or with gentle pressure on the lower eyelid to move the lens. A tight lens will not move at all, and a loose lens will move too much. By evaluating a patient's vision and comfort, slit-lamp findings (eg, lens movement, lens edge, limbal injection), and keratometry mires, the clinician can determine whether the fit is adequate (see Table 4-4).

Once a fit is deemed adequate, an overrefraction is performed to check the contact lens power. The power is changed if necessary, while other parameters are kept the same.

Table 4-4 Basic Soft Contact Lens Fitting

Initial Lens Selection

Parameter	Description
Diameter	Approximately 2 mm larger than the horizontal corneal diameter
Base curve	0.2–0.6 mm greater (flatter) than the radius of the flattest K reading
Power	As close as possible to the patient's refraction corrected for the vertex distance

Evaluating Soft Contact Lens Fit

Loose Fit	Tight Fit
Excessive movement	No lens movement
Poor centration; lens easily dislocates off the cornea	Centered lens
Lens-edge standoff	"Digging in" of lens edge
Blurred mires after a blink	Clear mires with blink
Fluctuating vision	Good vision initially
Continuing lens awareness	Initial comfort, but increasing lens awareness with continued use
Air bubbles under the lens	Limbal–scleral injection at lens edge

Adjusting Soft Contact Lens Fit

Create a Looser Fit	Create a Tighter Fit
Decrease the sagittal depth	Increase the sagittal depth
Choose a flatter base curve (increase the radius of curvature)	Choose a steeper base curve (decrease the radius of curvature)
Choose a smaller diameter	Choose a larger diameter

When the initial fitting process is complete, the clinician should teach the patient how to insert and remove the contact lenses, how to care for them, and how to recognize the signs and symptoms of eye emergencies. Follow-up care includes assessment of symptoms and vision and performing a slit-lamp examination. The follow-up appointment is usually scheduled for 1 week after the initial fitting (for EW lenses, an additional visit is usually scheduled for 24–48 hours after the first use of the lens); a second office visit is often scheduled for 1–6 months later, depending on the type of lens, the patient's experience with contact lenses, and the patient's ocular status.

At the end of the soft contact lens–fitting process, the final lens parameters should be clearly identified (Table 4-5). Also, the medical record should note any signs and symptoms of eye infection, any recommendation for lens wear (eg, DW or EW lenses) and lens care, and any follow-up plans.

Rigid Gas-Permeable Contact Lenses

RGP lenses, given their small overall diameter, should center over the cornea but move freely with each blink to allow tear exchange. Unlike with soft contact lenses, the parameters of RGP lenses often are not determined by the manufacturer but are individualized for each patient, making RGP lens fitting more challenging. However, for a normal eye, standard parameters are typically used, and as with soft lenses, a patient is fit from trial lenses. The fit is optimized first; then the vision is optimized by over-refraction (Table 4-6). In the following subsections, some key issues in RGP lens fitting are briefly reviewed; however, a complete coverage of the topic is beyond the scope of this chapter.

Table 4-5 Soft Contact Lens Parameters

Parameter	Common Abbreviation (in the United States)	Typical Range of Values
Overall diameter	OAD	12.5–16.0 mm
Base curve	BC	8.0–9.5 mm
Center thickness	CT	0.04–0.20 mm (varies with the power of the lens and is set by the manufacturer)
Prescription	RX	Sphere and astigmatism, if any, in diopters
Manufacturer	Varies	Company name and lens style

Table 4-6 Rigid Gas-Permeable Lens Parameters

Parameter	Common Abbreviation (in the United States)	Range of Normal Values
Overall diameter	OAD	8.0–11.5 mm
Optic zone diameter	OZD	7.0–8.5 mm
Peripheral curve width	PCW	0.1–1.0 mm
Base curve	BC	7.0–8.5 mm
Center thickness	CT	0.08–0.30 mm
Prescription	RX	Any power required

Base curve

Unlike soft contact lenses, an RGP lens maintains its shape when placed on a cornea. As described earlier, a tear layer forms between the cornea and contact lens (in this case, the RGP lens) that varies in shape, depending on the base curve and whether there is corneal astigmatism. The tear layer, usually known as the *tear lens,* is one of the parameters used to determine the best contact lens fit as well as the required contact lens power.

The type of fit is determined by the relationship between the base curve and the curvature of the cornea *(K).* For selection of the initial base curve, the following options are available (see Fig 4-4):

- *Apical alignment* (on *K*). The base curve matches that of the cornea.
- *Apical clearance* (steeper than *K*). The base curve has a steeper fit (smaller radius of curvature and smaller number in millimeters, and thus more curved) than that of the cornea.
- *Apical bearing* (flatter than *K*). The base curve has a flatter fit (larger radius of curvature and larger number in millimeters, and thus less curved) than that of the cornea.

Position

The most common type of RGP lens fit is the *apical alignment fit* (see Fig 4-4), in which the upper edge of the lens fits under the upper eyelid (Fig 4-8). This fit allows the lens to move with each blink, enhances tear exchange, and decreases lens sensation because the eyelid does not strike the lens edge with each blink.

A *central* or *interpalpebral fit* is achieved when the lens rests between the upper and lower eyelids. To achieve this fit, the lens is given a steeper fit than *K* (apical clearance; see Fig 4-4) to minimize lens movement and keep the lens centered over the cornea. Typically, with this type of fit, the diameter of the lens is smaller than with an apical alignment fit, the base curve is steeper than *K*, and the lens has a thin edge. There is also greater lens sensation because the eyelid strikes the lens with each blink. The resulting sensation discourages normal blinking and often leads to an incomplete blinking pattern and a reduced blink rate. Peripheral corneal staining at the 3-o'clock and 9-o'clock positions may arise from poor wetting. This type of fit is best for patients who have any or all of the following: very large interpalpebral opening, astigmatism greater than approximately 1.75 D,

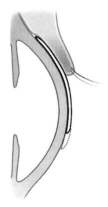

Figure 4-8 The most common and most comfortable type of rigid gas-permeable lens fit is apical alignment, in which the upper edge of the lens fits under the upper eyelid. *(Modified with permission from Albert DM, Jakobiec FA, eds.* Principles and Practice of Ophthalmology. *Philadelphia: Saunders; 1994;5:3630. Redrawn by Christine Gralapp.)*

and against-the-rule astigmatism. A *flatter-than-K fit* (apical bearing) is not typically used with normal eyes.

Other lens parameters

With an RGP lens, the diameter should be chosen so that when the lens moves, it does not ride off the cornea. Typically, the diameter is approximately 2 mm shorter than the corneal diameter. Central thickness and peripheral curves can also be selected, but often the lens laboratory assumes standard parameters. The lens edge is important for enhancing tear exchange and maintaining lens position, as well as for providing comfort. A thicker edge helps maintain the lens position under the upper eyelid in apical alignment fitting; a thin edge maintains centration and comfort for an interpalpebral fit.

Power

The tear lens, as previously noted, is the lens formed by the posterior surface of the RGP lens and the anterior surface of the cornea. Its power is determined by the base curve:

- *On* K. The tear lens has plano power.
- *Steeper than* K. The tear lens has plus power.
- *Flatter than* K. The tear lens has minus power.

The rule for calculating the needed contact lens power from the spectacle sphere power and the base curve of the RGP lens is SAM-FAP (steeper add minus; flatter add plus). For example, if the spectacle prescription is –3.25 –0.75 × 180, the *keratometry readings (K readings)* are 42.25/43.00 at 90°, and the base curve is slightly flatter than *K* at 41.75 D (ie, 0.50 D flatter), then according to the FAP rule, the contact lens power should be –3.25 + 0.50 = –2.75 D sphere. The tear lens will correct the corneal astigmatism.

The lens power can also be determined empirically. To do so, place a trial lens of known power on the eye, determine the overrefraction, and then add the lens power and the overrefraction power.

Fit

To evaluate the fit of a contact lens, the clinician considers vision quality, lens movement, and the fluorescein evaluation. Overrefraction determines whether a power change is needed. Vision should be stable before and immediately after a blink. Stable vision ensures that the lens covers the optical axis, even when it moves with normal blinking.

The peripheral zone of the cornea flattens toward the limbus; therefore, the central vault of a contact lens is determined by its base curve and diameter. Steepening the base curve (ie, decreasing its radius of curvature) obviously increases the vault of a contact lens. However, increasing the diameter of a lens also increases its central vault (ie, *sagittal depth*) (Fig 4-9).

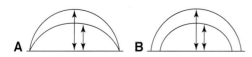

Figure 4-9 **A,** Changing the base curve of a contact lens changes the sagittal depth. **B,** Changing diameter with equal base curve also changes sagittal depth.

Lens position in the alignment fitting should be such that the lens rides high; approximately the upper one-third of the contact lens should be under the upper eyelid (see Fig 4-8). The lens should move as the eyelid moves. Insufficient movement suggests that the lens is too tight. To remedy this situation, the clinician may decrease the sagittal depth by either flattening the base curve (increasing the radius of curvature) or decreasing the lens diameter. Excessive movement, however, suggests that the lens is too loose. To tighten the lens, the clinician may increase its sagittal depth by either steepening the base curve (decreasing the radius of curvature) or increasing the diameter of the lens.

Evaluation of the fluorescein pattern with a cobalt blue light at the slit lamp can help in assessing RGP lens fit (Fig 4-10). If there is apical clearing of the cornea, pooling or a bright green area will be observed; if the RGP lens is touching the cornea, dark areas will be observed.

Once the lens parameters are determined, the information is given to a laboratory, which then makes the lens to these specifications, typically on a lathe. When the lens is received, the major parameters must be checked: base curve (by use of an optic spherometer), lens diameter, and lens power (by use of a lensmeter). Although RGP lens fitting can be more challenging than soft lens fitting, the use of trial lenses and consultation with the laboratory that will make the lens can yield a good fit on most patients with a normal anterior segment (Clinical Example 4-5).

Toric Soft Contact Lenses

An estimated 20% of the US population has significant astigmatism. With current contact lenses, however, such astigmatism can be corrected.

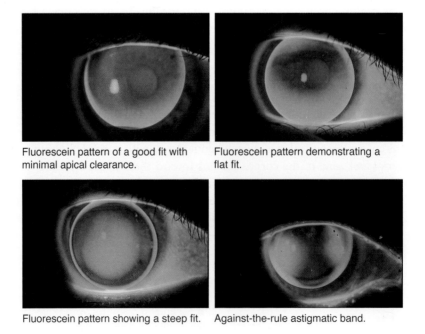

Fluorescein pattern of a good fit with minimal apical clearance.

Fluorescein pattern demonstrating a flat fit.

Fluorescein pattern showing a steep fit.

Against-the-rule astigmatic band.

Figure 4-10 Examples of fluorescein patterns in contact lens fitting. *(Courtesy of Perry Rosenthal, MD.)*

CLINICAL EXAMPLE 4-5

A patient with a refraction of –2.00 –2.00 × 180 desires contact lens correction. The keratometry measurement is 44.00 sphere. What is the residual refractive error if this eye is fitted with a spherical RGP contact lens? A spherical soft contact lens? A toric soft contact lens?

This eye has lenticular but not corneal astigmatism. Correction with spherical soft or rigid contact lenses will result in residual astigmatism. A soft toric contact lens may be used to correct the lenticular astigmatism.

When the clinician is considering a contact lens for a patient with astigmatism, the first question to ask is whether a toric lens is needed. The type of lens usually depends on the amount of astigmatism, although there is no infallible rule for when to correct astigmatism. In general, more than 0.75 D of astigmatism is significant enough to correct (Table 4-7).

Soft toric contact lenses are readily available in several fitting designs. In *front toric contact lenses,* the astigmatic correction is on the front surface; in *back toric contact lenses,* the correction is on the back surface. To prevent lens rotation, one of several manufacturing techniques is used:

- adding prism ballast, that is, placing extra lens material on the bottom edge of the lens
- truncating or removing the bottom of the lens to form a straight edge that aligns with the lower eyelid
- creating thin zones, that is, making lenses with a thin zone on the top and bottom so that eyelid pressure can keep the lens in the appropriate position

Most toric soft lenses use either prism ballast or thin zones to provide stabilization and comfort.

Fitting soft toric lenses is similar to fitting other soft lenses, except that lens rotation must also be evaluated. Toric lenses typically have a mark to note the 6-o'clock position. If the lens fits properly, it is in the 6-o'clock position. Note that the mark does not indicate the astigmatic axis; it is used only to determine proper fit. If a slit-lamp examination shows that the lens mark is rotated away from the 6-o'clock axis, the amount of rotation should be noted, in degrees (1 clock-hour equals 30°) (Fig 4-11). The rule for adjusting for lens

Table 4-7 Astigmatism and Lens Fitting

Degree of Astigmatism	First Choice of Lens
Less than 1 D	Spherical soft or RGP
1–2 D	Toric soft contact or spherical RGP
2–3 D	Custom soft toric or spherical RGP
More than 3 D	Toric RGP or custom soft toric

RGP = rigid gas-permeable.

If lens rotation is 10° to the left (clockwise)

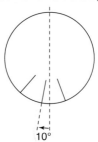

axis ordered is 180° + 10° = 190°

Figure 4-11 Evaluating lens rotation in fitting soft toric contact lenses using the LARS rule of thumb (left add; right subtract). The spectacle prescription in this example is −2.00 −1.00 × 180°. *(Modified with permission from Key JE II, ed. The CLAO Pocket Guide to Contact Lens Fitting. 2nd ed. Metairie, LA: Contact Lens Association of Ophthalmologists; 1998. Redrawn by Christine Gralapp.)*

If lens rotation is 10° to the right (counterclockwise)

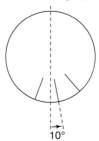

axis ordered is 180° − 10° = 170°

CLINICAL EXAMPLE 4-6

An eye with a refraction of −3.00 −1.00 × 180 is fitted with a toric contact lens with an astigmatic axis given as 180°. Slit-lamp examination shows that the lens is well centered, but lens markings show that the 6-o'clock mark is located at the 7-o'clock position. What axis should be ordered for this eye?

Because the trial contact lens rotated 1 clock-hour, or 30°, to the left, the contact lens ordered (recall the LARS rule: left add; right subtract) should be 180° + 30° = 210°, or −3.00 −1.00 × 30°.

---

rotation is *LARS (left add; right subtract)*. When ordering a lens, the clinician should use the adjusted axis (per LARS, adding or subtracting from the spectacle refraction axis), instead of the cylinder axis of the refraction (Clinical Example 4-6).

Contact Lenses for Presbyopia

Presbyopia affects virtually everyone older than 40 years. Thus, as contact lens wearers age, their accommodation needs must be considered. Three options are available for these patients: (1) use of reading glasses with contact lenses, (2) monovision, and (3) bifocal contact lenses.

The first option, using reading glasses over contact lenses, has the advantages of being simple and inexpensive. The second option, monovision, involves correcting one eye for distance and the other eye for near. Many patients tolerate this correction without difficulty, although some initially observe monocular blurring. Successful adaptation requires interocular suppression, which is easier to achieve with patients whose eyes differ by only 1.00 or 1.50 D. Typically, the dominant eye is corrected for distance, although trial and error are often needed to determine which eye is best for distance correction. For most tasks, no spectacle overcorrection is needed, but for driving and other critical functions, overcorrection is recommended to provide the best-corrected vision in each eye.

The third option for patients with presbyopia is to use bifocal contact lenses. There are 2 types of bifocal lenses: alternating vision lenses (segmented or concentric) and simultaneous vision lenses (aspheric or diffractive). *Alternating vision bifocal contact lenses* are similar in function to bifocal spectacles in that there are separate areas for distance and near, and the retina receives light from only 1 image location at a time (Fig 4-12). *Segmented contact lenses* have 2 areas, top and bottom, like bifocal spectacles, whereas *concentric contact lenses* have 2 rings (or *tines*), one for far and one for near. For segmented contact lenses, the position on the eye is critical and must change as the patient switches from distance to near viewing. The lower eyelid controls the lens position so that as a person looks down, the lens stays up and the visual axis moves into the reading portion of the lens. Maintenance of the proper lens position is crucial; therefore, such lens designs do not work for all patients.

Simultaneous vision bifocal contact lenses provide the retina with light from both distance and near points in space at the same time, requiring the patient's brain to ignore the reduction in contrast (Fig 4-13). Usually, either the distance or near vision is compromised; the compromise is greater for higher adds.

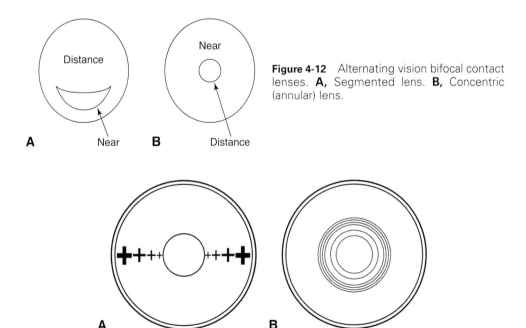

Figure 4-12 Alternating vision bifocal contact lenses. **A,** Segmented lens. **B,** Concentric (annular) lens.

Figure 4-13 Simultaneous vision bifocal contact lenses. **A,** Aspheric, or multifocal lens. **B,** Diffractive lens. *(Modified with permission from Key JE II, ed.* The CLAO Pocket Guide to Contact Lens Fitting. *2nd ed. Metairie, LA: Contact Lens Association of Ophthalmologists; 1998. Redrawn by Christine Gralapp.)*

These lenses have various optical designs. One type is *aspheric,* or *multifocal,* as are intraocular lenses. Aspheric surfaces change in power from the center to the periphery: minus lenses decrease in power from the center to the periphery, whereas plus lenses increase (see Fig 4-13A). Another type of simultaneous vision lens is *diffractive* (see Fig 4-13B). Such lenses have concentric grooves on the back surfaces, such that the light rays are split into 2 focal packages: near and far. The diffractive surfaces reduce incoming light by 20% or more, thereby reducing vision in dim lighting. These lenses are less sensitive to pupil size than are aspheric multifocal designs, but they must be well centered for best vision.

No single style works for all patients, and most require highly motivated patients and fitters for success. Despite the availability of contact lenses for presbyopia, monovision is still the most common approach. A trial of monovision contact lenses may be beneficial when considering a permanent correction such as laser refractive surgery or lens implant surgery.

Jain S, Arora I, Azar DT. Success of monovision in presbyopes: review of the literature and potential applications to refractive surgery. *Surv Ophthalmol.* 1996;40(6):491–499.

Keratoconus and the Abnormal Cornea

Contact lenses often provide better vision than do spectacles by *masking* irregular astigmatism (higher orders of aberration). For mild or moderate irregularities, soft spherical, soft toric, or custom soft toric contact lenses are used. Large irregularities typically require RGP lenses to mask the abnormal surface; the anterior surface of the contact lens creates a new optic surface, and the tear lens corrects the corneal irregularities. As with nonastigmatic eyes, fitters should first find the best alignment fit and then determine the optimal power. Three-point touch can be successfully used for larger cones to ensure lens centration and stability: slight apical and paracentral touch or bearing (dark areas on the fluorescein evaluation; Fig 4-14). The ophthalmologist may use the apical clearance fitting technique to place a lens vault slightly over the cone. Fitting the abnormal cornea requires experience, an understanding patient, and willingness on the part of both the patient and the fitter to spend the time necessary to optimize the fit. When the lenses are ordered, it is best to request a warranty or exchange option; typically, several lenses are fitted before the final lens parameters are determined.

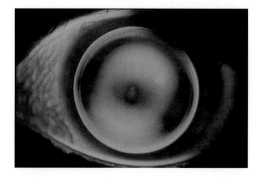

Figure 4-14 Three-point touch in keratoconus. *(Courtesy of Perry Rosenthal, MD.)*

Some specialized RGP lenses have been developed specifically for keratoconus. Most provide a steep central posterior curve to vault over the cone and flatter peripheral curves to approximate the more normal peripheral curvature. Larger RGP contact lenses with larger optical zones (diameters > 11 mm) are available for keratoconus and posttransplant fitting; they are known as intralimbic contact lenses. Some RGP lenses designed for keratoconus are made of new materials that have high oxygen permeability, allowing a more comfortable fit.

An alternative approach is to use a hybrid contact lens that comprises a rigid center and a soft skirt. The hybrid lens theoretically provides the good vision of an RGP lens and the comfort of a soft lens.

Hybrid contact lenses, including one designed specifically for patients with keratoconus (SynergEyes-KC, SynergEyes Inc, Carlsbad, CA), became available in the United States in January 2008. In addition to their use in patients with keratoconus or other degenerative conditions, SynergEyes lenses, which are the first hybrid contact lenses approved by the US Food and Drug Administration (FDA), can be used for patients with all types of refractive errors, in patients with corneal trauma, and in patients following refractive surgery (SynergEyes-PS) or penetrating keratoplasty. The lens has an RGP center ($Dk = 145$) and an outer ring whose material is similar to that of a soft lens.

Piggyback lens systems involve the fitting of a soft contact lens with an RGP lens fitted over it. This system may allow comfort benefits similar to those offered by hybrid lenses, as well as a greater choice of contact lens parameters.

Contact Lens Overrefraction

Patients with reduced vision and irregular corneas may be difficult to evaluate. Examination techniques such as *potential acuity measurement* and retinal imaging techniques such as *optical coherence tomography* and *fluorescein angiography* may not be helpful. Corneal irregularity may be corrected diagnostically with a rigid contact lens if the cornea is clear and there are no other significant media opacities. The examiner should choose a rigid contact lens that will center appropriately on the cornea, then perform an overrefraction. The resulting visual acuity will give the examiner the proportion of vision loss that is accounted for by the irregular cornea. This technique may be useful even in patients who are not contact lens candidates, as it helps direct other diagnostic and therapeutic modalities to the correct portion of the eye.

Gas-Permeable Scleral Contact Lenses

Scleral lenses have unique advantages over other types of contact lenses in rehabilitating the vision of eyes with damaged corneas. These lenses are entirely supported by the sclera; their centration and positional stability are independent of distorted corneal topography; and they avoid contact with a damaged corneal surface. Moreover, these lenses create an artificial tear-filled space over the cornea, thereby providing a protective function for corneas suffering from ocular surface disease.

Scleral lenses consist of a central optic that vaults the cornea and a peripheral haptic that rests on the scleral surface (Fig 4-15). The shape of the posterior optic surface is chosen so as to minimize the volume of the fluid compartment while avoiding corneal contact after

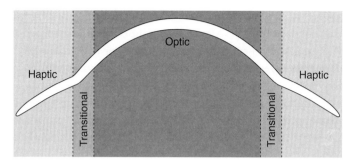

Figure 4-15 Scleral contact lens. *(Redrawn with permission from Albert DM, Jakobiec FA, eds.* Principles and Practice of Ophthalmology. *Philadelphia: Saunders; 1994;5:3643. Redrawn by Christine Gralapp.)*

the lenses have settled. The posterior haptic surface is configured to minimize localized scleral compression; the transitional zone that joins the optic and haptic surfaces is designed to vault the limbus. Historically, these lenses were composed of oxygen-impermeable PMMA. Currently, scleral lenses are composed of highly oxygen-permeable polymers.

A complication of scleral contact lenses occurs when some of the fluid behind the lens is squeezed out during eye movement and forceful blinking, thereby generating negative pressure that pulls the lens onto the eye. Unless the pressure is immediately relieved, this process becomes self-perpetuating and can lead to massive chemosis and corneal edema.

In traditional scleral lenses, holes drilled in the periphery of the optic enabled suction to be avoided. These holes permit the aspiration of air bubbles that replace the volume of fluid lost by lens compression and thereby prevent suction. These lenses are known as *air-ventilated lenses.* However, air bubbles desiccate the underlying corneal epithelium, which is especially damaging to corneas affected by ocular surface disease. Furthermore, air-ventilated scleral lenses require a more precise lens–cornea relationship to avoid the intrusion of air bubbles in the visual axis.

Fluid-ventilated gas-permeable scleral lenses depend on tear–fluid interchange to prevent suction. Their posterior haptic surfaces are designed to create channels large enough to allow tears to be aspirated into the fluid compartment of the lens between the haptic and scleral surfaces but small enough to exclude air. In every case, the requisite tear–fluid interchange must be confirmed via observation of fluorescein dye placed outside the lens seeping under the haptic into the fluid compartment after the lenses have been worn for at least 2 hours. The fitting method for these lenses uses a series of diagnostic lenses with known vaults, diameters, powers, and haptic design.

Gas-permeable scleral lenses have 2 primary indications: (1) correcting abnormal regular and irregular astigmatism in eyes that preclude the use of rigid corneal contact lenses, and (2) managing ocular surface diseases that benefit from the constant presence of a protective, lubricating layer of oxygenated artificial tears. It is more convenient and less costly to correct irregular astigmatism with rigid corneal contact lenses, whenever possible. However, the abnormal corneal topography of many eyes may preclude adequate corneal centration, stability, or tolerance. Conditions under which these problems may occur include pellucid degeneration, Terrien marginal degeneration, keratoconus, Ehlers-Danlos syndrome, elevated corneal scars, and astigmatism following penetrating keratoplasty.

Fluid-ventilated gas-permeable scleral contact lenses are especially useful in managing ocular surface diseases, many of which have no other definitive treatment options. These conditions include complications of neurotrophic corneas, ocular complications of Stevens-Johnson syndrome, graft-vs-host disease, tear layer disorders, and ocular cicatricial pemphigoid. The improvement in the quality of life that these lenses offer is most dramatic for these patients. When the fragile epithelium of diseased corneas is protected from the abrasive effects of the keratinized eyelid margins associated with distichiasis and trichiasis and from exposure to air, the disabling photophobia is remarkably attenuated. Moreover, these lenses are especially valuable in accelerating the healing of persistent epithelial defects that are refractory to all other available treatment strategies. For patients with such defects, the accompanying improvement in vision is a bonus.

Therapeutic Lens Usage

Therapeutic, or *bandage, contact lenses* are used to enhance epithelial healing, prevent epithelial erosions, or control surface-generated pain; they are not used for their optical properties. Usually, soft contact lenses with plano power are employed. They are worn on an extended basis without removal to decrease irritation to the ocular surface. Because the lenses are used on an EW basis and fit on abnormal corneas, oxygen permeability is high to prevent hypoxia. Fitting principles are similar to those of other soft lenses, although for therapeutic use, a tighter fit is usually sought—any lens movement could injure the healing epithelium further. Some fitters prefer high-water-content lenses, but high oxygen permeability is probably the critical factor in lens selection. The use of disposable lenses allows for easy lens replacement, such as during follow-up examinations.

Conditions and circumstances in which bandage contact lenses might be useful include

- bullous keratopathy (for pain control)
- recurrent erosions
- Bell palsy
- keratitis, such as filamentary or post–chemical exposure
- corneal dystrophy with erosions
- postsurgery, such as corneal transplant, laser in situ keratomileusis, or photorefractive keratectomy
- nonhealing epithelial defect, such as geographic herpes keratitis, slow-healing ulcer, or abrasion
- eyelid abnormalities, such as entropion, eyelid lag, or trichiasis
- bleb leak posttrabeculectomy

During fitting, patients should be made aware of the signs and symptoms of infection because the risk of infection will be increased, given the abnormal surface covered by a foreign body (the lens).

McDermott ML, Chandler JW. Therapeutic uses of contact lenses. *Surv Ophthalmol.* 1989; 33(5):381–394.

Orthokeratology and Corneal Reshaping

Orthokeratology generally refers to the process of reshaping the cornea and thus reducing myopia by fitting RGP contact lenses designed to flatten the central cornea for a period after the lenses are removed. The shape change is similar to that resulting from laser procedures for myopia. Orthokeratology, however, is reversible and noninvasive, and no tissue is removed. Experience in the 1970s with this procedure was disappointing: orthokeratology was unpredictable, the amount of correction that resulted (up to 1.5 D) was small, the procedure induced irregular astigmatism, the lenses were difficult to fit, multiple lenses were needed per patient per eye, and extensive follow-up was required. These problems led to unfavorable publicity about this procedure, and it was only rarely used.

However, advances in the 1990s in lens design and material led to a resurgence of interest in orthokeratology, and the FDA approved lenses for myopia correction. The introduction of so-called *reverse-geometry designs* and the strategy of overnight wear improved results. The shape of the central zone (molding surface) of these lenses is intentionally made somewhat flatter than is needed for the cornea to correct the eye's myopia. The intermediate zones are made steeper to provide a peripheral bearing platform, and the peripheral zones are designed to create the necessary clearance and edge lift.

Lens centration is key to the effectiveness of these lenses. It requires them to be supported by circumferential peripheral bearing at the junction of the intermediate and peripheral zones. It also requires that the lenses incorporate a design mechanism that enables the fitter to adjust the molding pressure independently of the central shape of the molding surfaces. Because the lenses are worn overnight, their oxygen transmissibility must be high; consequently, they are generally made of materials with very high oxygen permeability ($Dk \geq 100$).

In 2002, the FDA approved corneal refractive lenses for overnight wear to correct myopia up to 6.00 D. The fitting is simple and is based on manifest refraction and K readings as well as a nomogram. Typically, once a good fit is achieved—that is, centered, with a bull's-eye fluorescein pattern—that lens is the right one for the patient. Refractive change is rapid, usually occurring within 2 weeks of wear. The lens is worn only during sleep and provides good vision at night, if needed, and good vision all day without correction. It is not entirely clear how these lenses work, but central corneal thinning is observed with epithelial thinning or compression. Although corneal refractive lenses are approved for all ages, and FDA data show a high safety and efficacy record, corneal ulcers have been reported with other overnight orthokeratology lenses.

A development in the field of orthokeratology is the use of soft contact lenses as a means of reshaping the corneal curvature. In traditional orthokeratology, the reverse-geometry lens design creates positive pressure in the center of the cornea and negative pressure in the midperiphery. With the soft lens, however, the reverse occurs: negative pressure is created in the corneal center and positive pressure in the midperiphery. This pressure balance is achieved by the reverse-geometry soft lens design, which flattens the midperiphery and steepens the central curvature, making these lenses suitable for patients interested in hyperopic orthokeratology. See also BCSC Section 13, *Refractive Surgery.*

Bennett E. Contemporary orthokeratology. *Contact Lens Spectrum.* February 2005. www.clspectrum.com. Accessed September 30, 2012.

Laibson PR, Cohen EJ, Rajpal RK. Conrad Berens Lecture. Corneal ulcers related to contact lenses. *CLAO J.* 1993;19(1):73–78.

Custom Contact Lenses and Wavefront Technology

A normal cornea is generally steepest near its geometric center; beyond the center, the surface flattens. The steep area is known as the *apical zone* (or *optic cap*), and its center is the *corneal apex.* Outside the apical zone, which is approximately 3–4 mm in diameter, the rate of peripheral flattening can vary significantly in the different corneal meridians of the same eye, between the eyes of the same patient, and between the eyes of different patients. This variation is important because peripheral corneal topography significantly affects the position, blink-induced excursion patterns, and, therefore, wearing comfort of corneal contact lenses, especially gas-permeable lenses. In addition to addressing contact lens fitting in relation to corneal shape, custom contact lenses can address the correction of optical aberrations, especially higher-order aberrations, in much the same way that custom laser surgery attempts to improve the optics of the eye.

The availability of corneal topographers and wavefront aberrometers, together with desktop graphics programs, enables the design of contact lenses that are unique for each eye. Combining these unique designs with computerized lathes that can produce customized, nonsymmetrical shapes may permit the creation of contact lenses that are individualized to each specific cornea, thus offering patients better vision and increased comfort. However, before contact lenses can be made to order, significant obstacles need to be overcome:

- *Vertical lens movement.* Some contact lens movement is considered integral to good lens fit. With each blink, however, such movement may negate or even worsen custom optics. Because less movement typically occurs with soft as opposed to rigid lenses, soft contact lenses may be more suitable for customization.
- *Rotational movement.* A wavefront-designed contact lens needs rotational stability to maintain the benefit of aberration correction, but even toric contact lenses rotate by approximately 5° with each blink.
- *Variability of the optical aberration.* Variations in aberrations occur on the basis of pupil size, accommodation, lens changes, age, and probably other factors. Deciding which aberrations to correct may be yet another challenge.
- *Maintenance of corneal health.* Tear-film exchange is important for good, long-lasting contact lens health, but it is contrary to the stability and nonmovement requirements for optimal correction of optical aberrations.
- *Manufacturing issues.* Even with custom lathes and the ability to make nonsymmetrical curves, challenges remain in creating lens shapes that can correct aberrations, provide comfortable lenses, and allow identical copies to be made on demand.

Despite these challenges, there has been significant interest in using novel technology to evaluate aberrations and in new methods of lens manufacturing and design to deliver custom contact lenses—perhaps first for patients with abnormal eyes, such as those with keratoconus, and then for patients who have standard refractive errors and desire "super-vision." For a more extensive discussion of wavefront technology, see Chapter 6 in this volume and BCSC Section 13, *Refractive Surgery.*

Contact Lens Care and Solutions

Most contact lenses are removed after use, cleaned, stored, and used again (1-day dispos-able lenses are the exception). Lens-care systems have been developed to remove deposits and microorganisms from lenses, enhance comfort, and decrease the risk of eye infection and irritation associated with lens use. Although the specific components of these systems vary with the type of lens (soft or RGP), most include a lens cleaner, a rinsing solution, and a disinfecting and storage solution (Table 4-8). Multipurpose solutions, which perform several of these functions, are popular because of their ease of use and convenience. En-zymatic cleaners, which remove protein deposits from the lens surface, provide additional cleaning. These cleaners typically include papain, an enzyme derived from papaya; pan-creatin, an enzyme derived from pancreatic tissue; or enzymes derived from bacteria. In addition, lubricating drops can be used when the lenses are on the eyes. In 2007, cases of serious infectious keratitis (caused by the pathogens *Fusarium* and *Acanthamoeba*) related to the use of certain contact lens solutions were reported; these products were withdrawn from the market. Note that serious eye infections may occur with any chemical disinfec-tion system.

Several methods have been developed for disinfecting lenses, including the use of

- heat
- chemicals
- hydrogen peroxide
- ultraviolet light exposure

The care system selected depends on the personal preference of the fitter and patient, the simplicity and convenience of use, cost, and possible allergies to solution components. Currently, multipurpose solutions are the most popular care systems in the United States.

Table 4-8 Contact Lens–Care Systems

Type	Purpose	Lens Use	Comments
Saline	Rinsing and storing	All types	Use with disinfecting systems
Daily cleaner	Cleaning	All types	Use with disinfecting and storage systems
Multipurpose solution	Cleaning, disinfecting, rinsing, and storing	All types	May not be ideal for rigid gas-permeable lens comfort
Hydrogen peroxide solution	Cleaning, disinfecting, rinsing, and storing	All types	Lenses should be rinsed with saline before use

The fitter should instruct the patient in the care of contact lenses. The following are important guidelines:

- Clean and disinfect a lens whenever it is removed.
- Follow the advice included with the lens-care system that is selected; do not "mix and match" solutions.
- Do not use tap water for storing or cleaning lenses because it is not sterile.
- Do not use homemade salt solutions; they too are not sterile.
- Do not use saliva to wet a lens.
- Do not reuse contact lens–care solutions.
- Do not allow the dropper tip to touch any surface; close the bottle tightly when not in use.
- Clean the contact lens case daily and replace it every 2–3 months; the case can be a source of contaminants.
- Pay attention to labels on contact lens–care solutions because solution ingredients may change without warning to the consumer.

In addition to teaching appropriate contact lens and case care, the fitter should instruct the patient in proper lens insertion and removal techniques, determine a wear schedule (DW or EW), and decide if and when the lens should be disposed of or replaced. Insertion and handling vary significantly between soft and RGP lenses, and many manufacturers provide written information and videos to instruct professional staff and patients in appropriate insertion and removal techniques.

Chang DC, Grant GB, O'Donnell K, et al. Multistate outbreak of *Fusarium keratitis* associated with use of a contact lens solution. *JAMA.* 2006;296(8):953–963.

Contact Lens–Related Problems and Complications

Ocular problems related to contact lenses are uncommon but potentially serious. A wide spectrum of problems may arise secondary to contact lens wear, but they can be categorized as follows: infectious, hypoxic/metabolic, toxic, mechanical, inflammatory, and dry eye–related complications (Table 4-9).

Infections

Corneal infections secondary to lens use are rare, but when they occur, they are potentially serious and vision threatening. To reduce risk, the clinician and patient should ensure that the contact lenses are fitted properly, contact lens–care systems are used regularly, and follow-up care is provided. In addition, patients should understand the signs and symptoms of serious eye problems and know when to seek medical assistance. With the increased use of disposable lenses, better patient education, more convenient care systems, and the availability of more-oxygen-permeable lens materials, serious eye infections from lens use have become uncommon. However, practitioners should be aware of unusual infections that can occur, such as *Acanthamoeba* keratitis. Diagnosis

Table 4-9 Contact Lens–Related Problems and Complications

Category	Problem or Complication
Infectious	Conjunctivitis
	Keratitis
	Bacterial
	Fungal
	Acanthamoebal
Hypoxic/metabolic	Metabolic epithelial damage
	Corneal neovascularization
Toxic	Punctate keratitis
	Toxic conjunctivitis
Mechanical	Corneal warpage
	Spectacle blur
	Ptosis
	Corneal abrasions
	3-o'clock and 9-o'clock staining
Inflammatory	Contact lens–induced keratoconjunctivitis (CLIK)
	Allergic reactions
	Giant papillary conjunctivitis (GPC)
	Sterile infiltrates
Dry eye	Punctate keratitis
	Keratitis sicca

and treatment of corneal infections are covered in BCSC Section 8, *External Disease and Cornea.*

Hypoxic/Metabolic Problems

Metabolic epithelial damage

Contact lens overwear syndromes can be manifested in several forms. *Central epithelial edema* (Sattler veil) may present after many hours of wear, more commonly with hard contact lenses. This epithelial edema causes blurred vision that may persist for many hours or, in rare instances, progress to acute epithelial necrosis. Physiologic stress as a result of hypoxia, with lactate accumulation and impaired carbon dioxide efflux, is responsible for these complications.

    Microcystic epitheliopathy, another condition caused by impaired metabolic activities in the corneal epithelium, shows fine epithelial cysts that are most easily observed with retroillumination. This condition is most common in patients who use EW soft contact lenses. The cysts may either be asymptomatic or cause recurrent brief episodes of pain and epiphora. It takes up to 6 weeks following discontinuation of contact lens wear for the cysts to resolve. In some cases, this epitheliopathy may have a dendritic appearance.

Corneal neovascularization

Corneal neovascularization is usually a sign of hypoxia. Refitting with lenses of higher-oxygen-permeability material or with a looser fit, requiring fewer hours of lens wear per day, or switching to disposable lenses can prevent further progression. If neovascularization is extensive, it can lead to corneal scarring and lipid deposition or intracorneal hemorrhage. Superficial pannus is rarely associated with hard or RGP contact lens wear but is encountered more frequently in patients who use soft EW or nonfrequent disposable lenses. This type of neovascularization is probably caused by hypoxia and chronic trauma to the limbus, which lead to the release of angiogenic mediators. Other causes of pannus, such as staphylococcal and chlamydial keratoconjunctivitis, should be considered in the presence of the appropriate accompanying signs.

Deep stromal neovascularization has been associated with EW contact lenses, especially in aphakia. This condition is not usually symptomatic unless there is secondary lipid deposition. Deep neovascularization of the cornea is often irreversible and is best managed by discontinuing contact lens wear and resorting to spectacle correction or scleral-fixated intraocular lenses.

Toxicity

Punctate keratitis
A finding of punctate keratitis may be related to a poor lens fit, a toxic reaction to lens solutions, or dry eye.

Toxic conjunctivitis
Conjunctival injection, epithelial staining, punctate epithelial keratopathy, erosions, microcysts, and limbal stem cell deficiency are all potential signs of conjunctival or corneal toxicity arising from contact lens solutions. Any of the proteolytic enzymes or chemicals used for cleaning contact lenses, or the preservative-containing soaking solution, may be the culprit. Cleaning agents such as benzalkonium chloride, chlorhexidine, hydrogen peroxide, and other substances used for chemical sterilization, if not properly removed from contact lenses, can cause an immediate, severe epitheliopathy with accompanying pain.

Mechanical Problems

Corneal warpage
Change in corneal shape from contact lens use has been reported with both soft and RGP lenses, but it is more commonly associated with hard lenses. Most warpage resolves after the patient discontinues wearing the lens. To evaluate corneal shape on an ongoing basis, the clinician should include a standard evaluation by keratometry or corneal topography and manifest refraction as part of the contact lens follow-up examination, and the findings should be compared with previous measurements.

Spectacle blur
Corneal warpage and more temporary changes in corneal shape can change normal spectacle-corrected vision immediately after lens removal. If a patient reports symptoms of spectacle blur, the contact lens fit should be reevaluated and discontinuation of lens use for a period should be considered.

Ptosis

Ptosis is related not to corneal changes but possibly to dehiscence of the levator aponeurosis, which is secondary to long-term use of RGP lenses.

Corneal abrasions

Corneal abrasions can result from foreign bodies under a lens, a poor insertion or removal technique, or a damaged contact lens. Therefore, contact lens use can increase the risk of infection. Most clinicians treat abrasions with antibiotic eyedrops and without patching.

3-o'clock and 9-o'clock staining

This specific superficial punctate keratitis staining pattern may be observed in RGP contact lens users and is probably related to poor wetting in the horizontal axis (Fig 4-16). Paralimbal staining is characteristic of low-riding lenses and is associated with an abortive reflex blink pattern, insufficient lens movement, inadequate tear meniscus, and a thick peripheral lens profile. Occasionally, refitting the lens and/or initiating regular use of wetting drops can decrease the finding.

Inflammation

Contact lens–induced keratoconjunctivitis

The pathogenesis of contact lens–induced keratoconjunctivitis (CLIK) is multifactorial (ie, can arise from allergies, dry eye, and infection). Patients with ocular prostheses and exposed monofilament sutures have shown reactions similar to those observed in patients with contact lens–induced conjunctivitis. A hypersensitivity reaction to the contact lens polymer itself (or to antigens or other foreign material adhering to it) has also been postulated but not formally demonstrated. Dry eye may be present in some cases. The histologic findings in contact lens–induced conjunctivitis are similar to those observed in vernal keratoconjunctivitis. An abnormal accumulation of mast cells, basophils, and eosinophils is observed in the epithelium and/or the substantia propria of the superior tarsus. Abnormally elevated concentrations of immunoglobulins—specifically IgE, IgG, and IgM—and complement components have been found in the tears of affected patients. These findings suggest a combined mechanical and immune-mediated pathophysiology for this condition. Surface deposits on worn contact lenses are a known risk factor for the development and persistence of CLIK.

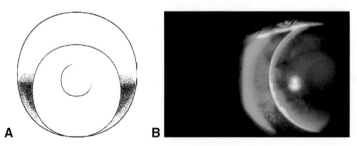

Figure 4-16 Three-o'clock and 9-o'clock corneal staining. **A,** Inferior corneal desiccation of the tear film. **B,** Peripheral corneal desiccation. *(Part B courtesy of Perry Rosenthal, MD.)*

Allergic reactions

The preservative *thimerosal* can produce a type IV delayed hypersensitivity response, resulting in conjunctivitis, keratitis, and even coarse epithelial and subepithelial opacities. Thimerosal was implicated in contact lens–induced superior limbic keratoconjunctivitis. This condition has become less common, probably as a result of the replacement of thimerosal by other preservatives in contact lens solutions and the introduction of disposable contact lenses.

Giant papillary conjunctivitis

At the more severe end of the spectrum of contact lens–related inflammation is giant papillary conjunctivitis (GPC). GPC tends to develop earlier and more frequently in EW soft contact lens wearers in the setting of dry eye and meibomian gland dysfunction. It may also be induced by other irritants, such as loose sutures or prosthetics. Symptoms include contact lens intolerance, itching, excessive mucus discharge, and blurred vision from mucus coating of the contact lens; contact lens decentration; and conjunctival redness. In rare instances, bloody tears and ptosis secondary to inflammation of the superior tarsal conjunctiva may be observed.

The signs of GPC consist of hyperemia, thickening, and abnormally large papillae (diameter > 0.3 mm) on the superior tarsal conjunctiva due to disruption of the anchoring septae. The morphologic appearance of the superior tarsal papillae may be variable in GPC. In some cases, the giant papillae cover the entire central tarsus from the posterior eyelid margin to the upper border of the tarsal plate; involvement in other cases may be less extensive. Long-standing or involuted giant papillae on the superior tarsus may resemble follicles. The symptoms of GPC generally resolve when contact lens wear is discontinued. The tarsal conjunctival hyperemia and thickening may resolve in several weeks, but papillae or dome-shaped scars on the superior tarsus can persist for months to years.

If GPC persists, the clinician should consider changing the lens to a different polymer or to DW disposable lenses. Some patients prefer low-water-content lenses. Nevertheless, some patients continue to experience symptoms of GPC as a result of soft contact lens wear despite these measures. In these cases, consider fitting the patient with RGP contact lenses, which are associated with a lower incidence of GPC. In some patients, GPC recurs despite aggressive lens management and even RGP lens wear; these patients should be counseled about alternatives to contact lens wear.

Pharmacologic therapy can be helpful in managing patients with GPC. Many practitioners recommend discontinuing lens wear for 2–3 weeks while treatment is initiated. Mast-cell stabilizers, such as cromolyn sodium and dual-active agents with antihistamine and nonsteroidal activity, have been reported to improve early, mild GPC. However, once advanced cases of GPC have been brought under control, maintenance therapy with topical mast-cell inhibitors may prevent further exacerbations. Topical corticosteroids, though effective in GPC, generally are of limited use because of their potential side effects. Topical cyclosporine and tacrolimus may play a role in treatment.

Elhers WH, Donshik PC. Giant papillary conjunctivitis. *Curr Opin Allergy Clin Immunol.* 2008;8(5):445–449.

Sterile infiltrates

Typically, sterile infiltrates are observed in the peripheral cornea; often there is more than one spot, and the epithelium over the spots is intact. Discontinuing lens use can usually resolve the problem quickly, but clinicians often prescribe an antibiotic, even though cultures tend to show no growth. Sterile infiltrates are also characterized by their small size.

Dry Eye

Evaluating a patient for dry eye should be part of the prefitting eye examination. A properly fitting lens rides on the tear film, which is essential for comfort and allows fluid exchange under the lens to remove debris and bring in oxygen. Patients with severe dry eye probably are not candidates for contact lens use. However, patients with moderate to mild dry eye may do well with contact lenses. Some soft lenses are marketed for dry eye patients; these lenses often have lower water content and/or better wettability. They may be made of material that is less prone to lens deposit formation.

Some patients may respond to placement of punctal plugs. Occasionally, the signs and symptoms of dry eye result from incomplete or infrequent blinking (fewer than 12 times per minute). The clinician may diagnose this condition by simply observing the patient during the examination. Some fitters feel that it is helpful to instruct the patient in how to blink.

Stein HA, Freeman MI, Stein RM. *CLAO Residents Contact Lens Curriculum Manual.* New York: CLAO; 1996.

Suchecki JK, Donshik P, Ehlers WH. Contact lens complications. *Ophthalmol Clin North Am.* 2003;16(3):471–484.

Chapter Exercises

Questions

4.1. Following laser correction, a patient presents with blurred vision. The best spectacle-corrected visual acuity is 20/50. All of the following will be useful in defining the source of the blurred vision *except*
   a. rigid contact lens overrefraction
   b. potential acuity measurement
   c. soft contact lens overrefraction
   d. pinhole acuity measurement

4.2. A patient with keratoconus is unable to see adequately with spectacles or soft contact lenses. Standard RGP lenses allow adequate vision, but the discomfort is intolerable. An acceptable alternative in this situation would be any of the following *except*
   a. piggyback soft and rigid contact lenses
   b. corneal transplantation
   c. specialty RGP contact lenses for keratoconus
   d. hybrid contact lenses
   e. scleral contact lenses

4.3. A trial soft contact lens moves excessively with eyelid blinks. Which of the following would decrease lens movement?
a. flattening the base curve while maintaining the diameter
b. decreasing the diameter while maintaining the base curve
c. increasing the power of the contact lens
d. steepening the base curve while maintaining the diameter
e. flattening the base curve and decreasing the diameter

4.4. You fit a patient who has –3.50 D of myopia with an RGP contact lens that is flatter than K. If the patient's average K reading is 7.80 mm and you fit a lens with a base curve of 8.00 mm, what is the shape of the tear lens?
a. plano
b. teardrop
c. concave
d. convex

4.5. For the patient in question 4.4, what power RGP lens should you order?
a. –3.50 D
b. –4.00 D
c. –2.00 D
d. –2.50 D

4.6. You fit a toric soft contact lens on a patient with a refractive error of –2.50 D –1.50 × 175. The trial lens centers well, but the lens mark at the 6-o'clock position appears to rest at the 5-o'clock position when the lens is placed on the patient's eye. What power contact lens should you order?
a. –2.50 D –1.50 × 175
b. –2.50 D –1.50 × 145
c. –2.50 D –1.50 × 55
d. –2.50 D –1.00 × 175

Answers

4.1. **c.** A soft contact lens does not correct irregular astigmatism on the cornea and therefore would not provide any additional information beyond that found with a manifest refraction. The other options should aid in differentiating reduced vision secondary to irregular astigmatism and other causes such as retinal disease. Corneal topography would be an additional test that would be helpful in documenting the irregular astigmatism present.

4.2. **b.** There are many options for the correction of an irregular cornea beyond standard RGP contact lenses. Penetrating and anterior lamellar keratoplasty may leave significant residual regular and irregular astigmatism requiring contact lens use; therefore, this option should be used only when all contact lens solutions have been considered.

4.3. **d.** Increasing the sagittal depth of the contact lens tightens the fit and decreases lens movement, which may be achieved through steepening (decreasing) the base curve or increasing the diameter of the contact lens. Flattening (increasing) the base curve or decreasing the diameter of the lens decreases sagittal depth and increases the movement of the lens on the cornea. The power of the contact lens should not affect the fitting relationships.

4.4. **c.** The tear lens is formed by the posterior surface of the contact lens and the anterior surface of the cornea. If these 2 curvatures are the same, as with a soft lens, the tear lens is plano. If they are different (as is typical of RGP lenses), a plus or minus tear lens forms. In this case, the contact lens is flatter than K, so the tear lens is negative, or concave, in shape.

4.5. **d.** For every 0.05-mm radius-of-curvature difference between the base curve and K, the induced power of the tear film is 0.25 D. The power of the concave tear lens in this case is –1.00 D. The power of the RGP contact lens you should order is –3.50 D – (–1.00 D) = –2.50 D. An easy way to remember this formula is to use the following rule: SAM = steeper add minus and FAP = flatter add plus.

4.6. **b.** The amount and direction of rotation should be observed. In this case, they are, respectively, 1 clock-hour and rotation to the right. Each clock-hour represents 30° (360°/12 = 30°), so the adjustment should be 30°. Because the rotation is to the right, you should order a contact lens with axis 145° instead of 175°—that is, –2.50 D –1.50 × 145. An easy rule to remember is LARS = left add, right subtract.

Appendix 4.1

Transmission of Human Immunodeficiency Virus in Contact Lens Care

Human immunodeficiency virus (HIV) has been isolated from ocular tissues, tears, and soft contact lenses used by patients with AIDS. However, no documented case of HIV transmission through contact with human tears or contaminated contact lenses has been reported. A 1985 US Centers for Disease Control and Prevention (CDC) advisory recommended the following disinfection methods for trial contact lenses:

- *Hard lenses.* Use a commercially available hydrogen peroxide contact lens–disinfecting kit (the type used for soft lenses); other hydrogen peroxide preparations may cause lens discoloration. Heat disinfection (78°–80°C for 10 min), as used for soft lens care, can also be used but may damage a lens.
- *RGP lenses.* Same as above, but heat disinfection is not recommended, because it can cause lens warpage.
- *Soft lenses.* Same as above, although heat should be used only if the lens is approved for such a care system.

For additional information, see the healthcare-associated infections page on the CDC website (www.cdc.gov/hai/).

The most commonly used disinfection systems for contact lenses today are chemical. Published studies suggest that chemical disinfection is effective against HIV-contaminated contact lenses, but these studies have not been reviewed by the US Food and Drug Administration (FDA). As a result, although the FDA requires demonstration of virucidal activity in treatments for herpes simplex virus, there is no such requirement for HIV.

American Academy of Ophthalmology. Minimizing transmission of blood-borne pathogens and surface infectious agents in ophthalmic offices and operating rooms. Information Statement. San Francisco: AAO; 2002.

Centers for Disease Control. Recommendations for preventing possible transmission of human T-lymphotropic virus type III/lymphadenopathy-associated virus from tears. *MMWR Morb Mortal Wkly Rep.* 1985;34(34):533–534.

Slonim CB. AIDS and the contact lens practice. *CLAO J.* 1995;21(4):233–235.

Appendix 4.2

Federal Law and Contact Lenses

The Federal Fairness to Contact Lens Consumers Act (PL 108-164) was passed by the US Congress and became effective on February 4, 2004. This law is intended to make it easier for consumers to obtain contact lenses from providers other than the individual who fitted the lenses. Once the fitting process is complete, the patient must automatically be provided with a free copy of the prescription, regardless of whether the patient requested it. Also, the provider must verify the prescription information within a reasonable period (typically defined as 8 hours during the normal business day) to anyone designated to act on behalf of the patient (eg, an Internet contact lens seller). The Federal Trade Commission (FTC) can impose sanctions for noncompliance on both prescribers and sellers of up to $11,000 per offense. For further details of this law, see the FTC website: www.ftc.gov.

CHAPTER **5**

Intraocular Lenses

The history of intraocular lenses (IOLs) began in 1949, when English ophthalmologist Harold Ridley implanted the first polymethylmethacrylate (PMMA) IOL in London. Ridley made 2 decisions that were fortuitous for the development of IOL implantation: he used extracapsular cataract extraction (ECCE), and he placed the IOL in the posterior chamber. In addition, he experienced the first IOL complication, a power error of 16 D. Initially, other ophthalmologists strongly opposed the use of IOLs, and it took years of development and perseverance for the IOL to become the standard it is today. For his pioneering contributions to this technology, Ridley was knighted by Queen Elizabeth II in 2000, a year before his death.

Theoretically, implantation of an IOL is the optimal form of aphakic correction. Correction with aphakic spectacles can cause numerous difficulties, including image magnification, ring scotomata, peripheral distortion, a "jack-in-the-box" phenomenon (in which images pop in and out of view), and a decreased useful peripheral field. Most of these aberrations and distortions derive from placement of the spectacles anterior to the pupillary and corneal planes.

This chapter focuses on the optical considerations relevant to IOLs. For more surgical information with respect to IOLs, see BCSC Section 11, *Lens and Cataract.*

Intraocular Lens Designs

Classification

IOLs can be categorized by

- implantation site (anterior chamber, posterior chamber, or prepupillary [no longer used] plane; Fig 5-1)
- optic profile (biconvex, planoconvex, or meniscus; see Fig 5-1)
- optic material (PMMA, glass, silicone, acrylic, collamer, or hydrogel)
- haptic style (plate or loop)
- sphericity (spheric, aspheric) and toricity
- wavelength feature (UV- or blue-light blocking)
- focality (monofocal, bifocal, or multifocal)
- degree of accommodation
- edge finish (ridge, square, or sharp)
- power (plus, minus, or plano)
- type of correction (phakic IOL or aphakic IOL)

195

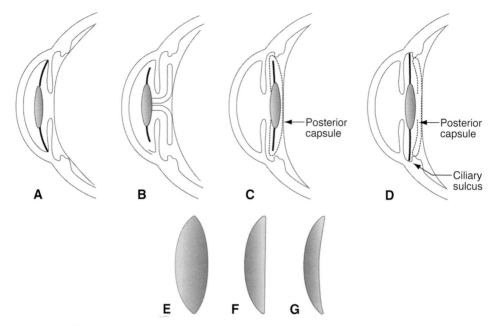

Figure 5-1 The major types of intraocular lenses (IOLs) and optics. **A,** Anterior chamber lens. **B,** Prepupillary lens (no longer used). **C,** Posterior chamber lens in the capsular bag. **D,** Posterior chamber lens in the ciliary sulcus. **E,** Biconvex optic. **F,** Planoconvex optic. **G,** Meniscus optic. *(Redrawn by C. H. Wooley.)*

The number of factors to consider requires that the surgeon know how to select the best IOL design for each patient's needs.

Background

In the 1970s, surgeons implanting IOLs included those who used *intracapsular cataract extraction (ICCE)* and those who used *small-incision phacoemulsification (phaco)*. The IOL optic was made from PMMA, with supporting haptics of metal, polypropylene, or PMMA. The rigidity of these materials required that the small phaco incision be enlarged for IOL insertion. However, following the introduction of a foldable optic (made from silicone) in the late 1980s, enlargement was no longer required, and the combination of phaco and IOL implantation became the standard of care.

The 2 basic lens designs currently in use are differentiated by the plane in which the lens is placed (posterior chamber or anterior chamber) and by the tissue supporting the lens (capsule/ciliary sulcus or chamber angle) (see Fig 5-1).

The effect of lens material on factors such as *posterior capsular opacification (PCO)* has been investigated. Earlier studies suggested that IOLs made from acrylic are associated with lower rates of PCO than are those made from silicone or PMMA. However, more recent studies suggest that lens edge design is a more important factor in PCO than is lens material, as Hoffer proposed in 1979 in the lens edge barrier theory. IOLs with an annular, ridge edge or a square, truncated edge create a barrier effect at the optic edge that reduces cell migration behind the optic and thus reduces PCO (Figs 5-2, 5-3, 5-4). The ridge concept led to the development of partial-ridge and meniscus IOLs, which were used for a time, and the sharp-edge designs now in use.

Plano IOLs are available for patients whose eyes require zero (or minimal) power in the aphakic state (ie, patients with very high myopia). The presence of an IOL helps maintain the structural integrity of the anterior segment and reduces the long-term incidence of retinal tears and detachments.

"Piggyback" lenses (ie, 2 IOLs in 1 eye; biphakia), implanted either simultaneously or sequentially, may be used in 2 situations: (1) when the postoperative IOL power is incorrect and (2) when the needed IOL power is higher than what is commercially available. Minus-power IOLs can be used to correct extreme myopia and (as piggybacks) to correct IOL power errors.

Current IOLs are foldable, injectable, aspheric, sharp edged, and single piece (or three piece), and they have higher refractive indices; together, these features allow for

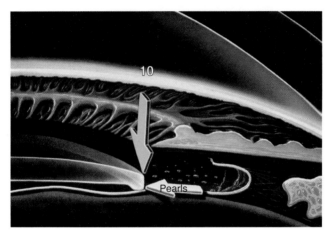

Figure 5-2 Schematic illustrating the concept of a tenfold increase in pressure *(green arrow)* at the edge of an IOL. *(Courtesy of Kenneth J. Hoffer, MD.)*

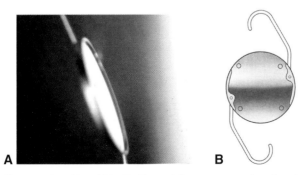

Figure 5-3 **A,** Hoffer annular ridge IOL. **B,** Kratz-Johnson posterior chamber IOL. *(Courtesy of Kenneth J. Hoffer, MD; part B redrawn by C. H. Wooley.)*

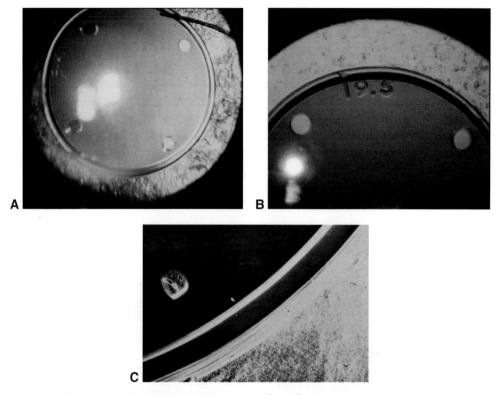

Figure 5-4 Increasing the pressure at the edge of an IOL leads to a blockage of cells to the central posterior capsule **(A, B). C,** The cell blockage as it appears on an electron micrograph. *(Courtesy of Kenneth J. Hoffer, MD.)*

implantation through smaller incisions than used for the earlier designs. The historical IOL designs and the alterations that led to the current IOL designs now in use are described in Appendix 5.1 at the end of the chapter.

Apple DJ. Influence of intraocular lens material and design on postoperative intracapsular cellular reactivity. *Trans Am Ophthalmol Soc.* 2000;98:257–283.

Hoffer KJ. Hoffer barrier ridge concept [letter]. *J Cataract Refract Surg.* 2007;33(7):1142–1143; author reply 1143.

Nagamoto T, Fujiwara T. Inhibition of lens epithelial cell migration at the intraocular lens optic edge: role of capsule bending and contact pressure. *J Cataract Refract Surg.* 2003;29(8):1605–1612.

Optical Considerations for Intraocular Lenses

Intraocular Lens Power Calculation

The aim of accurate power calculation is to provide an IOL that fits the specific needs and desires of an individual patient, rather than the surgeon's routine. It is the surgeon's responsibility to determine the patient's needs by examining and questioning the patient.

In IOL power calculation, a formula is used that requires accurate biometric measurements of the eye, the visual *axial length (AL),* and the *central corneal power (K).* The desired "target" postoperative refraction and the estimated vertical position of the IOL *(estimated lens position [ELP])* are added to these factors for use in power calculation. It is better to err slightly on the side of a myopic error (unless a multifocal IOL is to be implanted, in which case emmetropia is required). The advantage of selecting a slightly myopic lens power is that it allows for some degree of near vision and reduces image magnification.

Power prediction formulas

IOL power prediction formulas are termed *theoretical* because they are based on theoretical optics, the basis of which is the Gullstrand eye (see Chapter 2). In the 1980s, regression formulas (eg, Sanders, Retzlaff, Kraff [SRK] formulas I and II) were popular because they were simple to use. However, the use of these formulas often led to power errors that subsequently became the major reason IOLs were explanted. In the 1990s, regression formulas were largely replaced by more accurate, newer theoretical formulas.

Geometric optics was used to generate basic theoretical formulas for IOL power calculation, an example of which is shown below. The pseudophakic eye can be modeled as a 2-element optical system (Fig 5-5). Using Gaussian reduction equations, the IOL power that produces emmetropia may be given by

$$P = \frac{n_V}{AL - C} - \frac{K}{1 - K \times \dfrac{C}{n_A}}$$

where

P = power of the target IOL (in diopters [D])
n_V = index of refraction of the vitreous
AL = visual axial length (in millimeters)
C = ELP (in millimeters), the distance from the anterior corneal surface to the principal plane of the IOL
K = average dioptric power of the central cornea
n_A = index of refraction of the aqueous

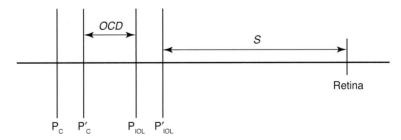

Figure 5-5 Schematic eye. P_C and P'_C are the front and back principal planes of the cornea, respectively. Similarly, P_{IOL} and P'_{IOL} are the front and back principal planes of the IOL. *OCD =* optical chapter depth; S = distance between back principal plane of the IOL and retina. (The drawing is not to scale.) *(Redrawn by C. H. Wooley.)*

Most of the advances in newer theoretical formulas (such as the Haigis, Hoffer Q, Hoffer H5, Holladay 1 and 2, Olsen, and SRK/T formulas) concerned improved methods of predicting the *ELP*, as described later in this chapter. These formulas are complex and cannot be used easily for calculation by hand. However, programmable calculators and applicable computer programs (eg, Hoffer Programs, Holladay IOL Consultant) are widely available, obviating this disadvantage. These formulas are also programmed into the IOLMaster, the Lenstar LS900 (discussed in the following section, "Biometric formula requirements"), and most modern ultrasonographic instruments, thereby eliminating any need for regression formulas. In all such cases, the surgeon must make sure that the formula author has verified the programming and accuracy of his or her particular formula.

Biometric formula requirements

Axial length The *AL* is the most important factor in these formulas. A 1-mm error in *AL* measurement results in a refractive error of approximately 2.35 D in a 23.5-mm eye. The refractive error declines to only 1.75 D/mm in a 30-mm eye but rises to 3.75 D/mm in a 20-mm eye. Therefore, accuracy in *AL* measurement is more important in short eyes than in long eyes.

ULTRASONIC MEASUREMENT OF AXIAL LENGTH When *A-scan ultrasonography* is used to measure *AL,* we either assume a constant ultrasound velocity through the entire eye or measure each of the various ocular structures at its individual velocity. A-scans measure not distance but rather the time required for a sound pulse to travel from the cornea to the retina. Sound travels faster through the crystalline lens and the cornea (1641 m/s) than it does through aqueous and vitreous (1532 m/s). Even within the lens itself, the speed of sound can vary in different layers of nuclear sclerosis. The measured sound transit time is converted to a distance by use of the formula

$$d = tV$$

where *d* is the distance in meters, *t* is the time in seconds, and *V* is the velocity in meters per second.

The average velocity through a phakic eye of normal length is 1555 m/s; however, it rises to 1560 m/s for a short (20-mm) eye and drops to 1550 m/s for a long (30-mm) eye. This variation is due to the presence of the crystalline lens; 1554 m/s is an accurate value for an aphakic eye of any length.

The following formula can be used to easily correct any *AL* measured with an incorrect average velocity:

$$AL_C = AL_M \times \frac{V_C}{V_M}$$

where AL_C is the *AL* value at the correct velocity, AL_M is the resultant *AL* value at the incorrect velocity, V_C is the correct velocity, and V_M is the incorrect velocity.

In eyes with *AL* values greater than 25 mm, *staphyloma* should be suspected, especially when numerous disparate readings are obtained. Such errors occur because the macula is located either at the deepest part of the staphyloma or on the "side of the hill." To measure such eyes and obtain the true measurement to the fovea, the clinician must use a *B-scan technique.* Optical methods (eg, IOLMaster, Lenstar) are very useful in such cases (see the following section).

When ultrasonography is used to measure the *AL* in *biphakic* eyes (ie, a phakic IOL in a phakic eye), it is difficult to eliminate the effect of the sound velocity through the phakic lens. To correct for this potential error, one can use the following published formula:

$$AL_{corrected} = AL_{1555} + C \times T$$

where

AL_{1555} = the measured *AL* of the eye at a sound velocity of 1555 m/s

C = the material-specific correction factor, which is +0.42 for PMMA, –0.59 for silicone, +0.11 for collamer, and +0.23 for acrylic

T = the central thickness of the phakic IOL

Published tables list the central thickness of phakic IOLs available on the market (for each dioptric power). The least degree of error (in terms of *AL* error) is associated with use of a very thin myopic collamer lens, and the greatest amount of error is associated with use of a thick hyperopic silicone lens.

The 2 primary A-scan techniques—*applanation* (contact) and *immersion* (noncontact)—often give different results (Figs 5-6, 5-7). The applanation method may yield a shorter *AL* measurement that is also inconsistent and unpredictable. An artificially short-ened *AL* measurement occurs with inadvertent corneal indentation. In the immersion method, which is accepted as the more accurate of the 2 techniques, space is maintained between the probe and the cornea, eliminating corneal indentation. See also Chapter 7 for more information on ultrasonography.

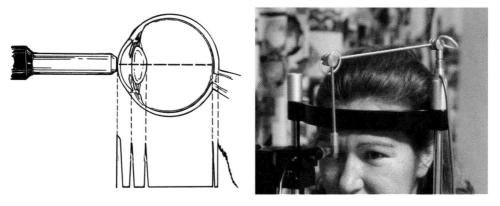

Figure 5-6 In applanation ultrasonography, the probe must contact the cornea, which causes corneal depression and shortening of the axial length reading. *(Courtesy of Kenneth J. Hoffer, MD.)*

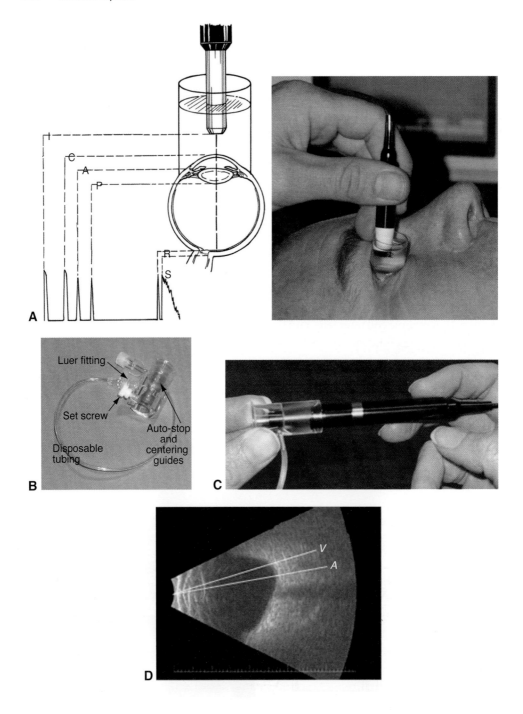

Figure 5-7 **A,** In immersion ultrasonography, the probe is immersed in the solution, placing it away from the cornea. **B,** Prager shell for immersion A-scan. **C,** Ultrasound probe and Kohn shell. **D,** B-scan of an eye with staphyloma, showing the difference between the anatomical length *(A)* and the visual length *(V)*. *(Courtesy of Kenneth J. Hoffer, MD.)*

OPTICAL MEASUREMENT OF AXIAL LENGTH Another method of measuring *AL* was introduced in 1999. The IOLMaster (Zeiss-Meditec, Jena, Germany) uses a partial coherence laser for *AL* measurement (Fig 5-8). In 2008, a similar optical measuring device was introduced, the Lenstar LS900 (Haag-Streit, Köniz, Switzerland). In a manner analogous to ultrasonography, this device measures the time required for infrared light to travel to the retina. Because light travels at too high a speed to be measured directly, light interference methodology is used to determine the transit time and thus the *AL*. This technique does not require contact with the globe, so corneal compression artifacts are eliminated. This instrument was developed such that its readings would be equivalent to those of the immersion ultrasound technique. Because this device requires the patient to fixate on a target, the length measured is the path the light takes to the fovea: the "visual" *AL*. The ocular media must be clear enough to allow voluntary fixation and light transmission. Thus, in dense cataracts (especially posterior subcapsular cataracts), ultrasound biometry is still necessary (in 5%–8% of cataract patients). Compared with ultrasonography, this technique provides more accurate, reproducible *AL* measurements. In addition, optical measurement is ideal in 2 clinical situations that are difficult to achieve using ultrasonography: eyes with staphyloma and eyes filled with silicone oil.

Corneal power The central corneal power, *K,* is the second most important factor in the calculation formula; a 1.0 D error in corneal power causes a 1.0 D postoperative refractive error. Corneal power can be estimated by keratometry or corneal topography, neither of which measures corneal power directly. The standard manual keratometer (Fig 5-9A) measures only a small central portion (3.2-mm diameter) of the cornea and views the cornea as a convex mirror. The corneal radius of curvature can be calculated from the size of the reflected image. Both front and back corneal surfaces contribute to corneal power, but the keratometer power "reading" is based on measurement of the radius of curvature of only the front surface and assumptions about the posterior surface.

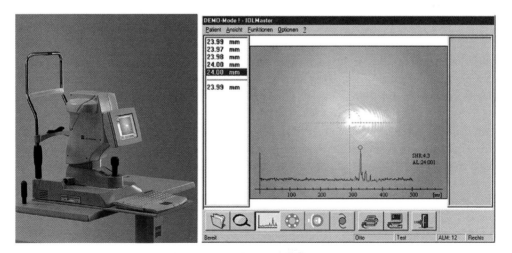

Figure 5-8 The IOLMaster *(left)* and view of the instrument's axial length screen *(right). (Courtesy of Kenneth J. Hoffer, MD.)*

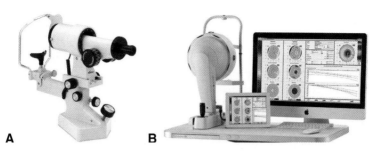

Figure 5-9 **A,** Manual keratometer. **B,** Oculus Pentacam. *(Part A courtesy of Reichert Technologies; part B courtesy of Oculus Optikgeräte GmbH.)*

The Pentacam (Oculus Optikgeräte GmbH, Wetzlar, Germany; Fig 5-9B) is a newer imaging system that uses a single Scheimpflug camera to measure the radius of curvature of the anterior and posterior corneal surfaces, as well as the corneal thickness, for the calculation of corneal power. Early studies have questioned the accuracy of the Pentacam in eyes that have undergone laser corneal refractive procedures. Newer software (2011) has made dramatic improvements. A later device, the Galilei (Ziemer Ophthalmic Systems AG, Port, Switzerland), measures corneal power by use of a dual Scheimpflug camera integrated with a Placido disk.

Estimated lens position All formulas require an estimation of the distance at which the principal plane of the IOL will be situated behind the cornea—a factor now known as the *ELP.* Initially, most IOLs were either anterior chamber (or prepupillary) IOLs. Thus, in the original theoretical formulas, this factor was called the *anterior chamber depth (ACD),* and it was a constant value (usually 2.8 or 3.5 mm). This value became incorporated in the *A* constant of the regression formulas of the 1980s.

In 1983, using pachymetry studies of posterior chamber IOLs as a basis, Hoffer introduced an *ACD* prediction formula for posterior chamber lenses that was based on the eye's *AL:*

$$ACD = 2.93 \times AL - 2.92$$

Other adjustments (second-generation formulas) were based on the *AL.* The Holladay 1 formula used the *K* reading and *AL* value as factors (in a corneal height formula by Fyodorov), as did the later SRK/T formula, whereas the Hoffer Q formula used the *AL* value and a tangent factor of *K* (all these formulas are third generation). Olsen added other measurements of the anterior segment, such as the preoperative *ACD,* lens thickness, and corneal diameter (this formula is fourth generation). Subsequently, Holladay used these factors, as well as patient age and preoperative refraction, in his Holladay 2 formula. Haigis eliminated *K* as a prediction factor and replaced it with the preoperative *ACD* measurement. These newer formulas are more accurate than those of the first and second generations, and all are currently in use.

The most accurate way to measure the preoperative *ACD* or the postoperative *ELP* is to use an optical pachymeter (Fig 5-10). Ultrasonography is usually less precise and provides a shorter reading. The IOLMaster is fairly accurate. The ACMaster (Zeiss-Meditec,

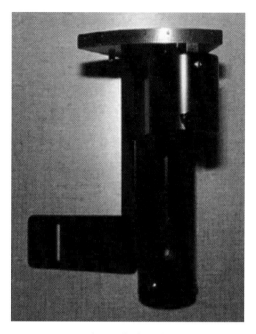
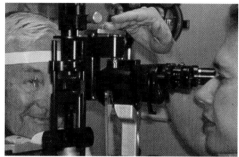
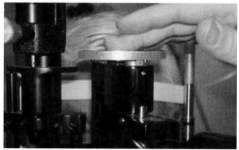

Figure 5-10 An optical pachymeter mounted on a slit lamp. *(Courtesy of Kenneth J. Hoffer, MD.)*

Jena, Germany), based on the partial coherence interferometry technique, has recently been introduced.

Most formulas use only one constant, such as the *ACD*, the *A* constant, or the *surgeon factor (SF)*. One exception is the Haigis formula, which uses 3 constants (a_0, a_1, a_2). The *A* constant, developed as a result of regression formulas, was widely used in the 1980s, so much so that manufacturers assigned each lens design a specific *A* constant, as well as an *ACD* value. Even though regression formulas (eg, SRK formula) are no longer recommended and rarely used for IOL calculation, the *A* constant still exists for the SRK/T formula.

Holladay developed 2 formulas that convert a lens's *A* constant to another factor. The first converts the *A* constant to an *SF* for the Holladay formula:

$$SF = (0.5663 \times A) - 65.6$$

where *A* is the IOL-specific *A* constant and SF is the Holladay surgeon factor. The second formula converts a lens's *A* constant to a personalized *ACD* (pACD) for the Hoffer Q formula:

$$pACD = \frac{(0.5663 \times A) - 62.005}{0.9704}$$

where *A* is the IOL-specific *A* constant and pACD is the Hoffer pACD *(ELP)*. So, for example, an *A* constant of 113.78, 116.35, or 118.92 converts to a pACD of 2.50 mm, 4.00 mm, or 5.50 mm, respectively.

It is prudent to calculate the power of an alternate IOL before surgery. If not calculated in advance, the power of an IOL intended for bag placement can be decreased for sulcus placement with subtraction of 0.75–1.50 D, depending on the *AL* value.

Formula choice

Several studies have indicated that the Hoffer Q formula is more accurate for eyes shorter than 24.5 mm; the Holladay 1, for eyes ranging from 24.5 to 26.0 mm; and the SRK/T, for eyes longer than 26.0 mm (very long eyes). A recent (2011) study conducted in the United Kingdom proved the statistical significance of these recommendations in more than 8000 eyes by use of optical *AL* values. For long eyes, the Haigis formula may achieve equivalent results.

The choice of formula is, of course, up to the surgeon, but whatever the method, every effort should be made to ensure that the biometry is as accurate as possible. The operating surgeon should review preoperative *AL* values and *K* readings. If a reading is suspect because it lies outside normal limits, biometry should be repeated during or immediately after the initial reading. Similarly, it is prudent to measure both eyes and recheck the readings if there is a large discrepancy between the 2 eyes. Great care should be taken in the measurement of eyes that have undergone previous refractive surgery (corneal or phakic IOL), as well as those that have undergone an encircling band treatment of a retinal detachment.

Piggyback and Supplemental Intraocular Lenses

When an IOL is inserted into an eye that already has an IOL, the second IOL is called a piggyback IOL. The piggyback IOL can be inserted at the time the first IOL is implanted to produce a high power that is commercially unavailable. It can also be inserted secondarily to correct a postoperative refractive error. Computer programs can be used to calculate the power of the second IOL and to make adjustments, which may be needed if the posterior IOL is displaced posteriorly. However, these adjustments are minor, and using one of the following formulas is the easiest way to calculate them:

Myopic correction: $P = 1.0 \times$ error
Hyperopic correction: $P = 1.5 \times$ error

where *P* is the needed power in the piggyback lens, and *error* refers to the residual refractive error that needs to be corrected.

Aristodemou P, Knox Cartwright NE, Sparrow JM, Johnston RL. Formula choice: Hoffer Q, Holladay 1, or SRK/T and refractive outcomes in 8108 eyes after cataract surgery with biometry by partial coherence interferometry. *J Cataract Refract Surg.* 2011;37(1):63–71.

Intraocular Lens Power Calculation After Corneal Refractive Surgery

IOL power calculation is a problem in eyes that have undergone *radial keratotomy (RK)* or laser corneal refractive procedures such as *photorefractive keratectomy (PRK), laser in situ keratomileusis (LASIK),* and *laser subepithelial keratomileusis (LASEK).* The difficulty stems from 3 sources of errors: (1) instrument error, (2) index of refraction error, and (3) formula error.

Instrument Error

Instrument error was first described by Koch in 1989. The instruments used by ophthalmologists to measure corneal power (keratometers and corneal topographers) cannot obtain accurate measurements in eyes that have undergone corneal refractive surgery. These instruments often miss the central, flatter zone of effective corneal power. The flatter the cornea is, the larger the zone of measurement is, and the greater the error. Topography units do not correct this problem, either; rather, they usually overestimate the corneal power, leading to a postoperative hyperopic refractive error in myopic eyes.

Index of Refraction Error

The assumed index of refraction (IR) of the normal cornea is based on the relationship between the anterior and posterior corneal curvatures. This relationship changes in eyes treated with PRK, LASIK, and LASEK. Ophthalmologists long believed that IR error did not occur in eyes that have undergone RK. This situation leads to an overestimation of the corneal power by approximately 1 D for every 7 D of correction obtained. A recent study showed that in eyes treated with RK, there is greater flattening of the posterior curvature than of the anterior curvature. A *manual keratometer* measures only the front surface curvature and converts the radius of curvature *(r)* obtained to diopters (D), usually by using an *IR* value of 1.3375. The following formula can be used to convert diopters to radius:

$$r = \frac{337.5}{D}$$

To convert *r* to D, use

$$D = \frac{337.5}{r}$$

Formula Error

With the exception of the Haigis formula, all of the modern IOL power formulas (eg, Hoffer Q, Holladay 1 and 2, and SRK/T) use the *AL* values and *K* readings to predict the postoperative position of the IOL *(ELP)*. The flatter-than-normal *K* value for eyes treated with RK, PRK, LASIK, or LASEK causes an error in this prediction because the anterior chamber dimensions do not actually change in these eyes commensurately with the much flatter *K*.

Power Calculation Methods for the Post–Keratorefractive Procedure Eye

In 2002, Aramberri developed the double-*K* method, which uses the pre-LASIK corneal power (or, if unknown, 43.50 D) to calculate the *ELP*, and the post-LASIK (much flatter) corneal power to calculate the IOL power. These calculations can be performed automatically with computer programs.

Aramberri's method is only one of more than 20 methods proposed over the years to either calculate the true corneal power or adjust the calculated IOL power to account for the errors discussed in the preceding sections. Some methods require knowledge of pre–refractive surgery values such as refractive error and *K* reading. Many of these methods have come in and out of favor on the basis of studies investigating their accuracy. It is up to the surgeon to keep abreast of the most accurate available methods.

It is not possible to describe all these methods in this chapter, but all of them are included in the Hoffer/Savini LASIK IOL Power Tool, which can be downloaded free of charge (see reference below). The tool requests the data needed to calculate each method, and the results are automatically calculated for every method for which complete data have been entered. The ultimate choice is left to the surgeon. The entire results can be printed on a single page and entered in the patient's chart. Calculations can also be performed through the American Society of Cataract and Refractive Surgery website, but it lacks the Hoffer Q formula in all calculations, especially needed in short eyes.

Perhaps in the future there will be a more satisfactory method of measuring true corneal power by use of topography and advanced measuring techniques. At present, the ideal method for use with post–refractive surgery patients has yet to be determined.

Hoffer KJ. The Hoffer/Savini LASIK IOL Power Tool. Available at www.iolpowerclub.org /post-surgical-iol-calc. Accessed June 3, 2013.

Koch DD, Liu JF, Hyde LL, Rock RL, Emery JM. Refractive complications of cataract surgery after radial keratotomy. *Am J Ophthalmol.* 1989;108(6):676–682.

Intraocular Lens Power in Corneal Transplant Eyes

It is very difficult to predict the ultimate power of the cornea after the eye has undergone penetrating keratoplasty. Thus, in 1987 Hoffer recommended that the surgeon wait for the corneal transplant to heal completely before implanting an IOL. The current safety of intraocular surgery allows for such a double-procedure approach in all but the rarest cases. Geggel has proven the validity of this approach by showing that posttransplant eyes have better uncorrected visual acuity (68% with 20/40 or better) and that the range of IOL power error decreases from 10 D to 5 D (95% within ±2.00 D).

If simultaneous IOL implantation and corneal transplant are necessary, surgeons may use either the *K* reading of the fellow eye or the average postoperative *K* value of a previous series of transplants, but these approaches are fraught with error. When there is corneal scarring in an eye but no need for a corneal graft, it might be best to use the corneal power of the other eye or even a power that is commensurate with the eye's *AL* and refractive error.

Geggel HS. Intraocular lens implantation after penetrating keratoplasty. Improved unaided visual acuity, astigmatism, and safety in patients with combined corneal disease and cataract. *Ophthalmology.* 1990;97(11):1460–1467.

Hoffer KJ. Triple procedure for intraocular lens exchange. *Arch Ophthalmol.* 1987;105(5): 609–610.

Silicone Oil Eyes

Ophthalmologists considering IOL implantation in eyes filled with silicone oil encounter 2 major problems. The first is obtaining an accurate AL measurement with the ultrasonic biometer. Recall that this instrument measures the transit time of the ultrasound pulse and, using estimated ultrasound velocities through the various ocular media, calculates the distance. This concept must be taken into consideration when velocities differ from the norm, for example, when silicone oil fills the posterior segment (980 m/s for silicone oil vs 1532 m/s for vitreous). Use of the IOLMaster to measure *AL* solves this problem somewhat. It is recommended that retinal surgeons perform an optical or immersion *AL* measurement before silicone oil placement, but doing so is not common practice. The second problem is that the oil filling the vitreous cavity acts like a negative lens power in the eye when a biconvex IOL is implanted. This problem must be counteracted by an increase in IOL power of 3–5 D.

Pediatric Eyes

Several issues make IOL power selection for children much more complex than that for adults. The first challenge is obtaining accurate *AL* and corneal measurements, which is usually performed when the child is under general anesthesia. The second is that, because shorter *AL* causes greater IOL power errors, the small size of a child's eye compounds power calculation errors, particularly if the child is very young. The third problem is selecting an appropriate target IOL power, one that will not only provide adequate visual acuity to prevent amblyopia but also allow adequate vision due to the large myopic shift that occurs after maturity.

A possible solution to the third problem is to implant 2 (or more) IOLs simultaneously: one IOL with the predicted adult emmetropic power placed posteriorly and the other (or others) with the power that provides childhood emmetropia placed anterior to the first lens. When the patient reaches adulthood, the obsolete IOL(s) can be removed (sequentially). Alternatively, corneal refractive surgery may be used to treat myopia that develops in adulthood. Most recent studies have shown that the best modern formulas do not perform as accurately for children's eyes as they do for adults.

Hoffer KJ, Aramberri J, Haigis W, Norrby S, Olsen T, Shammas HJ; IOL Power Club Executive Committee. The final frontier: pediatric intraocular lens power. *Am J Ophthalmol.* 2012;154(1):1–2.e1.

Image Magnification

Image magnification of as much as 20%–35% is the major disadvantage of aphakic spectacles. Contact lenses magnify images by only 7%–12%, whereas IOLs magnify images by 4% or less. An IOL implanted in the posterior chamber produces less image magnification than does an IOL in the anterior chamber. The issue of magnification is further complicated by the correction of residual postsurgical refractive errors. A Galilean telescope effect is created when spectacles are worn over pseudophakic eyes. Clinically, each diopter of spectacle overcorrection at a vertex of 12 mm causes a 2% magnification or minification (for plus or minus lenses, respectively). Thus, a pseudophakic patient with a posterior chamber IOL and a residual refractive error of –1 D would have 2% magnification from the IOL and 2% minification from the spectacle lens, resulting in little change in image size.

Aniseikonia is defined as a difference in image size between the 2 eyes and can cause disturbances in stereopsis. Generally, a person can tolerate spherical aniseikonia of 5%–8%. In clinical practice, aniseikonia is rarely a significant problem; however, it should be considered in patients with unexplained vision symptoms.

Lens-Related Vision Disturbances

The presence of IOLs may cause numerous optical phenomena. Various light-related visual phenomena encountered by pseudophakic (and phakic) patients are termed *dysphotopsias*. These phenomena are divided into positive and negative dysphotopsias. Positive dysphotopsias are characterized by brightness, streaks, and rays emanating from a central point source of light, sometimes with a diffuse, hazy glare. Negative dysphotopsias are characterized by subjective darkness or shadowing. Such optical phenomena may be related to light reflection and refraction along the edges of the IOL. High-index acrylic lenses with square or truncated edges produce a more intense edge glare (Fig 5-11A).

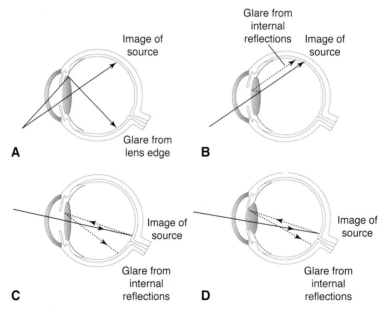

Figure 5-11 A, Light striking the edge of the IOL may be reflected to another site on the retina, resulting in undesirable dysphotopsias. These problems arise less often with smoother-edged IOLs. **B,** Light may be internally re-reflected within an IOL, producing an undesirable second image or halo. Such re-reflection may be more likely to occur as the index of refraction of the IOL increases. **C,** Light may reflect back from the surface of the retina and reach the anterior surface of the IOL. The IOL acts as a concave mirror, reflecting back an undesirable dysphotopsic image. When the anterior surface of the IOL is more curved, the annoying image is displaced relatively far from the fovea. **D,** When the anterior IOL surface is less steeply curved, the annoying image appears closer to the true image and is likely to be more distracting. *(Redrawn by C. H. Wooley.)*

These phenomena may also be due to internal re-reflection within the IOL itself; such re-reflection is more likely to occur with materials that have a higher IR, such as acrylic (Fig 5-11B). With a less steeply curved anterior surface, the lens may be more likely to have internal reflections that are directed toward the fovea and are therefore more distracting (Fig 5-11C, D).

Davison JA. Positive and negative dysphotopsia in patients with acrylic intraocular lenses. *J Cataract Refract Surg.* 2000;26(9):1346–1355.

Erie JC, Bandhauer MH. Intraocular lens surfaces and their relationship to postoperative glare. *J Cataract Refract Surg.* 2003;29(2):336–341.

Franchini A, Gallarati BZ, Vaccari E. Computerized analysis of the effects of intraocular lens edge design on the quality of vision in pseudophakic patients. *J Cataract Refract Surg.* 2003;29(2):342–347.

Nonspherical Optics

IOLs with more complex optical parameters are now available. It may be possible to offset the positive spherical aberration of the cornea in pseudophakic patients by implanting an IOL with the appropriate negative asphericity on its anterior surface. IOLs with a *toric* surface may be used to correct astigmatism. Rotational stability may be of greater concern when plate-haptic toric lenses are implanted in the vertical axis than when they are implanted in the horizontal axis. As a toric lens rotates from the optimal desired angular orientation, the benefit of the toric correction diminishes. A properly powered toric IOL that is more than 30° off-axis increases the residual astigmatism of an eye; if it is 90° off-axis, the residual astigmatism doubles. Fortunately, some benefit remains even with lesser degrees of axis error, although the axis of residual cylinder changes. Newer designs are more stable than earlier ones.

Recently, investigators have developed an IOL in which the optical power can be altered by laser after lens implantation. This feature would be useful for correcting both IOL power calculation errors and residual astigmatism.

Mester U, Dillinger P, Anterist N. Impact of a modified optic design on visual function: clinical comparative study. *J Cataract Refract Surg.* 2003;29(4):652–660.

Multifocal Intraocular Lenses

Conventional IOLs are *monofocal* and correct the refractive ametropia associated with removal of the crystalline lens. Because a standard plastic IOL has no accommodative power, its focus is essentially for a single distance only. However, the improved visual acuity resulting from IOL implantation may allow a patient to see with acceptable clarity over a range of distances. If the patient is left with a residual refractive error of simple myopic astigmatism, the ability to see with acceptable clarity over a range of distances may be further augmented. In this situation, one endpoint of the astigmatic conoid of Sturm corresponds to the distance focus and the other endpoint represents myopia and, thus, a near focus; satisfactory clarity of vision may be possible if the object in view is focused between these 2 endpoints. In bilateral, asymmetric, and oblique myopic astigmatism, the blurred axis images are ignored and the clearest axis images are chosen to form one clear image for distance vision; the opposite images are selected for near vision. It is difficult to replicate this process clinically. Thus, even standard IOLs may provide some degree of depth of focus and "bifocal" capabilities.

An alternate approach to this problem is to correct one eye for distance and the other for near vision; this approach is called *monovision*. Nevertheless, most patients who receive IOLs are corrected for distance vision and wear reading glasses as needed.

Multifocal IOLs are designed to improve both near and distance vision to decrease patients' dependence on glasses. With a multifocal IOL, the correcting lens is placed in a fixed location within the eye, and the patient cannot voluntarily change the focus. Depending on the type of multifocal IOL and the viewing situation, both near and far images may be presented to the eye at the same time. The brain then processes the clearest image, ignoring the other(s). Most patients, but not all, can adapt to the use of multifocal IOLs.

The performance of certain types of IOLs is greatly impaired by decentration if the visual axis does not pass through the center of the IOL. On the one hand, the use of modern surgical techniques generally results in adequate lens centration. Pupil size, on the other hand, is an active variable, but it can be employed in some situations to improve multifocal function.

Other disadvantages of multifocal IOLs are image degradation, "ghost" images (or *monocular diplopia*), decreased contrast sensitivity, and reduced performance in lower light (eg, decreased night vision). These potential problems make multifocal IOLs less desirable for use in eyes with impending macular disease.

Accuracy of IOL power calculation is very important for multifocal IOLs because their purpose is to reduce the patient's dependence on glasses. Preoperative and postoperative astigmatism should be low, given that visual acuity and contrast sensitivity degrade with against-the-rule astigmatism as low as 1.00 D.

Types of Multifocal Intraocular Lenses

Bifocal intraocular lenses

Of the various IOL designs, the bifocal IOL is conceptually the simplest. The bifocal concept is based on the idea that when there are 2 superimposed images on the retina, the brain always selects the clearer image and suppresses the blurred one. The first bifocal IOL implanted in a human was invented by Hoffer in 1982. The *split bifocal* was implanted in a patient in Santa Monica, CA, in 1990. In this simple design, which was independent of pupil size, half the optic was focused for distance vision and the other half for near vision (Fig 5-12A). This design was reintroduced in 2010 as the Lentis Mplus (Oculentis, Berlin, Germany) and is now showing encouraging results in Europe.

The additional power needed for near vision is not affected by the *AL* or by corneal power, but it is affected by the *ELP*. A posterior chamber IOL requires more near-addition power than does an anterior chamber IOL for the same focal distance. Approximately 3.75 D of added power is required to provide the necessary 2.75 D of myopia for a 14-inch reading distance.

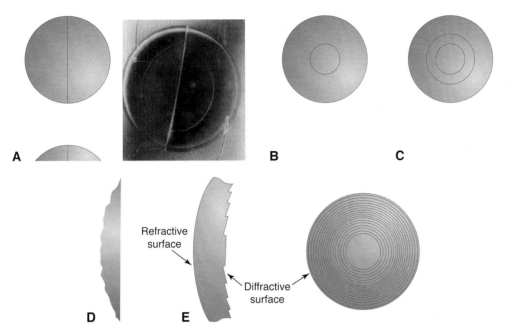

Figure 5-12 Multifocal IOLs. **A,** Hoffer split bifocal IOL *(left)* and photograph of a lens implanted in a patient in 1984 *(right)*. **B,** Bullet bifocal IOL. **C,** Three-zone multifocal design. **D,** Multifocal IOL with several annular zones. **E,** Diffractive multifocal IOL; the cross section of the central portion is magnified (the depth of the grooves is exaggerated). *(Photograph courtesy of Kenneth J. Hoffer, MD; all illustrations redrawn by C. H. Wooley.)*

A later design known as the *"bullet" bifocal IOL* (see Fig 5-12B) had a central zone for near power and an outer zone for distance. When the pupil constricted for near vision, its smaller size reduced or eliminated the contribution from the distance portion of the IOL. When the pupil dilated for distance vision, more of the distance portion of the IOL was exposed and contributed to the final image. Importantly, lens decentration could have a deleterious effect on the IOL's optical performance. A problem with the design itself was that the pupil size did not always correspond to the desired visual task. For this reason, the bullet bifocal IOL fell into disuse.

Multiple-zone intraocular lenses

To overcome the problems associated with pupil size, ophthalmologists developed a *3-zone bifocal lens* (Fig 5-12C). The central and outer zones are for distance vision; the inner annulus is for near vision. The diameters were selected to provide near correction for moderately small pupils and distance correction for both large and small pupils.

Another design uses several *annular zones* (Fig 5-12D), each of which varies continuously in power over a range of 3.50 D. The advantage is that whatever the size, shape, or location of the pupil, all the focal distances are represented on the macula.

Diffractive multifocal intraocular lenses

Diffractive multifocal IOL designs (Fig 5-12E) use Fresnel diffraction optics to achieve a multifocal effect. The overall spherical shape of the surfaces produces an image for distance vision. The posterior surface has a stepped structure, and the diffraction from these multiple rings produces a second image, with an effective add power. At a particular point along the axis, waves diffracted by the various zones add in phase, providing a focus for that wavelength. Approximately 20% of the light entering the pupil is absorbed in this process, and optical aberrations with diffractive IOLs can be troublesome.

Second-generation diffractive multifocal intraocular lenses

Currently, 3 second-generation diffractive multifocal IOLs are available. Each increases the patient's independence from spectacles and decreases the incidence of optical adverse effects.

The first of these IOLs, the AcrySof ReSTOR IOL (Alcon, Fort Worth, TX), is an apodized diffractive lens (Fig 5-13A). *Apodization* refers to the gradual tapering of the diffractive steps from the center to the outside edge of a lens to create a smooth transition of light between the distance, intermediate, and near vision focal points. This IOL is now available in an aspheric design. The second design, the ReZoom lens (Abbott Medical Optics [AMO], Santa Ana, CA) (Fig 5-13B), has 5 anterior surface zones for distance and near vision; grading between the zones provides intermediate vision. The third IOL, the TECNIS ZM 900 lens (AMO), adds an aspheric surface, whereas the ReZoom lens does not.

Clinical Results of Multifocal Intraocular Lenses

Some multifocal IOLs perform better for near vision; others, for intermediate. Studies have shown a benefit to using a combination of these lenses in the same patient.

The best-corrected visual acuity may be less with a multifocal IOL than with a monofocal IOL; this difference increases in low-light situations. However, the need for additional spectacle correction for near vision is greatly reduced in patients with multifocal

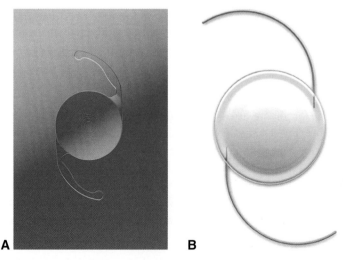

A　　　　**B**

Figure 5-13 **A,** The AcrySof ReSTOR lens. **B,** The ReZoom lens. *(Part A courtesy of Alcon Laboratories; part B courtesy of Abbott Medical Optics.)*

IOLs. Some patients are quite pleased with multifocal IOLs; others request their removal and replacement with monofocal IOLs. Interestingly, patients with a multifocal IOL in one eye and a monofocal IOL in the other often seem to be less tolerant of the multifocal IOLs than are patients with bilateral multifocal IOLs.

Patient selection is crucial for successful adaptation to multifocal IOLs. Selected patients must be willing to accept the trade-off—particularly in low-light situations—between decreased performance at distance vision (and at near vision, compared with that of a monofocal IOL and reading glasses) and the possibility of seeing well enough at all distances to be able to dispense with spectacles altogether. This technology will continue to evolve.

Ford JG, Karp CL. *Cataract Surgery and Intraocular Lenses: A 21st-Century Perspective.* 2nd ed. Ophthalmology Monograph 7. San Francisco: American Academy of Ophthalmology; 2001.

Hoffer KJ. Personal history in bifocal intraocular lenses. In: *Current Concepts of Multifocal Intraocular Lenses.* Maxwell WA, Nordan LT, eds. Thorofare, NJ: Slack; 1991:chap 12, pp 127–132.

Accommodating Intraocular Lenses

These lenses are essentially monofocal IOLs designed to allow some degree of improved near vision. Usually, such designs involve linking accommodative effort to an anterior movement of the IOL, thereby increasing its effective power in the eye. This mechanism may be more effective with higher-power IOLs because their effective powers are more sensitive to small changes in position than are those of lower-power IOLs. The US Food and Drug Administration (FDA) has approved one design that has shown some degree of accommodation, and other designs are awaiting FDA approval. At this time, there is no clinical evidence that "accommodating" IOLs actually change axial position in the eye during near-vision tasks.

Findl O, Kiss B, Petternel V, et al. Intraocular lens movement caused by ciliary muscle contraction. *J Cataract Refract Surg.* 2003;29(4):669–676.

Langenbucher A, Huber S, Nguyen NX, Seitz B, Gusek-Schneider GC, Küchle M. Measurement of accommodation after implantation of an accommodating posterior chamber intraocular lens. *J Cataract Refract Surg.* 2003;29(4):677–685.

Matthews MW, Eggleston HC, Hilmas GE. Development of a repeatedly adjustable intraocular lens. *J Cataract Refract Surg.* 2003;29(11):2204–2210.

Matthews MW, Eggleston HC, Pekarek SD, Hilmas GE. Magnetically adjustable intraocular lens. *J Cataract Refract Surg.* 2003;29(11):2211–2216.

Intraocular Lens Standards

The American National Standards Institute (ANSI) and the International Standards Organization (ISO) set standards for IOLs. Among these standards is one for IOL power labeling; it requires that IOLs with powers labeled as less than 25 D be within ±0.40 D of the labeled power and have no axial-power variations of more than 0.25 D. IOLs labeled 25–30 D must be within ±0.50 D of the labeled power, and those labeled greater than 30 D must be within ±1.0 D. Most ophthalmologists are unaware of this wide range allowed for the labeling of high-power IOLs. Although controversial, attempts are being made to narrow this allowed range so that all IOL powers would be within ±0.25 D of the labeled powers. Actual mislabeling of IOL power is rare but still occurs.

In addition to the labeling standards, the ANSI, ISO, and US Food and Drug Administration have set various other IOL standards for *optical performance,* a term that refers broadly to the image quality produced by an IOL. Lenses are also tested for biocompatibility, the absence of cytotoxicity of their material, the presence of any additives (such as UV filters), genotoxicity, and photostability, as well as for their safety with YAG lasers. There are also standards for spectral transmission. Physical standards exist to ensure adherence to the labeled optic diameter, haptic angulation, strength, and mechanical fatigability of the components, as well as to ensure sterility and safety during injection.

Chapter Exercises

Questions

5.1. *Error in sound velocity.* An ophthalmologist discovers that a measured axial length *(AL)* was taken using an incorrect AL. What should be the next course of action?

a. The patient should be scheduled for a return visit and the ultrasound repeated using the correct sound velocity.

b. A simple correction factor can be added algebraically to the incorrect-measure AL value.

c. The incorrect AL is likely due to an incorrect velocity. The incorrect AL can be corrected by dividing the AL by the incorrect velocity and multiplying by the correct velocity.

d. The sound velocity is so negligible that it does not need to be corrected.

5.2. *Error in corneal power.* Which option below is *not* a major contributing factor to errors in measuring the corneal power of eyes that have had corneal refractive surgery?

a. instrument error due to flattening of the anterior corneal surface

b. a change in the cornea from oblate to prolate

c. a change in the index of refraction from the standard 1.3375 used for normal eyes

d. the use in modern theoretic formulas of the very flat K reading to calculate the estimated lens position *(ELP)*

5.3. Select the best option to follow. Multifocal intraocular lenses (IOLs)

a. offer increased image clarity and contrast for both near and far viewing.

b. are independent of pupil size if they are well centered.

c. offer a trade-off between decreased image quality and increased depth of focus.

d. are indicated for all patients.

5.4. Which one of the following statements about piggyback IOLs is true?
   a. Piggyback IOLs modify the vergence of light entering the eye after it exits the incorrectly powered primary IOL.
   b. Piggyback IOLs can be used in a second operation only if the original IOL power was too low and additional dioptric strength is indicated.
   c. A piggyback IOL may be useful after removal of an incorrectly powered IOL.
   d. Piggyback IOLs may be less necessary as standard IOL power ranges increase.

5.5. Select the best option below with respect to biometric formulas for IOL calculation:
   a. The AL is the least important factor in the formula.
   b. The refractive error resulting from an error in AL measurement is more consequential in long eyes than in short eyes.
   c. Accuracy in AL measurement is relatively more important in short eyes than in long eyes.
   d. During ultrasonic measurement of AL (A-scan), sound travels faster through the aqueous and vitreous than through the crystalline lens and cornea. Therefore, there is a need to make adjustment to the AL "measurement" by correcting for the incorrect velocity of sound.
   e. The velocity of sound in an aphakic eye varies significantly between short and long eyes.

Answers

5.1. **c.** The formula to correct the AL is $AL \times V_C/V_I$, where V_C is the correct velocity and V_I is the incorrect velocity. This correction eliminates the need for the patient to undergo the procedure again. There is no factor that can be added to the AL to correct such an error, and the error is not negligible and thus cannot be ignored.

5.2. **b.** This corneal change has no effect on errors caused by refractive surgery.

5.3. **c.** Multifocal IOLs present both near and distant foci to the retina at the same time. This leads to an unavoidable decrease in image quality and contrast sensitivity, particularly at low levels of illumination. Pupil size may be a factor, particularly with certain types of multifocal IOLs. (Smaller pupil size results in increased depth of focus regardless!)

5.4. **d.** Piggyback IOLs have been used to reach a total dioptric power that was unavailable in a single lens. As IOLs are becoming available in a wider range of powers, however, it is less likely that a piggyback IOL will be needed to reach an unusually high or low power. Piggyback IOLs are placed anterior to the primary lens and thus modify the light vergence before the light reaches the primary IOL. These IOLs may be used to correct inaccurate primary IOLs in a second operation if the original IOL power was too low or too high. They are not used after removal of an incorrectly powered IOL—"piggyback" implies that a second IOL is present in the eye.

5.5. **c.** Note the following comments for each option:

    a. The axial length *(AL)* is the *most* important factor in the formula.

    b. The refractive error resulting from an error in *AL* measurement is more consequential in *short* eyes than in long eyes.

    c. Accuracy in *AL* measurement is relatively more important in short eyes than in long eyes. *Correct answer.*

    d. During ultrasonic measurement of *AL* (A-scan), sound travels faster through the *crystalline lens and cornea* than through the aqueous and vitreous. Therefore, there is a need to make adjustment to the *AL* "measurement" by correcting for the incorrect velocity of sound.

    e. The velocity of sound in an aphakic eye varies *insignificantly* between short and long eyes (ie, it is almost comparable).

Appendix 5.1

History of Intraocular Lens Design

Knowledge of the history of intraocular lens (IOL) design is important for understanding the reasons for the designs currently in use. Since IOLs were first developed, their designs and the location of IOL fixation have changed considerably. The early success of prepupillary lens designs in the 1970s was sufficient to allow IOL implantation to progress. An early IOL design for intracapsular cataract extraction (ICCE), known as the prepupillary Binkhorst *iris clip lens,* floated freely but maintained centrality by pupil fixation of its anterior and posterior loops (Fig 5-14A). The Binkhorst prepupillary *iridocapsular 2-loop lens* had posterior loops fixated in the capsular bag after extracapsular cataract extraction (ECCE) (Fig 5-14B). Later designs (eg, the Epstein lens, Fig 5-15; the Medallion and Platina lenses, Fig 5-16A) were sutured or clipped to the iris for fixation. The Fyodorov Sputnik was an extremely popular lens (Fig 5-16B). Prepupillary IOLs are no longer used because of their tendency to dislocate; however, one early loopless design, the Worst *"lobster claw" lens* (Fig 5-17; renamed the Artisan lens in 1997), which imbricates the iris stroma, has been

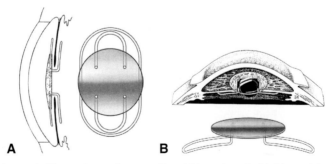

A   **B**

Figure 5-14 Schematic illustrations of prepupillary IOL styles. **A,** Binkhorst iris clip lens and its position in the eye. **B,** Iridocapsular 2-loop IOL by Binkhorst. *(Courtesy of Kenneth J. Hoffer, MD; IOLs redrawn by C. H. Wooley.)*

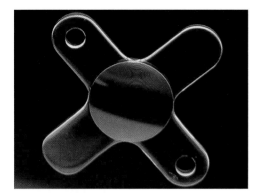

Figure 5-15 Prepupillary Epstein lens by Cope-land. *(Courtesy of Robert C. Drews, MD.)*

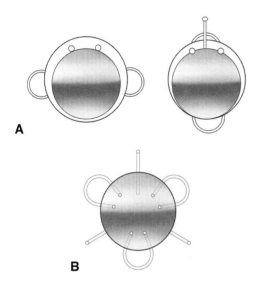

A

B

Figure 5-16 A, Prepupillary Medallion *(left)* and Platina *(right)* lenses by Worst. **B,** Sputnik lens by Fyodorov. *(Courtesy of Kenneth J. Hoffer, MD. Redrawn by C. H. Wooley.)*

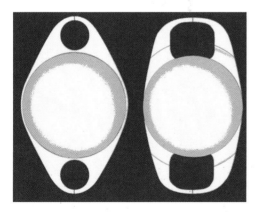

Figure 5-17 "Lobster claw" aphakic and pha-kic intraocular lenses by Worst. *(Courtesy of Kenneth J. Hoffer, MD.)*

approved by the US Food and Drug Administration for insertion in phakic eyes to correct high degrees of ametropia. The 2 basic lens designs currently in use are differentiated by the plane in which the lens is placed (posterior chamber or anterior chamber) and by the tissue supporting the lens (capsule/ciliary sulcus or chamber angle) (see Fig 5-1).

Posterior chamber lenses

The Ridley lens (Fig 5-18) and other early IOL styles were associated with serious complications, prompting ophthalmologists in the 1950s to turn their attention to anterior chamber IOLs, as well as prepupillary lenses. In the late 1970s, posterior chamber IOLs were reintroduced with a planar 2-loop design and continued to evolve, resulting in numerous successful designs. The first 2 design changes were (1) angulation of the loop haptics to prevent pupillary capture, which remains a feature of current designs, and (2) addition of a peripheral posterior annular ridge to prevent posterior capsular opacification. Today, posterior chamber IOLs are by far the most widely used IOLs and are generally employed following phacoemulsification (Fig 5-19).

With a posterior chamber IOL, the optic and supporting haptics are intended to be placed entirely within the capsular bag; in patients with a torn or an absent posterior capsule, the IOL is placed in the ciliary sulcus. The posterior chamber IOL may also be sutured in place (with a *nonabsorbable* suture) in cases with poor or no remaining capsular support. Alternatively, some surgeons prefer to use a well-placed, properly sized, high-quality modern anterior chamber lens.

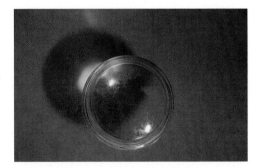

Figure 5-18 Original Ridley lens. *(Courtesy of Robert C. Drews, MD.)*

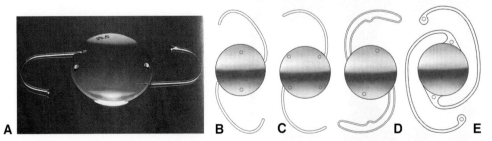

Figure 5-19 Posterior chamber IOLs. **A,** J-loop design. **B,** Kratz-Sinskey modified J-loop lens. **C,** Simcoe modified C-loop lens. **D,** Knolle lens. **E,** Arnott lens. *(Part A courtesy of Robert C. Drews, MD; parts B–E courtesy of Kenneth J. Hoffer, MD, and redrawn by C. H. Wooley.)*

Anterior chamber lenses

Anterior chamber IOLs (eg, Strampelli and Mark VIII lenses; Fig 5-20) sit entirely within the anterior chamber, but the optical portion of the lens is supported by solid "feet" or loops resting in opposite sides of the chamber angle. Anterior chamber IOLs are a popular style for secondary lens insertion in ICCE aphakic eyes. A particular problem with the use of rigid anterior chamber IOLs is inaccurate estimation of the size of the lens required to span the anterior chamber. The haptics must rest lightly in the chamber angle without tucking the iris (which would indicate that the lens is too large) or "propellering" in the anterior chamber from unstable fixation (too small). The "one-size-fits-all" (eg, Azar 91Z and Copeland lenses; Fig 5-21) and closed-loop designs of the 1970s and 1980s were associated with many complications (persistent uveitis, hyphema, cystoid macular edema, iris atrophy, corneal decompensation, and glaucoma), and poor manufacturing led to the *UGH* (uveitis-glaucoma-hyphema) *syndrome.*

These severe problems led to a bias against anterior chamber IOLs that persists to this day. One change manufacturers made that helped improve the status of these IOLs was to provide a supply of these lenses in several diameter sizes. Charles Kelman, MD, resolved

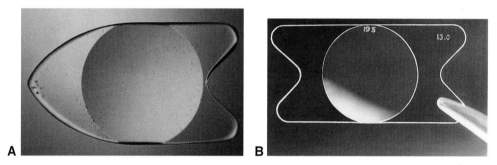

Figure 5-20 Anterior chamber IOLs. **A,** Angle-supported lens by Strampelli. **B,** Mark VIII lens by Choyce. *(Courtesy of Robert C. Drews, MD.)*

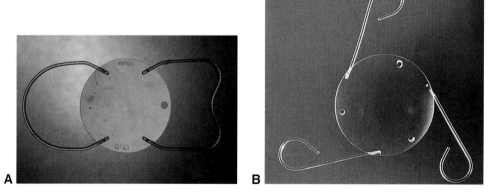

Figure 5-21 One-size-fits-all anterior chamber IOLs. **A,** Azar 91Z lens. **B,** Copeland lens. *(Courtesy of Robert C. Drews, MD.)*

other, more crucial problems by designing lathe-cut, single-piece polymethylmethacrylate anterior chamber IOLs with haptics that absorbed minor compression in the plane of the optic; in previous designs, the optic moved anteriorly, toward the cornea, to absorb compression. The original Kelman Tripod (Fig 5-22A) was replaced by the present-day quadripodal Multiflex II (Fig 5-22B) and other, similar designs (Fig 5-23).

In addition, Kelman strongly urged surgeons to measure horizontal corneal diameter carefully and to check the status and position of the haptics using *gonioscopy* in the operating room immediately after lens placement. When properly followed, these procedures make modern anterior chamber IOL implantation an excellent alternative when the use of a posterior chamber IOL is not advisable. One drawback is that an eye implanted with an anterior chamber IOL will be tender if rubbed vigorously. Thus, rubbing the eye should be discouraged.

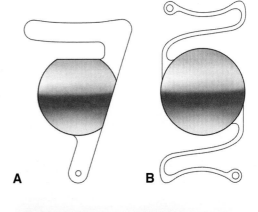

Figure 5-22 Anterior chamber lens designs by Kelman. **A,** Original Kelman tripod, also known as the "Pregnant 7." **B,** Multiflex II. *(Courtesy of Kenneth J. Hoffer, MD. Redrawn by C. H. Wooley.)*

A   **B**

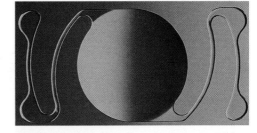

Figure 5-23 Kelman open-looped lens. *(Courtesy of Robert C. Drews, MD.)*

CHAPTER 6

Optical Considerations in Keratorefractive Surgery

This chapter provides an overview of the optical considerations specific to keratorefractive surgery. Refractive surgical procedures performed with the intent to reduce refractive errors can generally be categorized as *corneal* (keratorefractive) or *lenticular*. Keratorefractive surgical procedures include radial keratotomy (RK), astigmatic keratotomy (AK), photorefractive keratectomy (PRK), laser subepithelial keratomileusis (LASEK), epithelial laser in situ keratomileusis (epi-LASIK), laser in situ keratomileusis (LASIK), implantation of intracorneal ring segments and corneal inlays, laser thermal keratoplasty (LTK), and radiofrequency conductive keratoplasty (CK). Lenticular refractive procedures include cataract and clear lens extraction with intraocular lens implantation, phakic intraocular lens implantation, multifocal and toric intraocular lens implantation, and piggyback lens implantation. Although all of these refractive surgical techniques alter the optical properties of the eye, keratorefractive surgery is generally more likely than lenticular refractive surgery to produce unwanted optical aberrations. This chapter discusses only keratorefractive procedures and their optical considerations. For a discussion of optical considerations in lenticular refractive surgery, see BCSC Section 11, *Lens and Cataract.*

Various optical considerations are relevant to refractive surgery, both in screening patients for candidacy and in evaluating patients with vision complaints after surgery. The following sections address optical considerations related to the change in corneal shape after keratorefractive surgery, issues concerning the angle kappa and pupil size, and the various causes of irregular astigmatism.

Corneal Shape

The normal human cornea has a prolate shape (Fig 6-1), similar to that of the pole of an egg. The curvature of the human eye is steepest in the central cornea and gradually flattens toward the periphery. This configuration reduces the optical problems associated with simple spherical refracting surfaces, which produce a nearer point of focus for peripheral rays than for paraxial rays—a refractive condition known as *spherical aberration. Corneal asphericity,* the relative difference between the pericentral and central cornea, is represented by the factor *Q*. (Note that the asphericity *Q* factor is a geometric factor, distinct from the *Q* factor that characterizes a resonator such as a laser cavity.) In an ideal visual system, the curvature at the center of the cornea would be steeper than at the periphery (ie, the cornea would

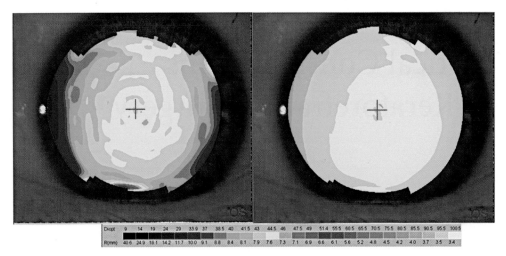

Figure 6-1 An example of meridional (tangential, *left*) and axial *(right)* maps of a normal cornea. *(Used with permission from Roberts C. Corneal topography. In: Azar DT, ed. Gatinel D, Hoang-Xuan T, associate eds. Refractive Surgery. 2nd ed. St Louis: Elsevier-Mosby; 2007:103–116.)*

be prolate), and the asphericity factor Q would have a value close to –0.50; at this value of negative Q, the degree of spherical aberration would approach zero. However, in the human eye, such a Q value is not anatomically possible (because of the junction between the cornea and the sclera). The Q factor for the human cornea has an average value of –0.26, allowing for a smooth transition at the limbus. The human visual system, therefore, suffers from minor spherical aberrations, which increase with increasing pupil size.

Following keratorefractive surgery for the treatment of myopia, the cornea becomes less prolate and has a shape resembling that of an egg lying on its side. The central cornea becomes flatter than the periphery. This flattening results in a change in the spherical aberration of the treated zone.

To demonstrate this change, consider the point spread function produced by all rays that traverse the pupil from a single object point. Generally, keratorefractive surgery for myopia reduces spherical refractive error and regular astigmatism, but it does so at the expense of increasing spherical aberration and irregular astigmatism (Fig 6-2). Keratorefractive surgery moves the location of the best focus closer to the retina but, at the same time, makes the focus less stigmatic. Such irregular astigmatism is what underlies many visual complaints after refractive surgery.

A basic premise of refractive surgery is that the cornea's optical properties are intimately related to its shape. Consequently, manipulation of the corneal shape changes the eye's refractive status. Although this assumption is true, the relationship between corneal shape and the cornea's optical properties is more complex than is generally appreciated.

Ablative procedures, incisional procedures, and intracorneal rings change the natural shape of the cornea to reduce refractive error. Keratometry readings in eyes conducted before they undergo keratorefractive surgery typically range from 38.0 D to 48.0 D. When refractive surgical procedures are being considered, it is important to avoid changes that may result in excessively flat (<33.0 D) or excessively steep (>50.0 D) corneal powers. A 0.8 D change in keratometry value (K) corresponds to approximately a 1.00 D change of

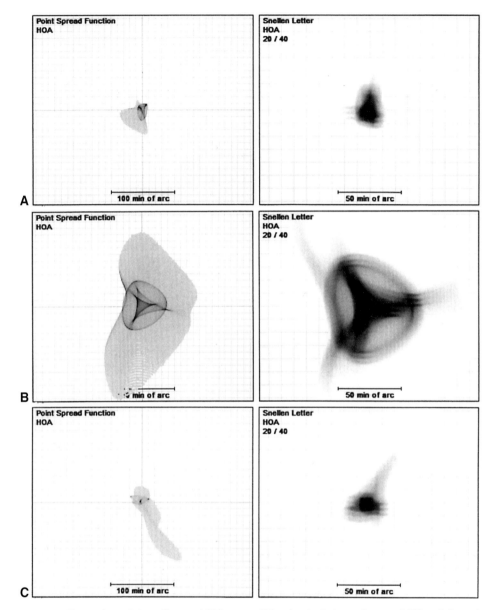

Figure 6-2 Examples of the effects of **(A)** coma, **(B)** spherical aberration, and **(C)** trefoil on the point spread functions of a light source and a Snellen letter E. *(Courtesy of Ming Wang, MD.)*

refraction. The following equation is often used to predict corneal curvature after keratorefractive surgery:

$$K_{postop} = K_{preop} + (0.8 \times RE)$$

where K_{preop} and K_{postop} are preoperative and postoperative K readings, respectively, and RE is the refractive error to be corrected at the corneal plane. For example, if a patient's preoperative keratometry readings are 45.0 D (steepest meridian) and 43.0 D (flattest meridian), then the average *K* value is 44.0 D. If the amount of refractive correction at the corneal plane is –8.50 D, then the predicted average postoperative *K* reading is 44.0 + (0.8 × –8.50) = 37.2 D, which is acceptable.

The ratio of dioptric change in refractive error to dioptric change in keratometry approximates 0.8:1 owing to the change in posterior corneal surface power after excimer ablation. The anterior corneal surface produces most of the eye's refractive power. In the Gullstrand model eye (see Table 2-1), the anterior corneal surface has a power of +48.8 D and the posterior corneal surface has a power of –5.8 D, so the overall corneal refractive power is +43.0 D. Importantly, standard corneal topography instruments and keratometers do not measure corneal power precisely because they do not assess the posterior corneal surface. Instead, these instruments estimate total corneal power by assuming a constant relationship between the anterior and posterior corneal surfaces. This constancy is disrupted by keratorefractive surgery. For example, after myopic excimer surgery, the anterior corneal curvature is flattened. At the same time, the posterior corneal surface remains unchanged or, owing to the reduction in corneal pachymetry and weakening of the cornea, the posterior corneal surface may become slightly steeper than the preoperative posterior corneal curvature, increasing its negative power. The decrease in positive anterior corneal power and the (minimal) increase in negative posterior corneal power cause an increase in the relative contribution to the overall corneal refractive power of the posterior surface.

The removal of even a small amount of tissue (eg, a few micrometers) during keratorefractive surgery may cause a substantial change in refraction (Fig 6-3). The Munnerlyn formula approximates these 2 parameters:

$$t = \frac{S^2 D}{3}$$

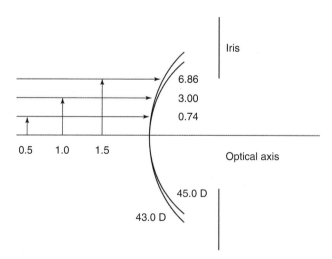

Figure 6-3 Comparison of a 43 D cornea with a 45 D cornea. Numbers below the *vertical arrows* indicate distance from the optical axis in millimeters; numbers to the right of the *horizontal arrows* indicate the separation between the corneas in micrometers. A typical pupil size of 3.0 mm is indicated. A typical red blood cell has a diameter of 7 μm. Within the pupillary space (ie, the optical zone of the cornea), the separation between the corneas is less than the diameter of a red blood cell. *(Courtesy of Edmond H. Thall, MD. Modified by C. H. Wooley.)*

where *t* is the depth of the central ablation in micrometers, *S* is the diameter of the optical zone in millimeters, and *D* is the degree of refractive correction in diopters.

An ideal LASIK ablation or PRK removes a convex positive meniscus in corrections of myopia (Fig 6-4A) and a concave positive meniscus in simple corrections of hyperopia (Fig 6-4B). A toric positive meniscus is removed in corrections of astigmatism. In toric corrections, the specific shape of the ablation depends on the spherical component of the refractive error.

Azar DT, ed. Gatinel D, Hoang-Xuan T, associate eds. *Refractive Surgery.* 2nd ed. St Louis: Elsevier-Mosby; 2007.

Azar DT, Primack JD. Theoretical analysis of ablation depths and profiles in laser in situ keratomileusis for compound hyperopic and mixed astigmatism. *J Cataract Refract Surg.* 2000;26(8):1123–1136.

Klyce S. Night vision after LASIK: the pupil proclaims innocence. *Ophthalmology.* 2004;111(1):1–2.

Munnerlyn CR, Koons SJ, Marshall J. Photorefractive keratectomy: a technique for laser refractive surgery. *J Cataract Refract Surg.* 1988;14(1):46–52.

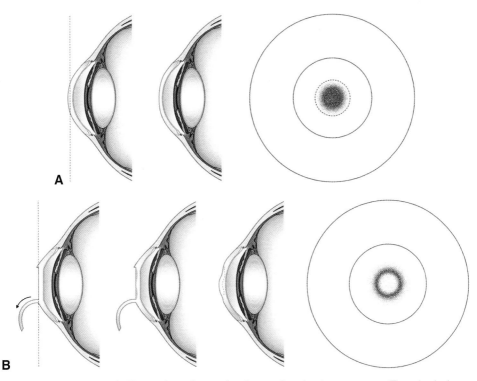

Figure 6-4 **A,** Schematic illustration of myopic photorefractive keratectomy. The shaded area refers to the location of tissue subtraction. More stromal tissue is removed in the central than in the paracentral region. **B,** Schematic illustration of hyperopic laser in situ keratomileusis. A superficial corneal flap is raised. The shaded area refers to the location of tissue subtraction under the thin flap. After treatment, the flap is repositioned. *(Used with permission from Poothullil AM, Azar DT. Terminology, classification, and history of refractive surgery. In: Azar DT, ed. Gatinel D, Hoang-Xuan T, associate eds. Refractive Surgery. 2nd ed. St Louis: Elsevier-Mosby; 2007:5–6. Figs 1-4, 1-5.)*

Angle Kappa

As discussed in Chapter 2, the pupillary axis is the imaginary line that is perpendicular to the corneal surface and passes through the midpoint of the entrance pupil. The visual axis is the imaginary line that connects the point of fixation to the fovea. The angle kappa (κ) is defined as the angle between the pupillary axis and the visual axis. A large angle kappa results from a significant difference between the pupillary axis and the central corneal apex. If the angle kappa is large, centering an excimer ablation over the geometric center of the cornea will effectively result in a decentered ablation. This can be particularly problematic in a hyperopic correction, in which a large angle kappa can result in a refractively significant "second corneal apex," causing monocular diplopia and decreased quality of vision. A large angle kappa must be identified before surgery to reduce the likelihood of a poor visual outcome.

Freedman KA, Brown SM, Mathews SM, Young RS. Pupil size and the ablation zone in laser refractive surgery: considerations based on geometric optics. *J Cataract Refract Surg.* 2003;29(10):1924–1931.

Pupil Size

Pupil size measurement is becoming the standard of care in preoperative evaluations, prompted by observations that some patients with large pupils (>8 mm) reported difficulties with night vision after undergoing keratorefractive surgery. Typical symptoms included the appearance of glare, starbursts, and halos; decreased contrast sensitivity; and poor overall quality of vision. Night-vision problems tended to occur in patients with both large pupils and small treatment zones (≤6 mm). The algorithms used in third-generation lasers, however, incorporate larger optical and transition zones, enabling surgeons to perform refractive procedures on patients with larger pupils. Use of these algorithms has dramatically decreased the incidence and severity of night-vision problems.

Many surgeons use default ablation zones during excimer procedures. The accepted standard transition zone between ablated and unablated cornea is 0.5–1.0 mm larger than the pupil; use of this zone helps minimize night-vision problems. To conserve corneal tissue, smaller optical zones are typically used in higher myopic corrections. In patients who require such corrections, the incidence of night-vision problems increases in part because of the mismatch between the size of the pupil and that of the optical zone.

Although pupil size does not affect surgical outcome as significantly as it once did, pupil size measurement continues to be the standard of care in preoperative evaluation. Patients with extremely large pupils (≥8 mm) should be identified and counseled about the potential for increased risk of complications. Spherical aberration may be increased in these patients. Clinical management of postoperative night-vision problems includes the use of a miotic such as brimonidine (0.2%) or pilocarpine (0.5%–1%).

Freedman KA, Brown SM, Mathews SM, Young RS. Pupil size and the ablation zone in laser refractive surgery: considerations based on geometric optics. *J Cataract Refract Surg.* 2003;29(10):1924–1931.

Klyce S. Night vision after LASIK: the pupil proclaims innocence. *Ophthalmology.* 2004;111(1):1–2.

Lee YC, Hu FR, Wang IJ. Quality of vision after laser in situ keratomileusis: influence of dioptric correction and pupil size on visual function. *J Cataract Refract Surg.* 2003;29(4):769–777.

Schallhorn SC, Kaupp SE, Tanzer DJ, Tidwell J, Laurent J, Bourque LB. Pupil size and quality of vision after LASIK. *Ophthalmology.* 2003;110(8):1606–1614.

Irregular Astigmatism

The treatment of postoperative irregular corneal astigmatism is a substantial challenge in refractive surgery. The diagnosis of irregular astigmatism is made by meeting clinical and imaging criteria: loss of spectacle best-corrected vision but preservation of vision with the use of a gas-permeable contact lens, coupled with topographic corneal irregularity. An important sign of postsurgical irregular astigmatism is a refraction that is inconsistent with the uncorrected visual acuity. For example, consider a patient who has –3.50 D myopia with essentially no astigmatism before the operation. After keratorefractive surgery, the patient has an uncorrected visual acuity of 20/25 but a refraction of +2.00 –3.00 × 060. Ordinarily, such a refraction would be inconsistent with an uncorrected visual acuity of 20/25, but it can occur in patients who have irregular astigmatism after keratorefractive surgery.

Another important sign is the difficulty of determining axis location during manifest refraction in patients with a high degree of astigmatism. Normally, determining the correcting cylinder axis accurately in a patient with significant cylinder is easy; however, patients with irregular astigmatism after keratorefractive surgery often have difficulty choosing an axis. Automated refractors may identify high degrees of astigmatism that are rejected by patients on manifest refraction. Because their astigmatism is irregular (and thus has no definite axis), these patients may achieve almost the same visual acuity with high powers of cylinder at various axes. Streak retinoscopy often demonstrates irregular "scissoring" in patients with irregular astigmatism.

Results of astigmatic enhancements (ie, astigmatic keratotomy, LASIK) are unpredictable for patients with irregular astigmatism. Avoid "chasing your tail" in keratorefractive surgery. For instance, a surgeon may be tempted to perform an astigmatic enhancement on a patient who had little preexisting astigmatism but significant postoperative astigmatism. If, however, the patient is happy with the uncorrected visual acuity (despite irregular astigmatism), avoiding further intervention may be preferable. In such cases, the stigmatic enhancement may cause the axis to change dramatically without substantially reducing cylinder power.

Irregular astigmatism can be quantified in much the same way as is regular astigmatism. We think of regular astigmatism as a cylinder superimposed on a sphere. Irregular astigmatism, then, can be thought of as additional shapes superimposed on cylinders and spheres. This approach is widely used in optical engineering.

Application of Wavefront Analysis in Irregular Astigmatism

Refractive surgeons derive some benefit from having a thorough understanding of irregular astigmatism, for 2 reasons. First, keratorefractive surgery may lead to visually significant irregular astigmatism in a small percentage of cases. Second, keratorefractive surgery may also be able to treat it. For irregular astigmatism to be studied effectively, it must be described quantitatively. Wavefront analysis is an effective method for such descriptions of irregular astigmatism.

An understanding of irregular astigmatism and wavefront analysis begins with stigmatic imaging. A stigmatic imaging system brings all the rays from a single object point to a perfect point focus. According to the Fermat principle, a stigmatic focus is possible only when the time required for light to travel from an object point to an image point is identical for all the possible paths that the light may take.

An analogy to a footrace is helpful. Suppose that several runners simultaneously depart from an object point (A). Each runner follows a different path, represented by a ray. All the runners travel at the same speed in air, just as all rays travel at the same (but slower) speed in glass. If all the runners reach the image point (B) simultaneously, the "image" is stigmatic. If the rays do not meet at point B, then the "image" is astigmatic.

The Fermat principle explains how a lens works. The rays that pass through the center of a lens travel a short distance in air but slow down when they move through the thickest part of the glass. Rays that pass through the edge of a lens travel a longer distance in air but slow down only briefly when traversing the thinnest section of the glass. The shape of the ideal lens precisely balances each path so that no matter what path the light travels, it reaches point B in the same amount of time. If the lens shape is not ideal, however, some rays reach point B at a certain time point and other rays do not; this focus is termed *astigmatic*.

Wavefront analysis is based on the Fermat principle. Construct a circular arc centered on the paraxial image point and intersecting the center of the exit pupil (Fig 6-5A). This arc is called the *reference sphere*. Again, consider the analogy of a footrace, but now think of the reference sphere (rather than a point) as the finish line. If the image is stigmatic, all runners starting from a single point will cross the reference sphere simultaneously. If the image is astigmatic, the runners will cross the reference sphere at slightly different times (Fig 6-5B). The *geometric wavefront* is analogous to a photo finish of the race. It represents the position of each runner shortly after the fastest runner crosses the finish line. The *wavefront aberration* of each runner is the time at which the runner finishes minus the time of the fastest runner. In other words, it is the difference between the reference sphere and the wavefront. When the focus is stigmatic, the reference sphere and the wavefront coincide, so that the wavefront aberration is zero.

Wavefront aberration is a function of pupil position. Figure 6-6 shows some typical wavefront aberrations. Myopia, hyperopia, and regular astigmatism can be expressed as wavefront aberrations. Myopia produces an aberration that optical engineers call *positive defocus*. Hyperopia is called *negative defocus*. Regular (cylindrical) astigmatism produces a wavefront aberration that resembles a cylinder. Defocus (myopia and hyperopia) and regular astigmatism constitute the lower-order aberrations.

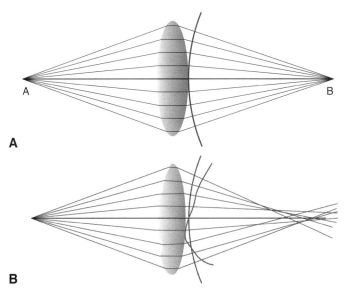

Figure 6-5 **A,** The reference sphere *(in red)* is represented in 2 dimensions by a circular arc centered on point B and drawn through the center of the exit pupil of the lens. If the image is stigmatic, all light from point A crosses the reference sphere simultaneously. **B,** When the image is astigmatic, light rays from the object point simultaneously cross the wavefront *(in blue),* not the reference sphere. *(Courtesy of Edmond H. Thall, MD; part B modified by C. H. Wooley.)*

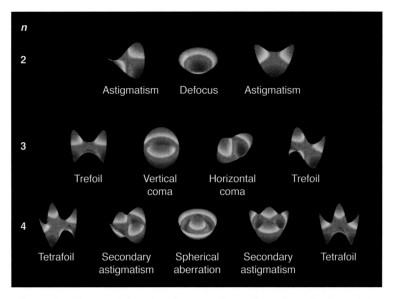

Figure 6-6 Second-, third-, and fourth-order wavefront aberrations (indicated by *n* values 2, 3, and 4, respectively) are most pertinent to refractive surgery. *(Reproduced with permission from Applegate RA. Glenn Fry Award Lecture 2002: wavefront sensing, ideal corrections, and visual performance. Optom Vis Sci. 2004;81(3):169.)*

When peripheral rays focus in front of more central rays, the effect is termed *spherical aberration*. Clinically, spherical aberration is one of the main causes of night myopia following LASIK and PRK.

Another important aberration is *coma*. In this aberration, rays at one edge of the pupil cross the reference sphere first; rays at the opposite edge of the pupil cross last. The effect is that the image of each object point resembles a comet with a tail (one meaning of the word *coma* is "comet"). Coma also arises in patients with decentered keratorefractive ablation. It is commonly observed in the aiming beam during retinal laser photocoagulation; if the ophthalmologist tilts the lens too far off-axis, the aiming beam spot becomes coma shaped.

Higher-order aberrations tend to be less significant than lower-order aberrations, but the higher-order ones may worsen in diseased or surgically altered eyes. For example, if interrupted sutures are used to sew in a corneal graft during corneal transplant, they will produce higher-order, clover-shaped aberrations. Also, in the manufacture of intraocular lenses, the lens blank is sometimes improperly positioned on the lathe; such improper positioning can also produce higher-order aberrations.

Optical engineers have found approximately 18 basic types of astigmatism, of which only some—perhaps as few as 5—are of clinical interest. Most patients probably have a combination of all 5 types.

Wavefront aberrations can be represented in different ways. One approach is to show them as 3-dimensional shapes. Another is to represent them as contour plots. Irregular astigmatism can be described as a combination of a few basic shapes, just as conventional refractive error represents a combination of a sphere and a cylinder. The approach used by ophthalmologists does not use graphs or contour plots to represent conventional refractive errors. Instead, ophthalmologists simply specify the extent of sphere and cylinder that make up the refractive error. Similarly, once ophthalmologists are comfortable with the basic forms of irregular astigmatism, they have little need for 3-dimensional graphs or 2-dimensional contour plots. They simply specify the degree of each basic form of astigmatism in a given patient. Prescriptions of the future may consist of 8 or so numbers: the first 3 may be sphere, cylinder, and axis; and the remaining 5 may specify the irregular astigmatism as quantitated by higher-order aberration.

Currently, wavefront aberrations are specified by *Zernike polynomials,* which are the mathematical formulas used to describe wavefront surfaces. *Wavefront aberration surfaces* are graphs generated using Zernike polynomials. There are several techniques for measuring wavefront aberrations clinically, but the most popular is based on the *Hartmann-Shack wavefront sensor.* In this device, a low-power laser beam is focused on the retina. A point on the retina then acts as a point source. In a perfect eye, all the rays would emerge in parallel and the wavefront would be a flat plane. In reality, the wavefront is not flat. An array of lenses sample parts of the wavefront and focus light on a detector. The wavefront shape can be determined from the position of the focus on each detector (eg, see Fig 1-6 in BCSC Section 13, *Refractive Surgery*).

Another method of measuring wavefront aberrations is a ray-tracing method that projects detecting light beams sequentially rather than simultaneously, as in a Hartmann-Shack device, further improving the resolution of wavefront aberration measurements. The application of Zernike polynomials' mathematical descriptions of aberrations to the human eye is less than perfect, however, and alternative methods, such as Fourier transform, are being utilized in many wavefront aberrometers.

To normalize wavefront aberration measurements and improve postoperative visual quality in patients undergoing keratorefractive surgery, ophthalmologists are developing technologies to improve the accuracy of higher-order aberration measurements and treatment by using "flying spot" excimer lasers. Such lasers use small spot sizes (<1-mm diameter) to create smooth ablations, addressing the minute topographic changes associated with aberration errors.

For a more detailed discussion of the topics covered in this subsection, see BCSC Section 13, *Refractive Surgery*.

Causes of Irregular Astigmatism

Irregular astigmatism may be present before keratorefractive surgery; it may be caused by the surgery; or it may develop postoperatively. Preoperative causes include keratoconus, pellucid marginal degeneration, contact lens warpage, dry eye, and epithelial basement membrane dystrophy (Fig 6-7). All these conditions should be identified before surgery. Common intraoperative causes include decentered ablations and central islands, and, less commonly, poor laser optics, nonuniform stromal bed hydration, and LASIK flap complications (a thin, torn, irregular, incomplete, or buttonhole flap; folds or striae of the flap; and epithelial defects). Postoperative causes of irregular astigmatism include flap displacement, diffuse lamellar keratitis and its sequelae, flap striae, posterior corneal ectasia, irregular wound healing, dry eye, and flap edema.

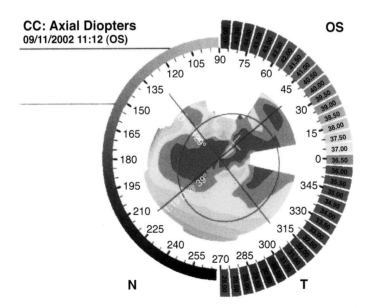

Figure 6-7 Irregular astigmatism in a corneal topographic map of the left eye of a patient with significant epithelial basement membrane dystrophy. The patient experienced glare and a general decline in quality of vision. Simulated *K* shows the flattest meridian at 39° and the steeper meridian at 129°. N = nasal; T = temporal. *(Courtesy of Ming Wang, MD.)*

Conclusion

Incorporating optical considerations into the treatment of patients undergoing keratore-fractive surgery is important to enhance the visual results. Patient dissatisfaction after surgery, albeit rare, often stems from the subjective loss of visual quality, the source of which can usually be identified through a sound understanding of how refractive surgery alters the optics of the eye. A good understanding of key parameters such as corneal shape, pupil size, the ocular surface, spherical and astigmatic errors, higher-order aberrations, laser centration and the angle kappa, and irregular corneal astigmatism can help optimize visual outcomes after keratorefractive surgery.

Chapter Exercises

Questions

6.1. The Munnerlyn formula approximates the depth of excimer laser tissue ablation:

$$t = \frac{S^2 D}{3}$$

where t is the central ablation depth in micrometers, S is the diameter of the optical zone in millimeters, and D is the degree of refractive correction in diopters. For a LASIK patient with a refractive correction of −6.00 D and a central corneal thickness of 520 μm, and for whom the LASIK flap thickness is 120 μm, an extremely conservative surgeon would not want to have a residual stromal bed (RSB) thickness of less than 300 μm. According to the Munnerlyn formula, what is the largest optical zone diameter that can be used for this treatment?

6.2. For the situation described in Question 6.1, what is the largest optical zone diameter that can be used if PRK, rather than LASIK, is planned? Assume an epithelium thickness of 58 μm and an RSB thickness of 300 μm.

6.3. A patient with a preoperative manifest refraction of −3.50 D, normal keratometry (K) readings, and a pachymetry measurement of 550 μm undergoes keratorefractive surgery. Three months postoperatively, the patient has an uncorrected visual acuity of 20/30 with a refraction of +2.00 −3.00 × 0.60 associated with postsurgical irregular astigmatism. What are the important signs that will aid in reaching a diagnosis?

   a. difficulty in determining axis location during manifest refraction
   b. discrepancy between automated refraction and manifest refraction
   c. no improvement or change in visual acuity with large powers of cylinder at markedly different axes
   d. all of the above

6.4. Corneal asphericity is represented by Q value. A spherical cornea with asphericity of $Q = 0$ is associated with
   a. better visual acuity than a prolate cornea
   b. improved optics if keratorefractive surgery results in postoperative $Q = -0.3$
   c. improved optics if keratorefractive surgery results in postoperative $Q = 0$
   d. improved optics if keratorefractive surgery results in postoperative $Q = +0.3$
6.5. A patient undergoing an evaluation for refractive surgery has K readings of 43.0 D/42.0 D and a manifest refraction of −9.50 D. If LASIK were performed, you would expect the postoperative average keratometry reading to be approximately
   a. 34.9 D
   b. 36.3 D
   c. 37.3 D
   d. 34.0 D

Answers

6.1. Pachymetry value = t + LASIK flap thickness + RSB thickness = t + 120 μm + 300 μm. This implies that t = 100 μm. Then, t = 100 = $S^2 \times 6/3$, which implies that S^2 = 50. Therefore, S = 7.1 mm; that is, the largest diameter that can be used for LASIK treatment in this situation by this surgeon is 7.1 mm.
6.2. Pachymetry value = t + epithelium thickness + RSB thickness. This implies that t = 520 μm − 58 μm − 300 μm = 162 μm. Because t = $S^2 \times 6/3$, this implies that S^2 = 162/2 = 81; thus, S = 9 mm, the largest diameter that can be used for PRK treatment in this situation by this surgeon.
6.3. **d.** all of the above
6.4. **b.** improved optics if keratorefractive surgery results in postoperative $Q = -0.3$
6.5. **a.** 34.9 D. The formula for keratometry change is approximately = 0.8 × refractive change. Here, the keratometry change = 0.8 × −9.50 D = −7.6 D, so the calculated final postoperative average is K = (43.0 D + 42.0 D)/2 − 7.6 D = 34.9 D.

CHAPTER 7

Optical Instruments and Low Vision Aids

In this chapter, we discuss magnification, telescopes, and other concepts of optical engineering and then explain the design of various instruments used to examine the eye. After that, the chapter describes various optical and nonoptical aids available to assist patients with impaired vision.

Magnification

The magnification an optical system provides may be defined several different ways. Three of these are as follows:

1. transverse magnification perpendicular to an optical axis
2. axial magnification along an optical axis
3. angular magnification, which is a measure of an instrument's ability to provide the viewer's retina with an enlarged image

Transverse (linear, lateral) magnification is the height of the image with respect to the optical axis divided by the height of the object with respect to the optical axis. *Axial magnification,* the change of depth along the axis, is the square of the transverse magnification. *Angular magnification* differs from transverse and axial magnification in that it is not a comparison of the size of an image to the size of an object. Angular magnification is a comparison of the size of the retinal image of an object viewed with and without an optical instrument; it is defined as the angle subtended at the nodal point of the viewing eye by an object viewed through an instrument, divided by the angle subtended by the same object when viewed by the naked eye. Increasing this angle proportionally increases the size of the image on the viewer's retina so that finer details can be discriminated.

The simple magnifier is a special case of angular magnification. An object is placed at the primary focal plane of a plus lens, so that a pencil of rays emanating from any point on the object emerges from the lens with its rays parallel, ready for viewing by the emmetropic eye (Fig 7-1). Magnification of the simple magnifier is defined to be the quotient of 2 angles. The numerator is the angle subtended at the eye by the object as seen through the magnifying glass, while the object is positioned at the focal length of the magnifier lens and the viewing eye is somewhere on the other side of the lens. The denominator is the angle subtended at the eye by the object when it is viewed 25 cm (one-fourth meter) from the eye without the magnifier (Fig 7-2). Assuming small angles, we therefore divide the

Figure 7-1 A plus lens used to view an object positioned in the focal plane of the lens. O = object; f = focal length. *(Redrawn from Basic and Clinical Science Course Section 2: Optics, Refraction, and Contact Lenses. San Francisco: American Academy of Ophthalmology; 1986–1987:73. Fig 43.)*

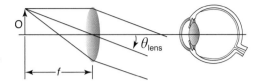

Figure 7-2 The reference viewing distance of 25 cm, used in the definition of magnification of simple magnifiers. *(Redrawn from Basic and Clinical Science Course Section 2: Optics, Refraction, and Contact Lenses. San Francisco: American Academy of Ophthalmology; 1986–1987:73. Fig 44.)*

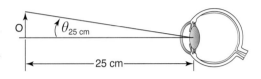

focal length of the lens by 4. Thus, a +10 D lens is considered a 2.5× magnifier and is held one-tenth of a meter, its focal length, from the object of interest. Note that rays coming from the object leave the magnifier with zero vergence, so that the user of the magnifier can gaze through it from any distance she prefers.

Telescopes

A telescope is an optical system designed to increase the angle subtended at the eye by distant objects. It is called *afocal* because pencils of light entering with zero vergence come out with zero vergence. The first lens, the *objective,* forms an image of the distant object. The second lens, the *eyepiece* or *ocular,* is then used to view the image formed by the objective. With small-angle approximations, a telescope's angular magnification (or "minification," if you look through the telescope turned the other way around) is the longer focal length of the objective divided by the shorter focal length of the ocular, with a minus sign to enable us to figure out whether the final image is upright or inverted:

$$\text{Angular Magnification of Telescope} = \frac{-f_{obj}}{f_{eye}}$$

$$= \frac{-P_{eye}}{P_{obj}}$$

where

f_{obj} = focal length of objective
f_{eye} = focal length of eyepiece
P_{eye} = power of eyepiece
P_{obj} = power of objective

Galilean Telescope

In a Galilean telescope, the objective is a plus lens, and the eyepiece is a minus lens. Bundles of rays with approximately zero vergence, emanating from various points on a distant object, pass through a low-power plus *objective lens.* Before the rays are able to arrive to focus at the secondary focal point of the first lens, they meet a higher-power minus lens, the eyepiece, which has been placed so that its primary focal point coincides with the secondary focal point of the first lens. Thus, the rays leave the second lens with no vergence, and the telescope is therefore said to be afocal (Fig 7-3). The image is magnified and upright.

The distance separating the eyepiece from the objective, which is the length of the telescope, equals the difference between the focal lengths of the objective and the eyepiece.

Astronomical Telescope

In an astronomical, or *Keplerian,* telescope, both the objective and the eyepiece are plus lenses. Light without vergence enters a low-power objective lens, just as in the Galilean telescope. Whereas in the Galilean telescope a minus lens is placed in the path before the light reaches its secondary focal point, in the astronomical telescope a stronger, convex lens is placed beyond the secondary focal point of the first convex lens, with its primary focal point coinciding with the secondary focal point of the first lens. The distance separating the eyepiece from the objective is the sum of the focal lengths of the objective and the eyepiece. Once again, we have an afocal system; rays that enter with zero vergence exit with zero vergence. A large low-power objective lens collects relatively large-angle pencils of light from a distant object; in particular, it collects more of the light coming from that object than would enter the viewer's smaller entrance pupil without the telescope (Fig 7-4).

The image seen through the astronomical telescope is inverted as well as magnified. If we wish to render the image upright, we must invert it again by passing the light path through at least one more lens or through a set of internally reflecting prisms such as those inside typical binoculars. Because they "fold" the light path, the prisms used in binoculars

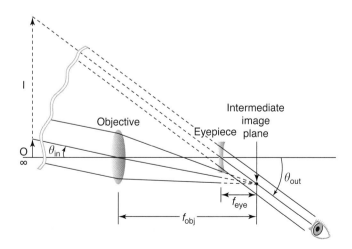

Figure 7-3 Galilean telescope. *(Redrawn from Guyton D, West C, Miller J, Wisnicki H. Ophthalmic Optics and Clinical Refraction. London: Prism Press;1999:39.)*

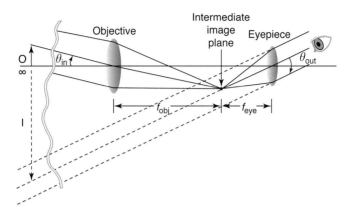

Figure 7-4 Astronomical telescope. *(Redrawn from Guyton D, West C, Miller J, Wisnicki H. Ophthalmic Optics and Clinical Refraction. London: Prism Press; 1999:39.)*

also enable the binoculars to be more compact and to have the right and left objective lenses spread farther apart than the viewer's eyes, enhancing the perception of depth. Note that the minus sign in the formula for the telescope's angular magnification yields, as it should, a positive power for the Galilean telescope's upright image and a negative power for the astronomical telescope's inverted image.

Accommodation Through a Telescope

If you look at an object one-third of a meter away, your otherwise emmetropic eye must accommodate 3 diopters. If you look at the same object one-third of a meter away through an afocal telescope, you have to accommodate much more: the accommodation required through the telescope is the usual amount, 3 D, multiplied by the square of the magnification of the telescope. For instance, the accommodation required through a 2× telescope would be $3 \times (2)^2 = 12$ D, which is too difficult for an adult to achieve. Therefore, in order to enable us to see near objects through a telescope, we need to alter the telescope, in the manner we next describe, to form a loupe.

Surgical Loupe

We can make an afocal telescope into a surgical loupe with a working distance of one-third meter by adding a +3 D lens to the front of the telescope. The +3 D lens is called a *collimating lens* because its purpose is to redirect the rays of pencils of light diverging from an object one-third of a meter away so that they have zero vergence, before they enter the telescope. Because the telescope is afocal, the pencils of light will have zero vergence again when they exit the telescope, and a surgeon with emmetropic vision can effortlessly view the object and see it as larger, thanks to the angular magnification. The +3 D additional power can be added to the power of the objective lens instead of adding an additional lens in front of the afocal telescope (Fig 7-5).

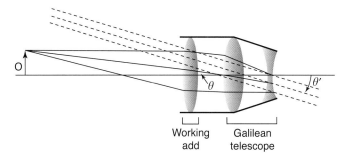

Figure 7-5 The surgical loupe. The working add first collimates the light from the tip of the object, O. This bundle of collimated light enters the Galilean telescope at a particular angle, θ, to the optical axis. The same bundle emerges from the telescope still collimated but at an increased angle, θ', where the magnifying power of the telescope is equal to the ratio of θ' to θ. The tip of the object is seen by the eye as if it were at infinity, with the entire object subtending the angle θ'. *(Redrawn from Basic and Clinical Science Course Section 2: Optics, Refraction, and Contact Lenses. San Francisco: American Academy of Ophthalmology; 1986–1987:74. Fig 45.)*

General Principles of Optical Engineering

More-elaborate designs of telescopes and microscopes use additional lenses, perhaps aspheric, to adjust the distance to the object (working distance) and combat the blurring caused by monochromatic and chromatic aberrations and diffraction. Apertures and antireflective lens coatings serve to eliminate undesirable rays.

Terminology

This section introduces some terminology you are likely to encounter elsewhere.

The *aperture stop* of an optical system is the opening—which could be the rim of one of its lenses or an empty diaphragm—whose edges limit the angular breadth of the pencils of light that are allowed to pass through the system to form the image of an object. For instance, the pupil of the eye serves as its aperture stop and opens in dim conditions to allow broader pencils of light to enter.

The *field of view* of a multi-element optical system is the visible extent of the image plane. For example, a typical pair of binoculars might have a field of view of 7 degrees—objects outside that field cannot be seen without turning the binoculars toward them. When a 2× condensing lens is used with the indirect ophthalmoscope, the field of view is 2 times larger in degrees than with a 4× condensing lens of the same diameter. Twice the diameter of the field viewed gives 4 times as much area.

When you look at someone's pupil through the cornea and aqueous, the pupil appears to be larger and closer than it truly is. What you are seeing is the *entrance pupil* of the eye's optical system—the image of the eye's aperture stop, the pupil, viewed through the optical elements that precede it in the system. Rays that do not pass through the eye's entrance pupil cannot reach the retina because they are unable to pass the aperture stop, which is the pupil of the eye.

For an observer to see the entire field of view of an optical instrument, his or her entrance pupil needs to be located at the instrument's exit pupil, which is the image of its aperture stop formed by the optical elements following it in the system. The distance from the last surface of the eyepiece to that exit pupil is called the *eye relief* of the instrument.

In the preceding section, we discussed the adjustment of working distance to form a loupe. Suppose an object is well focused on the loupe's image plane; how much closer or farther away can we move the object without noticeable blurring of the image? The distance the object can be moved is the system's *depth of field. Depth of focus,* on the other hand, is the amount of leeway on the image side of the system; for example, it refers to how near or far you can move a screen relative to a focused projector before the image becomes noticeably out of focus.

Measurements of Performance of Optical Systems

The *f-stop* of a lens, familiar to photographers, and a related concept, the *numerical aperture,* are measures of light gathering. Light gathering is important not only in generating a bright image of a dim source; it is also related to the resolving power of an instrument—how close together 2 points can be on an object before they become indistinguishable in the image. If a higher-power instrument does not take in a wide-angled pencil of light from each of the 2 nearby points, no matter how carefully the instrument is constructed, the diffraction patterns coming from the 2 points will overlap too much to be distinguished from each other. For example, the oil immersion objective of a microscope has a higher numerical aperture than a dry objective, which means that it can gather a wider angle of light from each point source and therefore have the potential for better resolution.

Light beginning at a point source and passing through a focused optical system does not all focus to the same image point because of aberrations and diffraction. The spread-out luminance that is detected is called the *point spread function.* The *modulation transfer function (MTF)* of an optical system is a measure of its ability to preserve an object's contrast, such as that of a sinusoidal pattern of light and dark, in the image that comes out of the system. This ability varies with the spatial frequency of the pattern being imaged, and the MTF helps a designer choose the best optical elements for the purpose at hand.

Optical Instruments and Techniques Used in Ophthalmic Practice

Direct Ophthalmoscope

Suppose you want to look at my retina and that we both have eyes that are emmetropic and not accommodating. A pencil of rays coming from a point on my retina leaves my eye with zero vergence, and the pencil continues to have no vergence until it reaches your eye, which focuses it exactly on your retina. When you look through the peephole of a direct ophthalmoscope with no lenses in place, just past the edge of a mirror that reflects light into my eye, almost coaxial to your view, you will see an upright, virtual, magnified image of a small portion of my retina; our retinas are on conjugate planes. The optics of the eye are approximately +60 D, so the magnification is 60/4, or 15×, as we have defined

magnification for a simple magnifier. In case either of us has an uncorrected spherical refractive error, a wheel of spherical lenses is available to dial into the path. If the subject eye
is myopic, the extra plus power of the eye's optics and the minus power dialed into place
in the ophthalmoscope together form a Galilean telescope, increasing magnification and
decreasing the field of view. Similarly, the retina of a hyperopic eye will be magnified less
than 15× because of the reverse Galilean telescope created by the optics of the eye and the
lens of the direct ophthalmoscope. A retinal lesion elevated 1 mm will be approximately
3 D out of focus when viewed with the direct ophthalmoscope (Fig 7-6).

Indirect Ophthalmoscope

In an indirect ophthalmoscope, mirrors direct a bright light toward the subject's retina
through, for instance, a 20 D lens and the subject's eye. The lens has an aspheric design on
one side and antireflective coatings to minimize aberrations and glare. Assuming that the
subject eye is emmetropic, a pencil of light coming from an illuminated point on the retina
leaves the eye with zero vergence (Fig 7-7A). The pencil of light is gathered and refracted
by the large +20 D "condensing" lens to focus to a point one-twentieth of a meter (5 cm)
closer to the observer, who therefore sees an optically real, inverted aerial image of the
retina that appears to be 5 cm closer to her eye than the 20 D lens in her hand (Fig 7-7B).

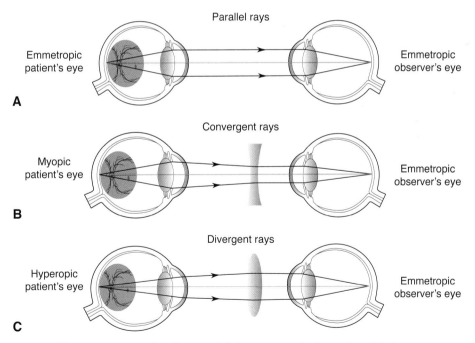

Figure 7-6 Viewing system of a direct ophthalmoscope. **A,** A bundle of light rays emerges
from the emmetropic eye with zero vergence. **B,** A bundle of light rays emerges converging
from the myopic eye with positive vergence; the corrective lens is minus. **C,** A bundle of rays
with negative vergence diverges coming out of the hyperopic eye; the corrective lens is plus.
(Developed by Neal H. Atebara, MD. Redrawn by C. H. Wooley.)

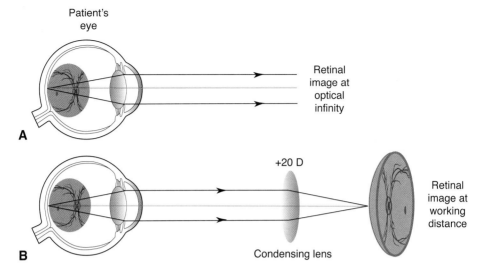

A

Patient's eye

Retinal image at optical infinity

B

+20 D

Retinal image at working distance

Condensing lens

Figure 7-7 Fundus image formation. **A,** A retinal image is formed at optical infinity. **B,** A condensing lens focuses a bundle of parallel rays to a place closer to the viewer than his or her hand. *(Developed by Neal H. Atebara, MD. Redrawn by C. H. Wooley.)*

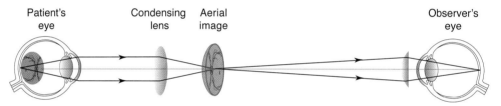

Patient's eye — Condensing lens — Aerial image — Observer's eye

Figure 7-8 The "aerial" image. The light rays focus and diverge, and they are brought to a new focus on the observer's retina by a condensing lens and the optics of the observer's eye. *(Developed by Neal H. Atebara, MD. Redrawn by C. H. Wooley.)*

If the aerial image is 50 cm from her eye, she will have to accommodate 2 D to see it, so a 2 D lens is added on the front of the ophthalmoscope (Fig 7-8).

Mirrors are used in the binocular instrument to bring an image to each of the observer's eyes, adjusting as needed for the observer's interpupillary distance. To avoid glare, it is important that the observer's pupils be conjugate with the pupil of the patient's eye, so that the illuminating and 2 viewing paths pass through the pupils of both people (Figs 7-9, 7-10). If the patient's pupil is small, the ingoing path and the 2 outgoing paths can be brought closer by varying the positions of mirrors (Fig 7-11).

This procedure can be conceived of as the observer viewing the retina through an astronomical telescope consisting of the 60 D optics of the patient's eye, which acts as the objective lens, and the 20 D lens held in the observer's hand, which acts as the eyepiece. In this case, the transverse magnification of the telescope would be 60/20 = 3×, and the axial magnification 9×.

The exaggerated depth is quartered by the mirrors, because they reduce the effective interpupillary distance from 60 mm to 15 mm, so the perception of axial magnification is only about 9/4. Condensing lenses of various powers may be used. For example,

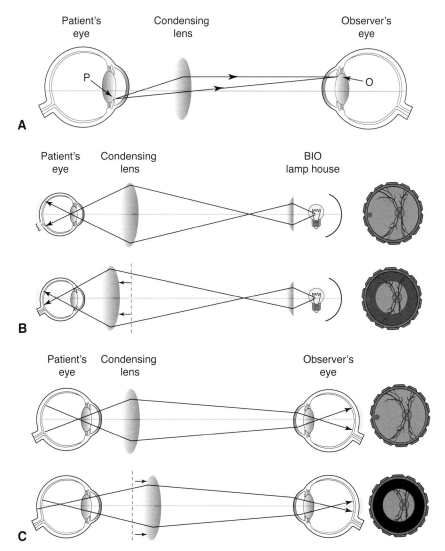

Figure 7-9 Conjugacy of pupils. **A,** In indirect ophthalmoscopy, the observer's pupil (O) and patient's pupil (P) are conjugate to avoid "wasting" light. **B,** If the condensing lens is too close to the patient's eye, the peripheral retina will not be illuminated. **C,** If the condensing lens is too far from the patient's eye, light from the patient's peripheral retina will not reach the observer's eye. *(Developed by Neal H. Atebara, MD. Redrawn by C. H. Wooley.)*

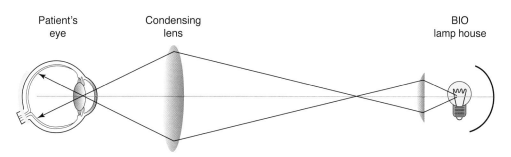

Figure 7-10 Indirect ophthalmoscope: illumination. *(Developed by Neal H. Atebara, MD. Redrawn by C. H. Wooley.)*

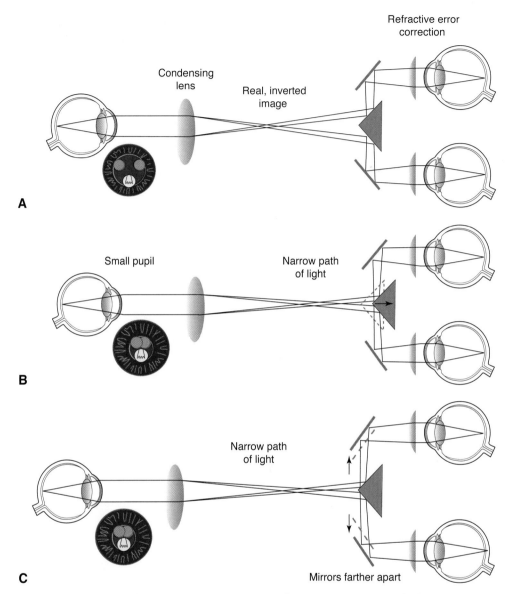

Figure 7-11 Indirect ophthalmoscope: mirrors used for binocular viewing. **A,** Binocular observation. **B,** To achieve binocularity when viewing through a small pupil, one can bring the light paths closer together by moving the triangular mirror closer to the observer. **C,** Alternatively, when viewing through a patient's small pupil, one can bring the light paths closer together by moving the eyepieces as far apart as the observer's interpupillary distance allows, or by moving the observer's head farther from the patient. *Orange circles* represent viewing paths, and *yellow circles* represent illumination paths in the black pupil. *(Developed by Neal H. Atebara, MD. Redrawn by C. H. Wooley.)*

a +30 D lens would give 2× transverse and 1× axial magnification, resulting in retinal features looking smaller and flatter and giving a larger field of view than that provided by the 20 D lens. Are the objects and images in this situation real or virtual? Rays reaching the observer's eye come from an "object" to the left of the direct ophthalmoscope's optics, so we consider that a "real" object. The indirect ophthalmoscope focuses a real image in the air to the right of itself, and the observer sees that aerial, real, inverted image with the assistance of a simple magnifier.

Fundus Camera

A fundus camera is nearly identical to the indirect ophthalmoscope; the aerial image is simply reimaged onto the camera's film or sensor array (Figs 7-12, 7-13).

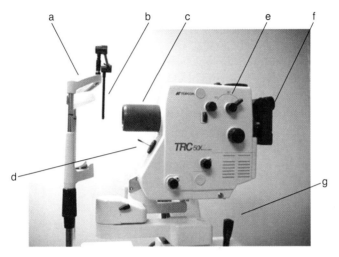

Figure 7-12 Photograph of a fundus and fluorescein angiography camera showing patient forehead rest (a), fixation light (b), objective lens (c), fixation pointer (d), magnification lever (e), camera housing and eyepiece (f), and joystick (g). *(Courtesy of Neal H. Atebara, MD.)*

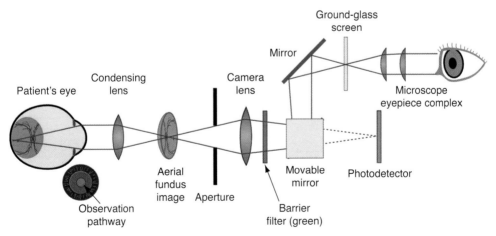

Figure 7-13 Observation system of a fundus camera. As in the observation system of an indirect ophthalmoscope, the condensing lens takes light rays from the illuminated fundus and creates an "aerial" image. A conventional single-lens reflex camera body, with its microscope eyepiece and ground-glass screen, is then used to focus on the aerial image. When the photograph is taken, a movable mirror flips up, exposing the film or photodetector. *(Courtesy of Neal H. Atebara, MD. Redrawn by C. H. Wooley.)*

Slit-Lamp Biomicroscope

In a slit-lamp biomicroscope, a system of lenses and apertures (known as *Koehler illumination*) is designed to collect the light from the device's bulb into a beam of homogeneous brightness, giving good contrast and minimal glare. The beam, limited by an adjustable slit to cut an optical section through the eye, can be rotated horizontally around the eye, as can the binocular microscope. The illuminating system and the microscope with its various levels of magnification are designed to be *parfocal*—the position of the slit lamp with respect to the eye being examined does not need to be changed as the power of the microscope is changed and the lamp and microscope are rotated around the eye.

Let's follow the outgoing light path. A pencil of rays diverging from the subject eye passes through a collimating lens so that its rays emerge parallel to each other before passing through an afocal Galilean telescope. Mirrors of internally reflecting prisms invert the image and reflect it into the eyepiece. The eyepiece is an astronomical telescope, which re-inverts the image. To vary the magnification of the system, there may be a rotating drum of Galilean telescopes that can be oriented either forward to provide higher magnification or backward to provide lower magnification, or there may be 2 sets of eyepieces. Another drum may enable the viewer, as with some indirect ophthalmoscopes, to choose a narrower angle between the microscope's 2 light paths, enabling a binocular view through a small pupil (Fig 7-14).

Features of the eye are examined in several ways (Fig 7-15):

- *Direct illumination.* Light is reflected from the object to the observer.
- *Retroillumination.* Light bouncing back toward the viewer silhouettes features, such as a cataract.
- *Sclerotic scatter.* The illumination is turned to shine a slit beam at the limbus, enabling the observer to look at the central cornea for features highlighted by the internally reflected light.
- *Specular reflection.* The corneal endothelial cell pattern can be seen by examining the partial specular reflection from the cornea–aqueous interface as a slit beam strikes it at an angle.

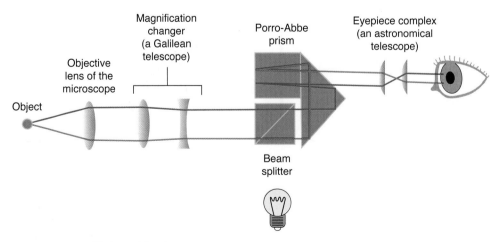

Figure 7-14 Slit-lamp biomicroscope. *(Developed by Neal H. Atebara, MD. Redrawn by C. H. Wooley.)*

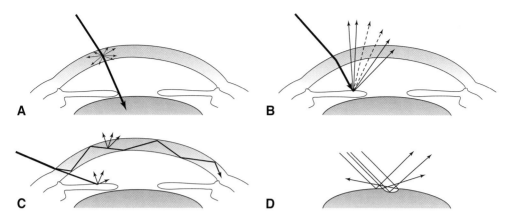

Figure 7-15 Diagram of how light rays interact with the eye in the 4 forms of slit-lamp biomicroscopic examination. **A,** Direct illumination. **B,** Retroillumination. **C,** Sclerotic scatter. **D,** Specular reflection. *(From Tasman W, Jaeger AE, eds. The slit lamp: history, principles, and practice. In:* Duane's Clinical Ophthalmology. *Philadelphia: Lippincott, 1995–1999:33. Redrawn by C. H. Wooley.)*

Auxiliary lenses for slit-lamp examination of the retina

The cornea and lens together provide so much convergence that we cannot look through them with the slit lamp and see the retina. We can overcome this problem by eliminating the corneal curvature with a flat-front contact lens (Fig 7-16). Mirrors inside such a lens provide views of more and less posterior portions of the eye (Fig 7-17). A high-minus

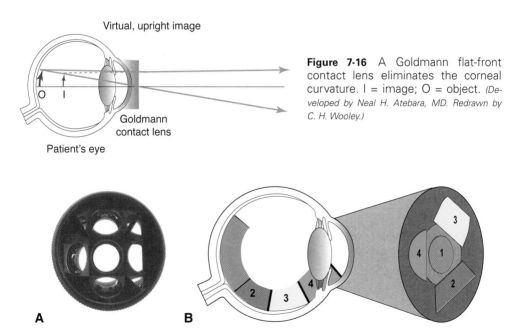

Figure 7-16 A Goldmann flat-front contact lens eliminates the corneal curvature. I = image; O = object. *(Developed by Neal H. Atebara, MD. Redrawn by C. H. Wooley.)*

Figure 7-17 Mirrors at various angles inside a flat-front contact lens for viewing different parts of the retina and the anterior chamber angle. **A,** Goldmann 3-mirror contact lens (observer's view). **B,** Schematic diagram of the part of the eye that can be seen with the central contact lens (1), midperipheral fundus mirror (2), peripheral fundus mirror (3), and iridocorneal angle mirror (4). *(Both parts courtesy of Neal H. Atebara, MD. Part B redrawn by C. H. Wooley.)*

(Hruby –55 D) lens is positioned in the air in front of the cornea (Fig 7-18) and yields a view that is not inverted. Indirect ophthalmoscopy at the slit lamp is accomplished either by holding a high-plus lens in front of the cornea to produce an inverted, aerial, real image (Fig 7-19) or by placing a panfundoscopic contact lens on the cornea (Fig 7-20), which produces an inverted, real image inside itself. Aspheric lenses are designed to minimize aberrations for their specific uses.

Gonioscopy

Unless a gonioscopy lens is placed on the eye, the anterior chamber angle is hidden from view by total internal reflection (TIR; see Chapter 1). This problem is solved by use of a contact lens with a mirror or a contact lens allowing direct viewing at an angle less than the critical angle (Fig 7-21).

Surgical Microscope

The viewing optics of an operating microscope are similar to those of the slit lamp. The illumination is "coaxial," running near the viewing paths.

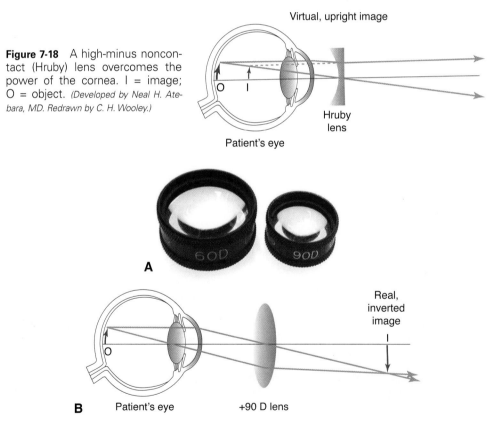

Figure 7-18 A high-minus noncontact (Hruby) lens overcomes the power of the cornea. I = image; O = object. *(Developed by Neal H. Atebara, MD. Redrawn by C. H. Wooley.)*

Figure 7-19 High-power plus lenses for slit-lamp indirect ophthalmoscopy. **A,** 60 D and 90 D fundus lenses. **B,** The lenses produce real, inverted images of the retina within the focal range of a slit-lamp biomicroscope. I = image; O = object. *(Both parts courtesy of Neal H. Atebara, MD. Part B redrawn by C. H. Wooley.)*

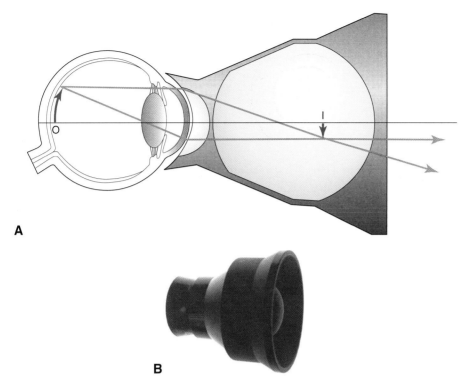

Figure 7-20 **A,** A panfundoscope lens consists of a corneal contact lens and a high-power, spherical condensing lens. A real, inverted image of the fundus is formed within the spherical glass element, which is within the focal range of a slit-lamp biomicroscope. I = image; O = object. **B,** Photograph of the panfundoscope lens. *(Both parts courtesy of Neal H. Atebara, MD. Part A redrawn by C. H. Wooley.)*

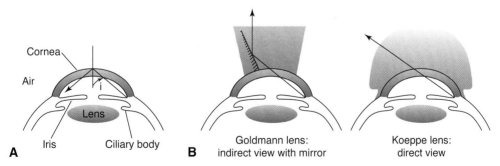

Figure 7-21 Gonioscopy. **A,** At the anterior corneal surface, rays from the anterior chamber angle are incident at greater than the critical angle of cornea in air. Therefore, these rays are totally internally reflected. **B,** The contact lens curvature approximately matches the cornea, the space between the lens and the cornea being filled with an aqueous solution of methylcellulose or with tears, which have a refractive index close to that of the cornea. Light can then traverse the interface with little lost to reflection, as the critical angle at the interface is now nearly 90°. On the left is a contact lens with an internal mirror, reflecting the image toward the observer. On the right is the Koeppe lens, which gives a direct rather than reflected view of the anterior chamber. *(Illustration by C. H. Wooley.)*

Geneva Lens Clock

The Geneva lens clock uses 3 pins to measure the curvature of a spectacle lens. It is calibrated for a specific refractive index (usually crown glass, n = 1.53), so the actual power reading will be incorrect for lenses made of other materials. For these lenses, the instrument is still useful to determine if there is front or back ground cylinder or if the lens is warped (Fig 7-22).

Lensmeter

To measure the power of a lens using a lensmeter, we place the lens on a nose cone at the top of a cylinder. Farther down, a convex lens is fixed in place such that its secondary focal point is just at the posterior vertex of the lens being measured. Still farther down the tube is a movable illuminated target; when the dial of the lensmeter reads 0, the target is at the primary focal point of the fixed lens. If the lens being measured has no power, then parallel rays arrive at the eyepiece, which is an astronomical telescope, and the target appears well focused to the emmetropic nonaccommodating observer. If the lens has power, the target is moved until it appears in focus, and the power of the unknown lens is read on the dial.

The fixed lens serves 2 purposes. First, the lensmeter does not have to be several meters long, and second, its scale becomes linear. That is, you turn the wheel the same amount to get from plus or minus 1 D to 2 D as you do to get from 11 D to 12 D. Badal suggested similar use of such a fixed lens in his version of the optometer, an instrument designed to measure the eye's refractive error (Fig 7-23). The observer looks into the lensmeter through an astronomical telescope, through which the image appears in focus only if the light entering it is collimated. This is a clever arrangement, as the measurement tends to be little affected by the observer's uncorrected refractive error. The spectacles are placed with the posterior vertex of the distance lens on the nose cone. Line bifocals are then turned around so that the front of the glasses rests on the nose cone, and the difference in power between the distance and near portions of the lens is measured to determine the reading add power. The lensmeter is calibrated by the manufacturer to measure the posterior vertex power of the distance spectacle lens. To measure the true power of the lens you would have to locate its principal planes, which is not feasible.

To summarize, the target is moved until the light that has passed through the fixed lens and spectacle lens is collimated (in the meridian being studied). The viewer then sees

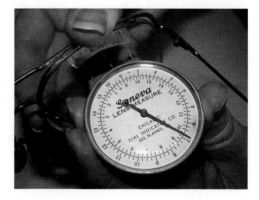

Figure 7-22 Geneva lens clock. Only the middle pin moves, measuring the curvature. *(Courtesy of Tommy S. Korn, MD.)*

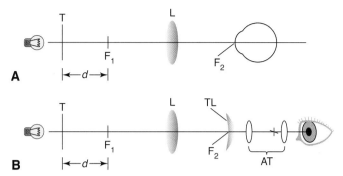

Figure 7-23 **A,** The optometer principle. T is an illuminated target. When the subject's eye is placed at the focal point (F_2) of the positive lens (L), the vergence at the eye is directly proportional to the distance *(d),* measured from the first focal point (F_1) of lens (L). **B,** The optometer principle applied to the lensmeter. The test lens (TL) is placed at F_2, and the target is viewed with an afocal telescope (AT) by the observer. The target is moved along the axis until the vergence at the test lens is equal and opposite to the vertex power of the test lens. The light will then emerge from the test lens with zero vergence (ie, collimated), and the target will be seen in sharp focus by the observer. The afocal telescope magnifies the target, increases the precision of the measurement, and reduces the effect of the observer's accommodation or refractive error. *(Redrawn from Basic and Clinical Science Course Section 2: Optics, Refraction, and Contact Lenses. San Francisco: American Academy of Ophthalmology; 1986–1987:252. Fig 13.)*

a sharp image of the target in the astronomical telescope, regardless of whether she tends to accommodate or has some uncorrected refractive error.

Automated lensmeters measure the deflection of a light path as it passes through various parts of the lens. Computerized compilation of this information then reveals how those regions of the lens bend the light.

Knapp's Rule

Suppose we have several eyes with the same anterior segment and, therefore, the same anterior focal plane determined by that cornea, anterior chamber depth, and lens. We suppose the eyes differ only in their axial lengths, and for each eye, we place at the anterior focal plane whatever power lens is needed to correct the refractive error of that eye, depending on how long the eye is. Knapp's rule, illustrated in Figure 1-41, says the size on the retina of the image of a distant object is the same for all those eyes, when each one's corrective lens is in place. Clinical application of this rule is limited. Eyes may have unequal myopia because of differences in their anterior segments rather than in their axial lengths. The retinal photoreceptors may be spaced farther apart in a longer eye, and spectacles are usually worn closer to the eye than the anterior focal point, which is approximately 17 mm in front of the cornea (see Chapter 1).

Optical Pachymeter

With the optical pachymeter, the thickness of the cornea or the depth of the anterior chamber is measured by lining up prism-split images in the focused slit lamp's optical section through the eye (Fig 7-24).

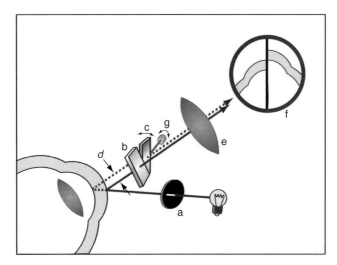

Figure 7-24 In the most common type of optical pachymeter, the cornea is illuminated with a slit beam (a). The image is viewed through a biomicroscope, half through a glass plate orthogonal to the path of light (b) and half through a glass plate rotated through an angle (c). The beam path through the plate is displaced laterally for a distance *(d)* that varies depending on the angle of rotation. Through the eyepiece (e), a split image is seen (f) wherein half the image comes from the fixed plate and the other half from the rotatable plate. The endothelial surface of one image and the epithelial surface of the other are aligned by the observer by adjustment of the rotatable plate (c), and the corneal thickness measurement is read off a calibrated scale (g). *(Courtesy of Neal H. Atebara, MD.)*

Applanation Tonometry

The head of the applanation tonometer contains a prism that splits the image of a fluorescing circle of tears to determine when that circle is precisely a certain size (Fig 7-25). Intraocular pressure is inferred from the amount of pressure required to flatten the cornea just enough to create that size circle of tears.

Specular Microscopy

Specular microscopy is a modality for examining endothelial cells that uses specular reflection from the interface between the endothelial cells and the aqueous humor. The technique can be performed using contact or noncontact methods. In both methods, the instruments are designed to separate the illumination and viewing paths so that reflections from the anterior corneal surface do not obscure the weak reflection arising from the endothelial cell surface.

Endothelial cells can also be visualized through a slit-lamp biomicroscope, if the illumination and viewing axes are symmetrically displaced on either side of the normal line to the cornea (Fig 7-26). A narrow illumination slit must be used; hence, the field of view is narrow. Photographic recording has been made possible by the addition of a long-working-distance microscope system on the viewing axis and flash capability to the illumination system. Patient eye motion is the chief problem with this technique.

In contact specular microscopy, the illumination and viewing paths traverse opposite sides of a special microscope objective, the front element of which touches the cornea.

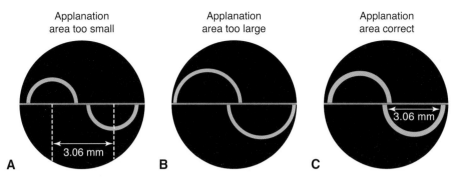

Figure 7-25 The split prism in the applanation head creates 2 offset images. **A,** When the area of applanation is smaller than 3.06 mm, the arms of the inner semicircles remain some distance apart. **B,** When the area of applanation is greater than 3.06 mm, the arms of the inner semicircles overlap. **C,** When the area of applanation is exactly 3.06 mm, the arms of the inner semicircles just touch each other. This is the endpoint for measuring intraocular pressure. The value of 3.06 mm was chosen to approximately balance tear-film surface tension and corneal rigidity. *(Courtesy of Neal H. Atebara, MD. Redrawn by C. H. Wooley.)*

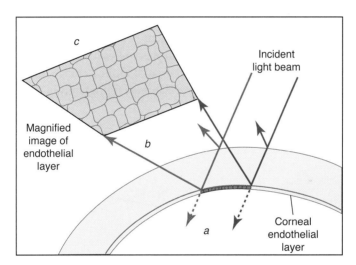

Figure 7-26 Specular reflection microscopy. When a beam of light passes through the transparent corneal structures, most of the light is transmitted *(a)*. However, at each optical interface, such as the corneal endothelium, a proportion of light is reflected *(b)*. This light (called *specular reflection*) can be collected to form a relatively dim image of the corneal endothelium *(c)*, where individual endothelial cells can be counted. *(Courtesy of Neal H. Atebara, MD. Redrawn by C. H. Wooley.)*

This reduces eye rotation and effectively eliminates longitudinal motion that interferes with focus. Contact specular microscopy allows for higher magnifications than slit-lamp biomicroscopy, making cellular detail and endothelial abnormalities more discernible.

Video recording of endothelial layer images makes it possible to document larger, overlapping areas of the endothelial layer. Also, it allows for the recording of high-magnification images, despite patient eye motion.

Wide-field specular microscopy employs techniques to ensure that reflections from the interface between the cornea and contact element do not overlap the image of the endothelial cell layer. Because scattered light from edema in the epithelium and stroma can degrade the endothelial image, variable slit widths are sometimes provided to reduce this problem.

Analysis of specular micrographs may consist simply of assessment of cell appearance together with notation of abnormalities such as guttae or keratic precipitates. Frequently, cell counts are desired; these are often obtained by superimposing a transparent grid of specific dimensions on the endothelial image (photograph or video) and simply counting the cells in a known area. Cell-size distribution can be determined by computer analysis after cell boundaries have been determined digitally. The normal cell density in young people exceeds 3000 cells/mm^2; the average density in the older age group susceptible to cataract is 2250 cells/mm^2, which suggests a gradual decline with age.

Specular microscopy has been important in studying the morphology of the endothelium and in quantifying damage to the endothelium produced by various surgical procedures and intraocular devices.

Keratometer

The keratometer is used to measure the curvature of the central outer corneal surface by measuring the size of a reflected image in each meridian (or only in the meridians of greatest and least curvature). The measurement is accomplished by lining up prism-doubled images at a distance regulated by sharpness of focus (Fig 7-27). This measurement is performed at only one diameter, 3 mm, in a limited choice of meridians, and is therefore lacking the detail provided by more elaborate topography.

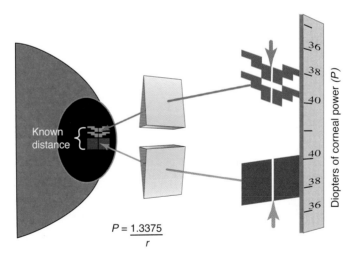

$$P = \frac{1.3375}{r}$$

Figure 7-27 Two prisms placed base to base produce doubled images separated by a fixed distance that are not affected by small movements of the eye. The observer varies the object size (ie, the distance between the red and green objects) until the doubled images touch. At this point, the images are a known distance from each other, and the object size can be measured to calculate the corneal radius of curvature. On most Javal-Schiøtz keratometers, the scale that measures the size of the object has already been converted to its corresponding estimates in diopters of corneal refractive power using the lensmaker's equation (p. 24): $P = (n' - n)/r$, where P is the refractive power of the cornea, r is the radius of the corneal curvature (in meters), 1.3375 is the "averaged" corneal refractive index, and $n = 1.000$ is the refractive index of air. *(Developed by Neal H. Atebara, MD. Redrawn by C. H. Wooley.)*

Topography

Computerized computations of measurements of the reflected image of a Placido disk of concentric circles painted inside a concavity enable corneal topography instruments to produce a detailed map of the shape of the entire outer corneal surface (Figs 7-28, 7-29).

Ultrasonography of the Eye and Orbit

In ultrasonagraphy, 8–15 million vibrations per second of a piezoelectric crystal are transmitted mechanically through the eye. The time of return of reflected sound waves is measured to create an A-scan graph. Using the presumed speeds of sound in the various parts of the eye, we can measure the location of the sound-reflective interfaces encountered.

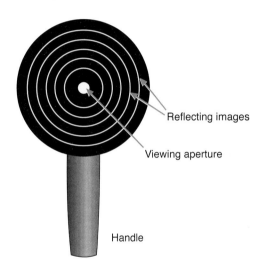

Reflecting images

Viewing aperture

Handle

Figure 7-28 A Placido disk. *(Courtesy of Neal H. Atebara, MD. Redrawn by C. H. Wooley.)*

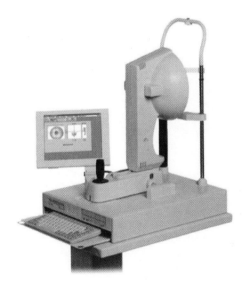

Figure 7-29 Photograph of a computerized corneal topography system. *(Courtesy of Neal H. Atebara, MD.)*

Their characteristic reflectance (the strength of the echoes) helps us identify the structures. Oscillations of the probe generate a B-scan 2-dimensional section. Scanning the eye while it is immersed in water gives better imaging of its anterior structures.

Macular Function Tests

When contemplating cataract surgery for a patient, we may want to know whether the macula is capable of better vision—so we wish we could let the patient see around the cataract to confirm this. The *potential acuity meter* does just that; it projects a vision chart into the eye, focusing the beam to be narrow as it passes through one of the clearer parts of the lens and spreading it out again to fall on the retina, where its pencils of light are in focus.

Alternatively, a *laser interferometer* can be used. It splits a laser beam into 2 parts, which meet and create interference fringes on the retina of variable spacing; the patient is then asked to identify the fringe patterns.

Scanning Laser Ophthalmoscopes

In a scanning laser ophthalmoscope, a rapidly scanning laser illuminates a small spot of retina, while a luminance detector measures the light that is reflected. An image is assembled from the data. The following sections describe a few types of scanning laser ophthalmoscopes.

Confocal scanning laser ophthalmoscopes and microscopes

Optical imaging devices may include a confocal aperture, a small opening through which pencils of light must pass in order to contribute to the device's image. Pencils of light that converge nearly to a point in the plane of the aperture are able to pass through the opening, but other pencils are mostly blocked (Fig 7-30). In this way, a particular tissue plane of a translucent organ can be imaged, while light reflected by other tissue planes as well as extraneous scattered and reflected light can be excluded.

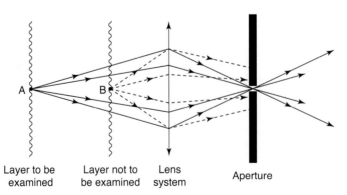

Layer to be examined   Layer not to be examined   Lens system   Aperture

Figure 7-30   Principle of confocal microscopy. The pencil of light from point A passes through the aperture. Most of the pencil of light emanating from point B is blocked by the aperture. *(Illustration developed by Leon Strauss, MD, PhD.)*

Scanning laser polarimeter

The nerve fiber layer is birefringent, which means that polarized light travels through it at different speeds depending on whether the polarization is along or across the fibers. The GDx (Carl Zeiss AG, Oberkochen, Germany), a scanning laser ophthalmoscope, calculates the thickness of the nerve fiber layer based on the phase shift between the slower-traveling light of one direction of polarization and the faster-traveling light polarized perpendicular to the first. The thicker the layer of nerve fibers is, the more the wave peaks of the 2 polarizations of light will be out of phase. Radial symmetry of the orientation of nerve fibers surrounding the fovea is used to correct calculations for the birefringence of the cornea, through which the light must pass twice.

Wide-field scanning laser ophthalmoscope

Mirrors arranged on a rotating polygon enable rapid wide-angle scanning of the retina with red and green lasers, the red being reflected more by the deeper layers and the green by the more superficial layers of the retina. Scanning of the retina far into its peripheral regions is achieved through the use of an ellipsoidal mirror (Fig 7-31).

Scheimpflug Camera

In a Scheimpflug camera, the image and object planes are tilted with respect to the instrument's optics. Although this tilting yields a distorted image, it allows for a greatly increased depth of focus. Thus, such a camera can image, in sharp focus, a slit lamp's optical section of the eye, which would not be feasible with an ordinary camera's more shallow depth of focus. This technique can be used to measure the curvature of the anterior and posterior corneal surface.

Autorefractors

Various optical principles have been used in the design of automated objective refractors, some of which will be discussed briefly here. Retinoscopy, also called dynamic skiascopy,

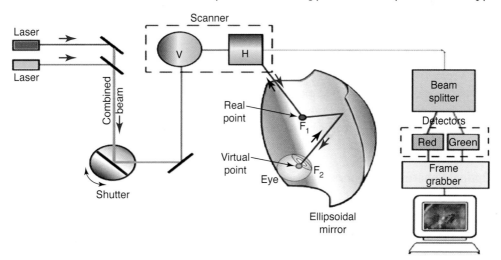

Figure 7-31 Optical principle of the Optos Optomap laser ophthalmoscope. V = vertical spinning polygonal mirror; H = horizontal spinning polygonal mirror. *(Courtesy of Optos, Inc.)*

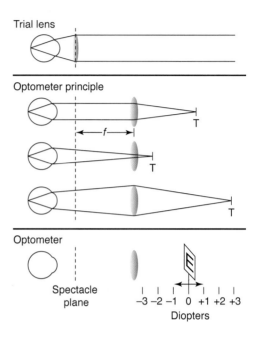

Figure 7-32 The optometer principle. Instead of using interchangeable trial lenses, a single converging lens is used, placed at its focal length *(f)* from the spectacle plane. Light from a target (T) on the far side of the lens enters the eye with vergence of different amounts (0, minus, or plus), depending on the position of the target. Vergence in the spectacle plane may thus be changed smoothly and is directly proportional to the axial displacement of the target. This arrangement exactly simulates a spherical trial lens having smoothly variable power. *(Modified from Duane TD, ed. Clinical Ophthalmology. Vol 1. Hagerstown, MD: Harper & Row; 1983:2.)*

is the analysis of the direction and speed of motion of the edges of shadows. The optometer principle is illustrated in Figures 7-23 and 7-32. Autorefraction may also be accomplished by illuminating a small patch of the retina, which reflects light to emerge from the eye, passing through the eye's optics. That emerging light, passing through the pupil, can then be imaged, and the image analyzed, in order to infer the optical power of the eye's optics. The final result is calculated based on repeating this measurement along numerous paths through the subject's pupil. The Scheiner principle gives another method of measuring the power of the eye's optics.

The Scheiner principle

Suppose that someone uses 1 eye to look at a small, distant light source. An occluder with 2 pinholes, one above the other, isolates 2 pencils of parallel rays coming from a distant small source. If the eye is emmetropic, the 2 pencils converge at the retina and the viewer sees 1 spot. If the eye is too short (ie, hyperopic) or too long (ie, myopic) for its optics, then 2 separate spots are illuminated on the retina. If we momentarily cover one of the holes, say the top one, which spot disappears? The myopic eye sees crossed images, which are projected mentally as uncrossed diplopia, so the patient says that the top spot disappears; conversely, the hyperopic eye sees the bottom spot disappear (Fig 7-33).

Optical Coherence Tomography

The resolution of ultrasound is limited by the long wavelength of sound. Light has much shorter wavelengths than sound, allowing for finer resolution, but direct electronic measurement of the extremely short time it takes light to bounce in and out of an eye is not feasible. Interferometry enables us to overcome this difficulty in the following manner. If we split a beam of light and bring the 2 parts back together after they have traveled paths that take very slightly different amounts of time, interference patterns are observable. In

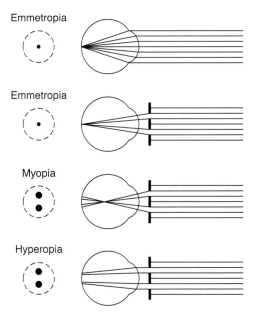

Figure 7-33 The Scheiner principle. Double pinhole apertures placed before the pupil isolate 2 small bundles of light. An object not conjugate to the retina appears doubled instead of blurred. *(Modified from Duane TD, ed. Clinical Ophthalmology. Vol 1. Hagerstown, MD: Harper & Row; 1983:2.)*

optical coherence tomography (OCT), a superluminescent diode emits a beam of light with long (red) wavelengths—reds being chosen because they are scattered in tissue less than is blue light. A superluminescent diode is used, rather than a laser, because it emits a broader spectrum of color, which gives the instrument greater sensitivity to the differences in time the 2 beams have traveled than would be achieved with only one frequency of light. When the beam is split, the reference beam is aimed at a mirror, and the other portion is aimed at one of the reflective interfaces within the tissue being examined (Fig 7-34).

In time-domain OCT, the position of the mirror is adjusted so that interference patterns show up whenever the 2 beams have traveled almost the same amount of time. Results similar to the ultrasound's A-scan are generated, as light is reflected at interfaces between layers of tissue. Scanning the plane of the retina yields 2-dimensional and hence 3-dimensional results like an ultrasound's B-scan.

In Fourier- (also called spectral- or frequency-) domain OCT, the reference beam mirror is fixed at one position. Interference fringe patterns, all mixed together, arise from the various tissue interfaces, but Fourier analysis enables them to be dissected apart. When the pattern arises from closer tissue interfaces, the fringe patterns' undulations are spaced farther apart than those arising from deeper tissue planes, which yield fringes spaced more closely together. The more highly reflective tissue plane interfaces yield higher-amplitude fringe patterns. Thus, the spacing of the fringe pattern tells us how deep in the tissue it comes from, and its amplitude tells us how much the light is reflected by that tissue plane interface. In this manner, the A-scan of all the depths is obtained instantly without moving the reference mirror. Scanning across the retina yields 2-dimensional and hence 3-dimensional images. A swept-source version of the Fourier-domain OCT replaces the superluminescent diode's band of frequencies with a laser; the laser emits different frequencies, one at a time, and the A-scan is performed for each frequency at each location.

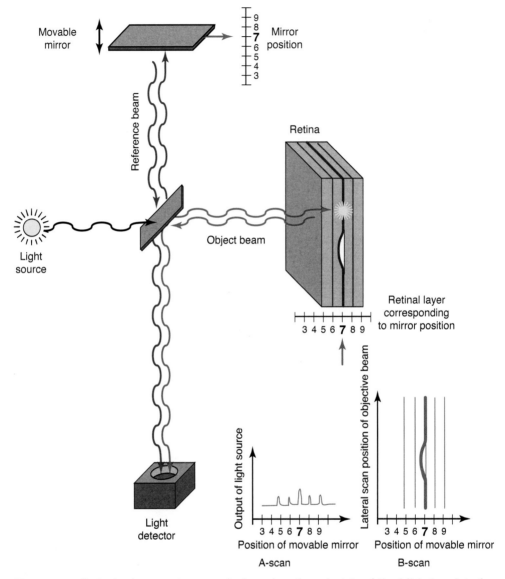

Figure 7-34 Optical coherence tomography based on the principle of the Michelson interferometer. *(Courtesy of Neal H. Atebara, MD. Redrawn by C. H. Wooley.)*

Optical Aids

A variety of optical devices, including handheld and stand magnifiers, high-add spectacles, and telescopes, are available to assist patients with impaired vision and normally sighted individuals.

Magnifiers

The simplest low vision aid is a handheld magnifying glass (Fig 7-35). Low- to medium-power magnifiers can make continuous text reading possible for patients with mild to

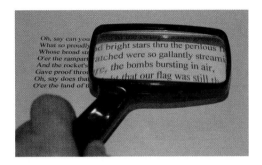

Figure 7-35 Simple hand magnifier. A +4 D lens mounted in a convenient handle, often described as a 2× magnifying glass. *(Courtesy of Scott E. Brodie, MD, PhD.)*

moderate vision loss. When function is more severely affected, stronger magnifiers may allow for shorter reading periods or for spot reading. However, the smaller field of view requires that the device be moved continuously along the reading material; this limits the feasibility of using a handheld magnifier for reading extended text passages for long periods of time. Newer magnifiers with LED illumination are excellent options for spot reading.

The most commonly prescribed powers range between +5 D and +20 D. Above +20 D, the higher magnification and reduced field of view make it more difficult for the patient to maintain a steady focus, although some patients may do very well with a +24 D or +28 D magnifier.

The "power" or "magnification factor" of a magnifier is usually specified in terms of the relative angular size of the magnified image compared with the angular size of the original object at a standard reading distance. Most commonly, the reference distance is taken as 25 cm. In general, the maximal magnification will be obtained when the object to be viewed is placed at the anterior focal point of the magnifier. When the magnifier is used this way, the magnification factor is equal to the dioptric power of the lens divided by 4 (the dioptric equivalent of the reference distance of 25 cm). For example, the power of a +24 D magnifier is 6× (24 D/4 D).

Simple low-power magnifiers (typically around +4 D) are rarely used in this way, as it is difficult to hold a lens steady so far from the page, and this magnification factor convention is no longer appropriate. If such a lens is held with the text at half the distance to the anterior focal point, the virtual image seen by the user will be located at the anterior focal point and will be twice as large as the original text. These magnifiers are often casually described as 2×.

Patients with tremors, arthritis, paralysis, or poor hand–eye coordination often have difficulty holding handheld magnifiers steady as they scan along lines of continuous text. Typically, they will have improved performance with the same lens in a stand magnifier that rests directly on the page (Fig 7-36).

Telescopes

Tasks that require magnification for distance viewing are less common than those for near viewing, especially in older patients. Handheld monoculars, binoculars, and spectacle-mounted telescopes are available and allow the benefit of magnification at a greater distance, with the drawback of reduction in field of view, a narrow depth of field, and reduced

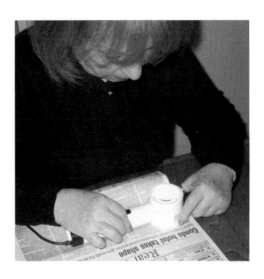

Figure 7-36 An illuminated stand magnifier placed flat against the page provides magnification, illumination, and stability. As with all magnifiers, the field of view decreases with increased magnification. *(Courtesy of Darren L. Albert, MD.)*

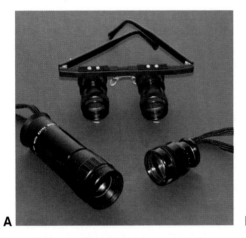

A

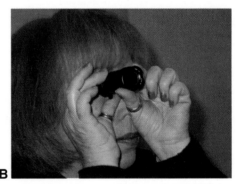

B

Figure 7-37 **A,** *Top:* Binocular, spectacle-mounted telescopes are available for prolonged distance tasks, such as watching a play in a theater, and/or near tasks such as reading. *Bottom left:* A high-power (6×), monocular, handheld Keplerian telescope may be difficult to hold steady and on target because of magnified motion and a narrow field of view. *Bottom right:* A low-power (2.8×), monocular, handheld Galilean telescope is ideal for intermittent distance tasks such as reading street signs or bus numbers. **B,** Both hand–eye coordination and training are required for successful use of telescopic and other visual aids. *(Courtesy of Darren L. Albert, MD.)*

contrast (Fig 7-37). In addition, patients cannot wear a telescopic device when walking. Autofocus telescope models are available. A simple telescopic spectacle without a casing is available commercially and has become very popular, as it is lightweight and relatively inexpensive.

Loupes are spectacle-mounted telescopes set to focus at near points. They can provide an escape from the trade-off between high magnification and short working distance inherent in simple high-add reading glasses. However, the visual field is narrow and the depth of field small.

Bioptic telescopes are spectacle-mounted telescopes set to focus at distance, mounted in the upper portion of the lenses of carrier spectacles. These are allowed in many states for use while driving. The telescopic portion of the spectacles is positioned superior to the line of sight and used only briefly to read signs or look into the distance. The rest of the time, the individual drives looking through the regular prescription portion of his or her spectacles. Driving with a bioptic requires prescription of the device as well as device training and driver training on an individual basis.

Prisms

A variety of designs of prisms have been proposed to compensate for field loss by projecting the visual image onto the functioning portion of the retina or by redirecting the image of the object of regard onto the preferred retinal location (PRL) in patients with central macular dysfunction. Research is currently evaluating the efficacy of such devices compared to, or in conjunction with, training in systematic scanning.

High-Add Spectacles

High-plus reading glasses are an option for patients who can adapt to the closer working distance required. As a starting point, the clinician may estimate the required reading add power by using the Kestenbaum rule, which states that the predicted add power, in diopters, to read 1 M type is the inverse of the visual acuity fraction. For example, a patient with 20/200 visual acuity may benefit from a +10 D lens (200/20 = 10), with the material held at the focal point of the lens, 1/10 m (ie, 10 cm, or 4 in). Very often, however, patients require different magnification from that predicted by the Kestenbaum rule (usually even stronger), including patients with poor contrast sensitivity, macular scotomas, or a requirement to read print that is smaller than 1 M (Clinical Example 7-1).

Bifocals or reading glasses can be prescribed in strengths greater than +3.00 D as long as the shortened working distance is understood and accepted by the patient. Such add powers are usually well tolerated binocularly up to approximately +4.50 D, and monocularly up to +16.00 D for the better-seeing eye. In binocular patients, prism is required

---

CLINICAL EXAMPLE 7-1

For purposes of vision rehabilitation, it is often convenient to describe the print size of reading materials using *M notation*. The M size of an optotype is the distance (in meters) at which the sample can be read by a person with normal acuity—thus, "1 M" print is normally legible at 1.0 m.

For example, a standard 20/20 optotype intended for viewing in a full-size refracting lane is approximately 6 M (20 ft ≈ 6 m). In practice, 1 M type is approximately 8 points, corresponding to a 20/50-equivalent letter on a standard 14-inch near card, and the 20/20-equivalent optotypes on such a card correspond to 0.4 M. The Kestenbaum rule then follows directly from the definition of the diopter.

to assist convergence and relax accommodation. The recommended prism strength is 2 prism diopters (Δ) more base-in (BI) than the numerical add power, in each eye. For example, if the distance prescription is plano OU and the appropriate add power for reading is +8.00 D, then the prescription should read as follows: OD: +8.00 sp with 10Δ BI; OS: +8.00 sp with 10Δ BI. Readers with prism are available ready-made in powers from +6.00 D to +14.00 D and allow a wide field of view. Aspheric spectacles, available from +6.00 D to +32.00 D, are suitable for monocular use and require a very short working distance, which may present difficulty in directing light onto the material.

Glasses with intermediate-strength add powers are important for tasks such as using a computer. The intermediate add power for viewing a computer monitor is often prescribed as the upper segment of a bifocal; some patients use a clip-on add lens. Single-vision glasses matched to the distance from the eyes to the screen may be better tolerated, and if the patient works mainly at a single computer workstation, these can be left there for use when needed.

Before reading glasses are prescribed, the patient should demonstrate proficiency with actual print material. In general, reading glasses allow hands-free magnification and a large field of vision; however, there is a shortened working distance, and they cannot be worn when walking or driving.

Nonoptical Aids

The armamentarium of tools to assist patients with impaired vision extends beyond optical devices. Many simple, practical, nonoptical devices are available through specialty stores, catalogs, and websites. These items include large-format watches, telephones, remote controls, playing cards, and checks. Bold-lettered computer keyboards, needle threaders, dark-lined writing paper, and felt-tip pens with black ink are also useful. Patients should be made aware of, and trained to use, such aids as appropriate. Medicare and other health insurers in the United States cover costs for occupational therapists to train patients in the use of such devices to achieve their individual goals but rarely cover costs for the actual devices.

Some of the more sophisticated devices and techniques available to assist patients are discussed in the following sections.

Electronic Devices

Many of the most exciting solutions for patients with reduced vision are found in new technologies (Fig 7-38). Video cameras combined with screens (video camera magnifiers) are available in many formats. These components allow variable magnification, comfortable reading positions, and enhanced or reversed contrast—features not available with optical magnifiers. Computer accessibility options on both Windows and Macintosh computers provide magnification, modified contrast, and audio screen readers.

A large-screen monitor is helpful in many cases. Screen-enlargement software (eg, AI Squared's ZoomText; see Fig 7-38H, I) provides sophisticated utilities for enlarging screen text and graphics and for integrating text-to-speech capabilities. In addition, smartphones, e-readers, and audio books have made reading possible for many patients with vision loss or even blindness. Cell phones are very accessible, and global positioning

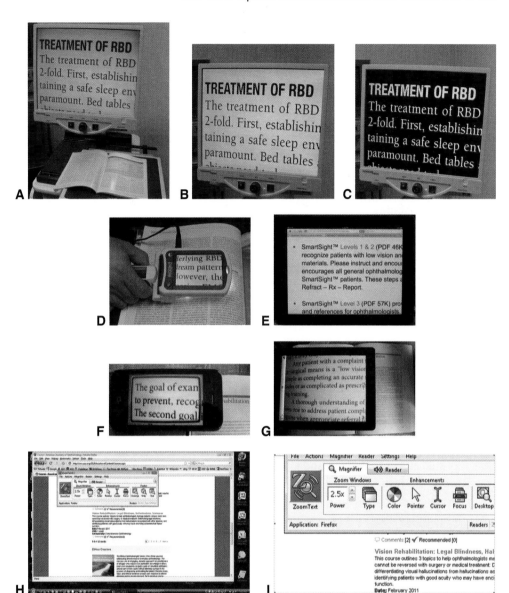

Figure 7-38 Electronic low vision aids. **A,** Desktop-model closed-circuit video magnifier. **B,** Same magnifier as in **A,** in high-contrast mode. **C,** Same magnifier as in **A,** in reverse-contrast mode. **D,** Handheld closed-circuit video magnifier. **E,** Tablet device used as a large-print e-reader. **F,** Smartphone used as a video magnifier. **G,** Tablet device used as a video magnifier. **H,** Standard-format Windows computer screen. **I,** Same computer screen as in **H,** magnified using screen enlargement tools. *(Courtesy of Scott E. Brodie, MD, PhD.)*

system (GPS) technology increasingly facilitates navigation for severely visually impaired individuals. Refreshable Braille displays are available for computers and tablet devices. They have small moving pins that rise up or down to create Braille patterns that can be read tactilely. These displays are connected to a computer or other device with a USB or serial cable.

Lighting, Glare Control, and Contrast Enhancement

Proper lighting is important for patients with reduced visual function, especially when contrast sensitivity is reduced. It is important to direct light onto the task, for example, with a gooseneck lamp or a head-worn light. Optimal types of lighting and positions of lights should be determined to minimize glare from light shining directly into the patient's face or reflecting off the page. Video magnifiers are important options for patients with decreased contrast sensitivity. Patients who experience glare from light reflected off the page may benefit from the contrast reversal feature available in many video magnifiers (see Fig 7-38C). Tinted lenses may also enhance contrast for some patients.

Nonvisual Assistance

As visual loss becomes more profound, vision enhancement may become less effective, and the importance of "visual substitution skills," such as tactile and auditory aids, increases. The following are some examples:

- *Tactile aids.* These range from raised dots on a kitchen appliance control knob to the use of Braille for reading.
- *Refreshable Braille displays.* As mentioned, these devices are available to connect to computers or portable electronic devices and create readable Braille output from electronic text.
- *Auditory aids.* Talking watches, audio output on computers and e-readers, audio books, and audio newspaper services are included in this category. In addition, voice recognition software is readily available for computers, and screen readers are built into computer operating systems, as well as being available separately. Optical character recognition (OCR) allows any printed text to be converted to audio format, and both desktop and handheld stand-alone devices are available that make use of this technology.
- *Orientation and mobility training.* This type of training offers instruction in using remaining visual cues, telescopes, white canes, and GPS devices for safe and independent ambulation.

Eccentric Viewing or Fixation Training

Eccentric fixation training can help patients improve eye–hand coordination, tracking, and scanning. Training may improve reading performance. As mentioned above, prisms may facilitate the use of an extrafoveal PRL. Research is evaluating best practices.

Instruction and Training

It should be emphasized that for most patients, some instruction, training, and practice will be needed for them to be successful at accomplishing tasks with any of the devices or techniques described here. The use of computer accessibility features, video magnifiers, hand magnifiers, high-add spectacles, and adaptations for activities of daily living is not intuitive. Training with respect to nonoptical strategies, including safety measures, is equally important. Training sessions should be given to the patient, and preferably also to a family member or friend, who can later reinforce the training.

Chapter Exercises

Questions

7.1. The basic design of a slit-lamp biomicroscope includes all of the following except
   a. a Galilean magnification changer
   b. an astronomical telescope
   c. a single monocular viewing system
   d. an illumination system

7.2. The corneal endothelium may be viewed using the slit-lamp biomicroscope by using which of the following techniques?
   a. sclerotic scatter
   b. direct illumination
   c. proximal illumination
   d. specular reflection

7.3. In what way is the manual (von Helmholtz) keratometer inaccurate for determining corneal power in intraocular lens calculations following myopic laser vision correction?
   a. The keratometer mire cannot be imaged at all following laser vision correction.
   b. The assumed relationship between the anterior and posterior surfaces, which is the basis of the assumed index of refraction, is no longer accurate.
   c. Significant irregular astigmatism is present in all corneas that have undergone keratorefractive surgery, and the keratometer is no longer accurate.
   d. The keratometry measurement of the posterior surface does not change and is still accurate.

7.4. You are planning cataract surgery to achieve emmetropia for a patient with the following measurements:

   Refraction: $-3.00 +2.00 \times 120$
   K: 42.50 D/42.75 D @ 120°

   Which of the following plans is the best option?
   a. toric IOL with minus cylinder axis at 120 degrees
   b. relaxing incision at 30 degrees
   c. relaxing incision at 120 degrees
   d. monofocal intraocular lens

7.5. What is the size, in M notation, of the optotypes that are just visible to a patient with 20/20 visual acuity at the standard reading distance of 40 cm?

    a. 0.2 M
    b. 0.4 M
    c. 0.6 M
    d. 0.8 M

7.6. According to the Kestenbaum rule, what is the appropriate reading add power for a patient with best-corrected visual acuity at a distance of 20/80 who wishes to read 1.0 M type?

    a. 2.0 D
    b. 3.0 D
    c. 4.0 D
    d. 5.0 D

7.7. The indirect ophthalmoscope employs one of the brightest light sources used in clinical ophthalmology. Why is such a bright light necessary?

7.8. The patient described in question 7.6 will read 1.0 M type at a distance of 25 cm, or approximately 10 inches, using his 4.0 D add spectacles. To alleviate the need to converge the eyes for extended periods when reading at such a close distance, what is the appropriate prism correction to incorporate into the high-add spectacles?

    a. 4Δ base-out OU
    b. 4Δ base-in OU
    c. 6Δ base-out OU
    d. 6Δ base-in OU

7.9. When a binocular indirect ophthalmoscope is used with a patient with small pupils, binocular visualization can be improved by

    a. moving the ophthalmoscope's mirror closer to the observer
    b. narrowing the observer's effective interpupillary distance
    c. moving the ophthalmoscope's eyepieces farther apart
    d. increasing the distance between the observer's head and the patient
    e. all of the above

7.10. Which of the following statements is not true for how keratometers work?

    a. They measure the radius of curvature of the central cornea.
    b. They assume the cornea to be a convex mirror.
    c. They directly measure the refractive power of the cornea.
    d. They use a mathematical formula to convert radius of curvature to approximate refractive power.

7.11. Which of the following devices is not an optical component of the slit-lamp biomicroscope?

    a. field lens
    b. astronomical telescope
    c. inverting prism
    d. Galilean magnification changer

7.12. Proper distance visual acuity testing for a low vision patient includes all of the following except
   a. a testing chart with an equal number of symbols on each line
   b. nonstandardized room illumination
   c. a Snellen visual acuity chart at 20 feet
   d. a test distance of 10 feet

7.13. A patient with moderately low vision (20/160 in each eye) requests a prescription to be able to read. Which of the following would be the best choice?
   a. a +8.00 D single-vision reading spectacle
   b. a +4.00 D half-glass reader with a total of 6Δ base-in (BI) prism
   c. a +8.00 D half-glass reader with a total of 10Δ BI prism
   d. a +8.00 D half-glass reader with 10Δ BI prism per lens
   e. an 8.0× magnifier

7.14. Which one of the following conditions does not *commonly* cause glare? (See Appendix 7.1.)
   a. iritis
   b. corneal scarring
   c. posterior subcapsular cataract
   d. albinism

Answers

7.1. **c.** The slit-lamp biomicroscope is a binocular instrument in which the viewing system and illumination system are coupled so that in ordinary viewing, the image remains clear despite changes in illumination angles and changes in magnifications (parfocal). The Galilean magnification changer is used in some, but not all, slit-lamp biomicroscopes. See also the answer to question 7.11.

7.2. **d.** With an ordinary slit lamp, the outlines of individual endothelial cells are best seen by viewing the specular reflection of a narrow slit beam at high magnification. A wider field can be viewed using a specular microscope, with a contact optical system to decrease surface reflections.

7.3. **b.** The 1.3375 index of refraction is calculated to compensate for the minus-powered posterior corneal surface that cannot be measured with the keratometer. Myopic keratorefractive surgery primarily flattens the anterior surface, and therefore the assumed index of refraction is no longer correct. Another problem following myopic keratorefractive surgery is that the extreme center of the cornea is usually flattened substantially more than the annulus measured by the manual keratometer (approximately 3 mm). Both of these errors will lead to overestimating the power of the cornea and a hyperopic postoperative result, if not corrected for in the calculation.

7.4. **d.** The cornea accounts for only 0.25 D of the astigmatic correction. The remainder must be in the lens, and therefore removal of the lens with cataract surgery will also correct the astigmatism. When considering toric lens implants or relaxing incisions with cataract surgery, it is prudent to verify the corneal astigmatism with at least 2 separate instruments.

7.5. **b.** By definition, 1.0 M optotypes are just visible to a patient with 20/20 visual acuity at a distance of 1.0 m. Print at a distance of only 40 cm needs to be only 4/10 as large to be equally visible.

7.6. **c.** According to the Kestenbaum rule, the add power needed to read 1.0 M type is the reciprocal of the Snellen fraction for the best-corrected distance acuity. This patient requires an add power of 1/(20/80) = 4.0 D. (In practice, higher add powers are often needed.)

7.7. The condensing lens images the observer's entrance pupils as 2 very small discs that fall within the patient's entrance pupil (along with the image of the ophthalmoscope bulb's filament, which must not coincide with the images of the observer's pupils to avoid obscuring the fundus with reflections from the patient's cornea). Of all the light the ophthalmoscope shines into the patient's eye, only the emergent light that passes through these pupillary images enters the eyes of the observer and is available to view the fundus. As these image discs occupy far less than 1% of the area of the patient's entrance pupil, the ophthalmoscope "wastes" over 99% of the light that enters the patient's eye in forming the image visible to the observer, requiring a very bright light source. (The small images of the observer's pupils create a strong "pinhole effect," which explains the extraordinary ability of the indirect ophthalmoscope to provide clear views of the fundus through inhomogeneous media, such as cataracts of moderate severity.)

7.8. **d.** The rule of thumb for adding prism to high-add spectacles is to incorporate base-in prism for each eye at a correction that is 2Δ greater than the required add power.

7.9. **e.** When looking through a small pupil, the observer can improve visualization by narrowing his or her effective interpupillary distance. This can be accomplished by several means. Moving the ophthalmoscope's mirror closer to the observer (the "small-pupil feature" available on some ophthalmoscopes) decreases the distance between the light paths to the observer's left and right eyes, effectively narrowing the observer's interpupillary distance. Moving the ophthalmoscope's eyepieces farther apart also decreases the distance between the light paths to the observer's eyes, similarly narrowing the observer's effective interpupillary distance. Increasing the distance between the observer and the patient decreases the angle formed by the observer's eyes and the patient's eye, thereby allowing the light paths from the observer's eyes to "squeeze through" a smaller pupil.

7.10. **c.** Keratometers approximate the refractive power of the cornea by measuring the radius of curvature of the central cornea and assuming the cornea to be a convex mirror. The formula $r = 2u(I/O)$ is then used to convert this radius of curvature into an approximate refractive power, where r is the radius of curvature of the reflective cornea, u is the distance from the object to the cornea, I is the size of the image, and O is the size of the object.

7.11. **a.** A slit-lamp biomicroscope is a high-power binocular microscope with a slit-shaped illumination source. Most of the microscope's magnifying power is produced by an astronomical telescope, and additional magnifying power is produced by a Galilean magnification changer. The resulting magnified image is inverted, so an inverting prism is used to create an upright image. An objective lens, which moves the working distance from infinity to a distance close enough to focus on the eye, is the last component of the slit-lamp biomicroscope. A field lens, which is often used in a lensmeter, is not a component of the slit-lamp biomicroscope.

7.12. **c.** For low vision patients, distance acuity testing is best done at a distance of 10 feet; standard projection charts, such as the Snellen chart, are not ideal for obtaining accurate visual acuity measurements for these patients. The Early Treatment Diabetic Retinopathy Study (ETDRS) chart has a geometric progression of optotypes, with letter sizes from 10 to 200 and with each line having the same number of letters. In contrast to a Snellen-type chart, the ETDRS chart has a 160 line and a 125 line between the 100 and 200 lines. Performance on visual function tests often varies depending on room illumination, which should be adjusted to obtain the patient's best response.

7.13. **d.** A patient with 20/160 visual acuity should still be able to maintain binocularity with reading despite requiring a reading add power of +8.00 D (see the Kestenbaum rule). This will require adding to each lens a base-in prism that is 2.0Δ more than the dioptric strength of the lens. A half-glass reader is the most convenient spectacle form for this type of lens because the lens bulk and weight are minimized.

7.14. **a.** Glare occurs when light is scattered by an optical medium, resulting in a reduction of contrast. This scattering of light can be caused by corneal scars and cataracts (especially posterior subcapsular cataracts). In albinism, the unpigmented iris allows too much light to pass, and light is scattered by the peripheral lens and zonules. In iritis, glare may in rare cases result from the presence of severe cell and flare in the anterior chamber. Although iritis patients are often photophobic, that is because of spasm of the ciliary body and is not a result of glare.

Appendix 7.1

Approach to the Patient With Low Vision

The ophthalmologist is in a unique position to support patients with vision loss by "recognizing and responding": *recognizing* that vision loss, even moderate vision loss, impacts patients' ability to successfully accomplish the things they need and want to do, and *responding* by facilitating access to vision rehabilitation. Although the ophthalmologist may not personally provide vision rehabilitation services, appreciation of the strategies and options in the vision rehabilitation "toolbox" allows you to understand why referring patients to such services is beneficial and to provide specific examples to your patients of what vision rehabilitation can offer.

Any patient with eye disease that cannot be improved with medical or surgical treatment, and who is not able to successfully accomplish the visual tasks necessary to perform the activities of daily living, has low vision and is a candidate for vision rehabilitation. Practitioners frequently err in referring only patients with severe vision loss for vision rehabilitation. In fact, rehabilitation is often most effective for patients with only moderate visual impairment. For example, a patient may have relatively good visual acuity but have significant difficulty associated with scotomas or with reduced contrast perception or glare. Patients whose only difficulty is in reading fine print can usually be assisted by routine eye-care services. However, when visual function cannot be restored to normal by routine eye care, and when low vision impacts activities beyond the ability to read fine print, the many practical options of vision rehabilitation are useful. Patients with less than 20/40 visual acuity or with central or peripheral field loss are typically excellent candidates for vision rehabilitation.

Evaluation of visual function

Vision rehabilitation begins with a low vision evaluation that includes both history and measurement of visual function. In contrast to an ophthalmic examination, in which visual function and ocular status are evaluated with the intent to diagnose and treat, the evaluation of the patient seeking vision rehabilitation focuses on vision as applied to task performance. This requires an in-depth assessment of visual function, an evaluation of current success in performing visual tasks, a detailed history of individual goals, and identification of interventions to maximize independent function.

Patient history As with other clinical encounters, the history provides important information that directs the remainder of the examination.

OCULAR HISTORY Correlate the patient's functional complaints to progression of disease and to any medical and surgical interventions. Miotic therapy and panretinal photocoagulation are 2 examples of treatments that may adversely affect visual function while conferring therapeutic benefits in treating ocular disease.

GENERAL MEDICAL HISTORY Systemic diseases can indirectly affect patient functioning in the completion of visual tasks in addition to directly affecting the visual system. For instance, orthopedic conditions, arthritis, tremors, or paralysis from a stroke can impair a patient's ability to hold a book or a handheld magnifier, and thus interfere with reading.

TASK ANALYSIS The goal of the task analysis is to determine which tasks the patient both values and finds difficult or impossible to perform. Enabling the patient to perform these tasks will be the goal of rehabilitation. Tasks may still be difficult after rehabilitation, but patients highly value success in accomplishing tasks that are important to them. The value of the task makes it worthwhile to put forth both the effort of rehabilitation and the continued effort of using devices or alternative strategies. The examiner should ask the patient about difficulties with a range of activities such as different forms of reading (eg, books, medication labels, newspapers, signs) and other activities of daily living (eg, shopping, cooking, dialing a phone, viewing a computer screen, shaving, watching television or sporting events), and patients should be encouraged to prioritize tasks that are most important to them as goals for their individual rehabilitation.

Questions about difficulty with independent travel, such as seeing steps and curbs, as well as driving, are important. In addition, it is useful to ask general questions about the adaptations that the patient has already made and to note the patient's observations about lighting requirements.

WELL-BEING As the history is obtained, most patients will describe the impact that vision loss has had on their lifestyle, family, vocation, and hobbies. Living situation, support systems, driving status, and personal responsibilities, such as being a caregiver for a chronically ill spouse, all bear consideration. It is helpful to inquire about the patient's current social participation, including vocation, attendance at a place of worship, volunteer activities, and/or travel. When asked directly, many patients with vision loss will report being depressed, and this can prompt referral to appropriate professionals.

It is also important to determine whether the patient has experienced falls, because fall prevention can be addressed.

CHARLES BONNET SYNDROME Patients who have Charles Bonnet syndrome, which causes them to see images of objects that are not real (and which affects one-third of visually impaired persons), are often relieved to discuss their hallucinations. Many patients are puzzled by this symptom. Some are anxious, as they do not understand what they are experiencing, and a small proportion are very upset. Most patients will not report the hallucinations unless the clinician inquires, for fear of being labeled as mentally unwell.

A diagnosis of the Charles Bonnet syndrome can be made if the patient has 4 clinical characteristics—vivid recurrent hallucinations, some degree of vision loss, insight into the unreal nature of the images when it is explained to them, and no other neurologic or psychiatric diagnosis to explain the hallucinations. Charles Bonnet syndrome is a diagnosis of exclusion, and patients should be referred for neurologic or psychiatric evaluation if they have any other neurologic signs or symptoms.

Measurement of visual function As in ophthalmology in general, visual acuity is an important and common measure of visual function in vision rehabilitation, as the task performance of a person with 20/70 visual acuity will differ from that of someone with 20/400 visual acuity. Other measures of visual function are also important, especially contrast sensitivity and central visual field. Three patients with 20/40 visual acuity might have different contrast perception and different central visual field, and hence have very different reading performance. For some patients, other measures such as peripheral visual field will also be important.

VISUAL ACUITY Accurate visual acuity measurements can be made to very low levels. Charts can be brought to closer-than-standard viewing distances (eg, 10 ft, or perhaps 1 m), extending the range of measureable acuities, compared to testing only at 20 ft. When evaluating a patient with low vision, an Early Treatment Diabetic Retinopathy Study (ETDRS) chart is commonly used at 1 or 2 m (Fig 7-39). For patients with very poor vision, the Berkeley Rudimentary Vision Assessment is available for quantifying visual acuity as low as 20/16,000.

Patients with normal vision fixate a visual acuity chart with their fovea. Patients with macular disease may fixate with other areas of the retina, and visual acuity can vary with different locations of fixation, as different retinal areas have different sensitivities. Some eye diseases, such as diabetic retinopathy, may cause fluctuating levels of visual acuity from one day to another. Some patients have very different visual function in different

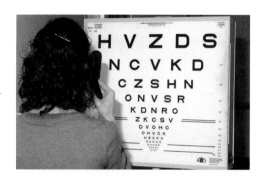

Figure 7-39 Measuring visual acuity with the ETDRS chart at 1 meter. *(Courtesy of Scott E. Brodie, MD, PhD.)*

levels of illumination. Patients with limited areas of central vision surrounded by a scotoma may be unable to read the larger letters on a visual acuity chart, causing the examiner to abandon the testing. More careful testing, however, may reveal that the patient can in fact discern smaller letters if he or she is able to align the limited central field with the targets on the eye chart.

CONTRAST SENSITIVITY The ability to discern contrast is a visual function separate from visual acuity. Although visual acuity and contrast sensitivity are frequently correlated, they may not be so in the presence of certain pathologies (eg, optic neuropathies, geographic atrophy). Patients with poor contrast sensitivity have difficulty seeing the edges of steps, reading light-colored print, driving in foggy or snowy conditions, and recognizing faces. Contrast sensitivity varies with target size (spatial frequency), and the relationship between contrast threshold and spatial frequency may be displayed as a contrast sensitivity curve (see Chapter 2). Formal tests of contrast sensitivity include the Vistech charts (available for distance or near), which map the contrast-sensitivity curve over a wide range of spatial frequencies (Fig 7-40A), and the Pelli-Robson chart, which presents large optotypes (containing a fixed mixture of spatial frequencies) over a wide range of contrasts (Fig 7-40B).

Patients whose visual impairment includes loss of contrast sensitivity may benefit from enhanced lighting, reduction of glare, or nonoptical strategies such as the use of black felt-tip markers.

CENTRAL VISUAL FIELD The largest group of patients referred for vision rehabilitation are patients with central field loss due to age-related macular degeneration (AMD). When central fixation is not reliable, traditional field testing with Goldmann or Humphrey perimeters is problematic, as such devices map the visual field relative to a central fixation point. Amsler grid tests may underestimate central field loss due to perceptual completion, or "filling in," much as the brain normally fills in the physiologic blind spot in each eye. The optimal device for evaluating central field vision in patients with central field loss is a macular perimeter that monitors fundus location and then determines the patient's direction of gaze before each target is presented. Macular perimetry documents the patient's retinal point of fixation, scotomas present in the central field, and the relationship of the fixation point to the scotomas (Fig 7-41). Most patients with central scotomas reliably

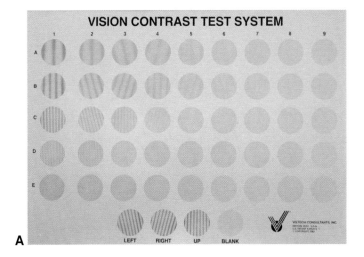

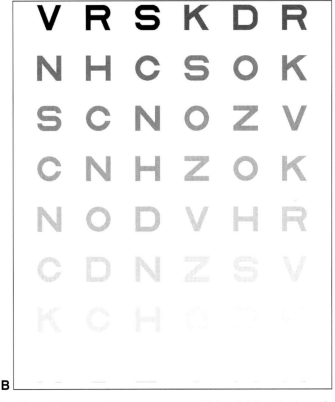

Figure 7-40 Eye charts for measuring contrast sensitivity. **A,** Vistech chart. Spatial frequency increases from top to bottom; contrast decreases in each row from left to right. Patient must detect whether grating pattern is tilted to left, vertical, or tilted to right; see samples in bottom row. **B,** Pelli-Robson chart. Contrast of large Sloan letters decreases in groups of 3 from top to bottom and left to right within each line. *(Part A courtesy of Scott E. Brodie, MD, PhD; part B reprinted with permission from Pelli DG, Robson JG, Wilkins AJ. The design of a new letter chart for measuring contrast sensitivity.* Clin Vision Sci. *1988;2(3):187–199. Copyright © 2002, Pelli DG, Robson JG. Distributed by Haag-Streit.)*

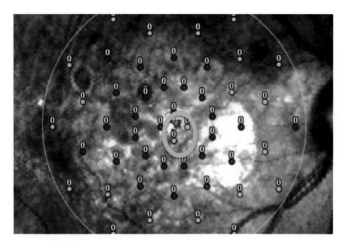

Figure 7-41 Macular microperimetry of paracentral scotoma: *green dots* indicate targets that are seen by patient; *red dots* indicate missed targets. *(Courtesy of Mary Lou Jackson, MD, and AAO Vision Rehabilitation Committee.)*

develop an eccentric functional *pseudofovea*, often called the *preferred retinal locus (PRL)*, for fixation. There may be several loci of eccentric fixation, and the PRL may change as the underlying disease progresses. Different eccentric fixation loci may be used for different tasks or in different levels of illumination.

Knowing the location of the PRL relative to the scotoma can assist the clinician in understanding specific difficulties the patient has in carrying out visual tasks. For example, scotomas to the right of fixation may obscure the ends of words; scotomas to the left of fixation may make it difficult to carry out an accurate saccade to the beginning of the next line of print. Ring scotomas may interfere with the recognition of large objects or long words (Fig 7-42).

Scotomas can vary widely in size, shape, number, and density, and they may not correspond to the fundus appearance of atrophy, scarring, or pigment alteration. This lack of correspondence is particularly important to consider in patients with wet AMD who receive anti–vascular endothelial growth factor (anti-VEGF) injections. Such patients may not exhibit obvious scars yet still have significant scotomas in their central field.

PERIPHERAL VISUAL FIELD The peripheral visual field is crucial for mobility and orientation. Typical symptoms of peripheral visual field defects include bumping into objects or people and difficulty navigating through unfamiliar territory, particularly in poor illumination or at night. Variable patterns of visual field loss can result from diseases of the retina, optic nerve, and central nervous system. Appreciating patterns of peripheral field loss, such as may occur in retinitis pigmentosa or glaucoma, or after cerebrovascular accidents, is useful in planning rehabilitation interventions such as orientation and mobility training or in counseling and training patients about strategies to compensate for the field defects.

Poor vision does not preclude peripheral visual field testing. Many older patients may be better able to work with the manual Goldmann perimeter than with computerized

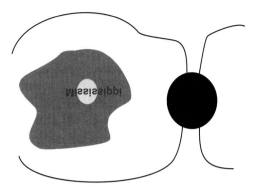

Figure 7-42 Effect of paracentral scotoma on visualization of large print. *(Courtesy of Mary Lou Jackson, MD, and AAO Vision Rehabilitation Committee.)*

static field instruments such as the Humphrey perimeter or Octopus. Unsteady central fixation can be steadied by using larger central fixation targets, if necessary using the tangent screen. Larger or brighter test targets should be used as needed. If formal perimetry testing is not possible, confrontation testing with fingers or flashlights may allow appreciation of large hemianopic or bitemporal field defects.

The common central visual field protocols such as the 24-2 and 30-2 programs on the Humphrey perimeter are not suitable for mapping peripheral scotomas. Goldmann perimetry is preferable when peripheral scotomas are an important visual limitation, such as in patients with retinitis pigmentosa or vigabatrin-induced retinal toxicity.

GLARE Glare is the discomfort or impairment of vision caused by scattered light. Common conditions resulting in glare include corneal edema, cataracts, cone–rod dystrophy, and albinism, but AMD or glaucoma may also cause glare. Patients with reduced contrast sensitivity often require increased illumination, which may, in turn, exacerbate glare. Therefore, determining sensitivity to glare is important so that you can advise patients about optimal lighting.

The simplest way to assess glare is through the history; however, clinicians can also informally perform visual acuity and contrast sensitivity testing with and without a source of light adjacent to the test target, directed toward the patient. One commercially available test is the Brightness Acuity Tester, a handheld device that allows the patient to view a distant target through a small dome that floods the eye with off-axis illumination. The clinician should also ask about the current and desired light sources and their positions in the patient's normal environments, as this information is useful for planning rehabilitation strategies.

COLOR VISION Acquired color vision deficits affect performance in tasks involving color identification or matching. Most acquired color vision defects in low vision patients are blue-yellow defects. The commonly used pseudoisochromatic plate tests (Ishihara test plates) do not provide assessment of blue-yellow defects; rather, they detect (typically) hereditary red-green color vision deficits. Tests suitable for detecting blue-yellow as well as red-green color vision abnormalities include the Hardy-Rand-Rittler plates and the Farnsworth D-15 panel. The "jumbo" version of the D-15 panel, with larger color discs, is a convenient color vision test for low vision patients, although it can miss mild deficits.

Performance of visual tasks In addition to formal assessment of visual function, evaluation of the patient for vision rehabilitation should include assessment of the performance of tasks requiring vision, such as reading. Reading charts are available to assess reading short segments of text, sentences, or paragraphs. Useful variables include the minimum size of print that can be seen with current glasses or devices, reading errors, and reading speed. Note that different patients with the same distance visual acuity may read different sizes of near print if they are using different powers of reading add. The reading add power used and the distance from the eye to the text should always be documented when measuring near vision (eg, 0.4 M at 40 cm, add +2.50). Observing a patient reading the actual material that he or she normally reads—such as the newspaper, medication labels, or directions on a package—is also informative, not only to determine success but also to note other factors such as head posture or strategies to manipulate the reading material. Close work such as sewing may be an issue as well.

Watching a patient write or attempt to perform a task such as dialing a cell phone or reading e-mail is informative. Adaptations that the patient has already made should be noted. Observing a patient ambulate provides valuable insight into the need for training in scanning or the use of devices such as a support cane and/or a white cane.

Computers offer both special challenges and opportunities for patients with visual impairment (as discussed in the section Electronic Devices). It is worthwhile to ask specifically about computer use and what strategies the patient may have already implemented. Other vision-dependent challenges may include intermediate distance tasks such as playing a musical instrument, reading labels in museums and grocery stores, and playing cards.

Interventions

Refraction A careful determination of refraction is required for all patients with reduced vision to uncover uncorrected refractive errors and assist with planning reading adds. A trial frame may be more effective for refraction than working with a phoropter.

Retinoscopy is frequently very helpful. In cases where the reflex is dull or motion of the reflex is difficult to see, retinoscopy can be conducted at half the customary distance from the retinoscope to the eye. This requires doubling the power of the working-distance lens. Be aware of the possibility of "pseudoneutralization" when performing retinoscopy on patients with very high myopia. In these cases, in which there is only a very dull, immobile retinoscopic reflex, reversing the sleeve of the retinoscope (creating the so-called concave-mirror effect) will reverse the reflexes, converting the pseudoneutral image to a readily perceptible "with" reflex, which should be neutralized with minus sphere power. As the reflex starts to broaden, return the sleeve to the normal position; the reflex will revert to a recognizable "against," and the retinoscopy can be completed in the usual way.

For patients with reduced visual function to perceive a change between choices shown in a binary comparison ("Which is better, 1 or 2?") during manifest refraction, the dioptric interval between the lenses must be increased. As a starting point, increase the interval from the usual 0.50 D (+0.25 D/−0.25 D) to 1.00 D (+0.50 D/−0.50 D) for patients with visual acuity from 20/50 to 20/100 and to 2.00 D (+1.00 D/−1.00 D) for patients with visual acuity worse than 20/100.

Occasionally, an automated refractor will detect a cylinder that is difficult to see with a retinoscope. In some cases, particularly patients with irregular optics, the stenopeic slit will clarify an astigmatic error better than will other tools.

In prescribing glasses for patients with anisometropia (unequal refractive errors), consider giving the correct lens power for the poorer seeing eye, rather than a balance lens, particularly if this will allow better peripheral vision in a patient with central visual field loss. Polycarbonate lenses are recommended for safety.

Watch for unreasonable expectations, which may lead patients to hope that new glasses can solve vision problems associated with the eye disease. As the complex spectacles often prescribed for low vision patients can be expensive, clinicians should ensure that patients' financial resources are not depleted on spectacles that offer little benefit, especially when that money could be put toward other devices that significantly improve function. If possible, a trial simulating the proposed spectacles in temporary frames should be used to help the patient anticipate the expected results.

Optical devices Traditional options for magnification include high-plus reading glasses, magnifiers, and telescopes, as discussed in the chapter. Recent, commercially available technological advances include an electronic device combining a camera and a head-worn display that allows both near and distance viewing and a surgically implanted miniature telescope.

It should be remembered, however, that patients may also simply move closer to distant targets such as the television or the blackboard. This strategy is much more common and practical, and less costly, than using a telescope.

Electronic devices The use of electronic low vision aids is described in the chapter text. These devices should be selected carefully to meet the patient's needs, and appropriate training in their use must be provided. Assistance with setup may be necessary for successful use by patients with low vision.

Education, counseling, and support groups Resource materials should be provided to all patients, because education is an important component of rehabilitation. Such materials may include information about their ocular disease; alternative transportation; free local and national services, such as the Library of Congress Talking Books Program and radio reading services; sources of large-print books and music; telephone information and dialing services; and contact information for support groups.

Vision loss has an impact on patients' quality of life, independence, and emotional well-being. Patients with vision loss experience fear, isolation, anger, and sometimes depression. Seniors with vision loss are at high risk for falls, injuries, medication errors, nutritional decline, social isolation, and depression at far higher rates than reported for sighted individuals. Vision loss also affects the patient's spouse and family. Psychological counseling and support groups may be part of the rehabilitation team's approach to helping patients and their families cope and adapt. Social workers and other counselors may be called upon to contribute to this rehabilitation process.

Pediatric low vision

Although vision loss is less frequent in the pediatric population, this cohort is an important group requiring the ophthalmologist's attention. Every child with loss of vision needs to be recognized, and the ophthalmologist's response should include recommending vision rehabilitation. Most adults with low vision have lost vision because of an ocular disease incurred later in life. Thus, they have already acquired many of the vision-aided skills (eg, reading, understanding social cues, cooking, self-care tasks) that are important for functioning in society. Children with low vision, however, need to learn these skills despite poor or no vision.

The most prevalent causes of visual impairment in children in the United States are cortical visual impairment, retinopathy of prematurity, optic nerve hypoplasia, albinism, optic atrophy, and congenital infections. Many of these children have coexisting physical and/or cognitive disabilities that create further challenges to successful integration into society.

In addition, skill acquisition is developmentally linked to vision, thus requiring different interventions at different ages. It is important to be aware of the needs of each age group and tailor the assistance to those needs. Rehabilitation of infants and children requires a team approach, often involving occupational and physical therapists, special educators, and physicians working with the child and family from the earliest stages possible. Ophthalmologists may be one of the most consistent contacts over many years for the parents of a visually impaired child, and, as such, they need to be aware of and support the rehabilitation process. (See BCSC Section 6, *Pediatric Ophthalmology and Strabismus.*)

Schwartz T. Causes of visual impairment: pathology and its implications. In: Corn AL, Erin JN, eds. *Foundations of Low Vision: Clinical and Functional Perspectives.* 2nd ed. New York: American Foundation for the Blind Press; 2010:chap 6.

Infants The ophthalmologist plays a key role in the examination and assessment of an infant with suspected low vision. A definite diagnosis, together with a clear and realistic prognosis, helps guide the rehabilitation plan. Early intervention by a skilled multidisciplinary team is critical during early development. Vision is the primary means by which infants interact with their world, and it drives motor development as well. Interventions must be individualized to each child's set of capabilities and challenges.

The role of vision stimulation training is controversial. Little evidence indicates that these activities actually improve visual function, but such classes may help parents prepare a visually impaired child to function in a seeing world and make best use of his or her remaining vision. That said, care should be taken not to put pressure on children to "see" things they cannot see or to stigmatize nonvisual strategies.

Preschool children For preschool children, more sophisticated low vision testing and more precise evaluation are possible. Near visual aids are usually not necessary owing to a child's high accommodative amplitude and the relatively large size of toys and images or text in printed books. However, early sensory stimulation to compensate for the lack of visual stimulation is important. For accommodation to be used effectively, large astigmatic errors, hyperopic errors, and anisometropia must be treated.

Kindergartners to preadolescents Simple devices may be of value for young children; devices include the dome-type magnifier (Fig 7-43) for near tasks or a handheld monocular telescope for viewing the blackboard (see Fig 7-37). Providing teachers with a bucket of

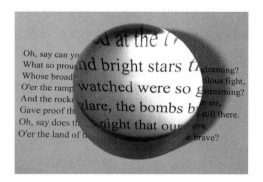

Figure 7-43 Bright-field dome ("paperweight") magnifier. Note how this type of stand magnifier gathers ambient light, avoiding the need for artificial illumination. *(Courtesy of Scott E. Brodie, MD, PhD.)*

thick chalk sticks ("sidewalk chalk"), may encourage them to write in larger letters on the blackboard.

It is a good idea to introduce new devices at home so that the child becomes comfortable with their use before trying them out among his or her peers. Children with low vision should acquire typing skills and learn to use the computer early, because the computer will probably become their main portal to the world of information, and many adaptations are possible through its use. In addition, Braille literacy is valuable and is most easily acquired in childhood.

As children mature, they begin to formulate and express personal goals. Parents and the vision rehabilitation team need to be sensitive to these goals, because the ultimate success of the rehabilitation program depends on the child's continued active participation.

Teenagers Low vision aids that were used at a younger age may be rejected by teenagers concerned about peer acceptance. However, new technologies such as smartphones or tablet devices may be readily accepted. (See the section Electronic Devices.) The clinician should be sensitive to the complex demands of the teenage years for patients with low vision.

Ongoing eye care

It is important to remember that referral of patients with impaired vision for visual rehabilitation should not mean the end of the therapeutic relationship between patient and ophthalmologist. Patients should continue to be monitored, including screening for glaucoma and diabetic retinopathy, and treatment implemented as indicated. Refractive errors may continue to evolve, and updates of prescriptions for glasses and/or contact lenses may be needed.

Treatment for disorders such as cataract and AMD should still be considered for patients with limited visual potential, even though normal or near-normal visual acuity may not be a potential outcome. For example, treatment of a disciform scar with anti-VEGF injections may stabilize macular function, protecting the patient's 20/200 or 20/400 vision against further deterioration and enlargement of the central scotoma. In this case, the difference between, say, 20/200 and 20/400 vision may substantially reduce the magnification required for reading and enhance the effectiveness of visual rehabilitation techniques.

Resources

The American Academy of Ophthalmology and the American Foundation for the Blind offer vision rehabilitation resources of use to ophthalmologists.

AAO SmartSight SmartSight is the American Academy of Ophthalmology's initiative in vision rehabilitation. It provides materials for ophthalmologists to give to patients to introduce them to the possibilities of vision rehabilitation, as well as guidelines and references for ophthalmologists. The SmartSight resources described here are available for download at http://one.aao.org/ce/educationalcontent/smartsight.aspx.

MATERIALS FOR PATIENTS The SmartSight Patient Handout is available for download (in PDF format) for you to give to patients. It provides essential tips for making the most of remaining vision and offers a list of resources where patients can locate local services using the Find Services Near You directory.

MATERIALS FOR OPHTHALMOLOGISTS Information and materials for ophthalmologists through the SmartSight link include the following:

- The SmartSight Levels 1 and 2 documents (in PDF format) provide easy guidelines for recognizing, assisting, and examining patients with low vision, including a patient handout and steps associated with the "4 R's of Rehabilitation"—Record, Refract, Rx, Report.
- The SmartSight Level 3 document (in PDF format) provides more extensive information on vision rehabilitation services and references.
- A sample letter (in Microsoft Word format) can be used to inform primary care physicians of a patient's vision loss and the possibility of Charles Bonnet syndrome.
- For questions about vision rehabilitation or the SmartSight program, contact the AAO at SmartSight@aao.org.

American Foundation for the Blind AFB's Senior Site (www.visionaware.org/section.aspx?FolderID=11) contains information about living with vision loss, including home adaptations, products, and connections to local services.

CHAPTER 8

Physical Optics

This chapter discusses the characteristics of light and some of the ways these characteristics can be put to clinical use.

The Corpuscular Theory of Light

The Greek philosophers Leucippus and Democritus (c 450 BC) proposed that light is a flow of miniscule particles or "corpuscles." Such particles, it was thought, travel instantaneously between points separated by any distance, which is to say at infinite speed.

According to the law of rectilinear propagation, light moves in straight lines and changes direction only if reflected or refracted (Fig 8-1). The law of reflection was established by observing light rebounding symmetrically from smooth surfaces (Fig 8-2). Refraction was also readily observed but, at the time, not as clearly understood (Fig 8-3). The angles of incidence and transmission (the latter also known as the angle of refraction) were thought to be proportional, which is not correct but is a good approximation for small angles.

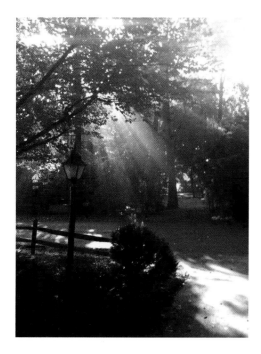

Figure 8-1 Sunlight passing through openings between partially overlapping leaves suggests that light moves in straight lines. However, such "rays" would be invisible without light scattering caused by mist in the air (eg, Tyndall effect). Likewise, the beam of a slit lamp is not normally visible in the anterior chamber but becomes so when light is scattered by the presence of abnormal proteins or cells. *(Illustration by Edmond H. Thall, MD.)*

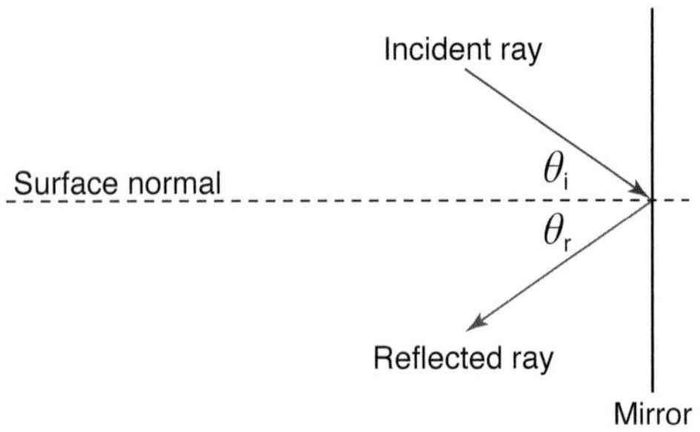

Figure 8-2 The law of reflection states that an incident ray rebounds symmetrically after striking a smooth surface. The angles of incidence (θ_i) and reflection (θ_r) are defined with respect to an imaginary line, the surface normal. The law states that (1) the incident ray, reflected ray, and surface normal are coplanar, and (2) θ_i equals θ_r. *(Illustration by Edmond H. Thall, MD.)*

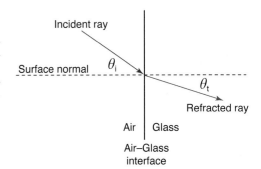

Figure 8-3 Light moving from one material to another abruptly changes speed (refraction) and usually direction. The angles of incidence (θ_i) and transmission (θ_t) are defined with respect to the surface normal. The incident ray, refracted ray, and surface normal are coplanar. θ_i and θ_t are related by the equation $n_1 \sin \theta_i = n_2 \sin \theta_t$. The approximation $n_1 \theta_i = n_2 \theta_t$ is sufficiently accurate for small angles. *(Illustration by Edmond H. Thall, MD.)*

The corpuscular hypothesis lacked supporting experimental evidence. Nevertheless, it was accepted essentially unchallenged for 2000 years.

Diffraction

According to the corpuscular theory, collimated light should remain so after traversing an aperture. Actually, the beam diverges, violating the law of rectilinear propagation (Fig 8-4). All apertures produce diffraction to some extent. The smaller the aperture is relative to the wavelength, the more pronounced is the consequent diffraction (Fig 8-5).

Some scientists believed that the discovery of diffraction (c 1665) offered sufficient justification to abandon the corpuscular theory completely, and they concluded that light was fundamentally a wave. Sir Isaac Newton and others, however, believed that the

Figure 8-4 Behavior of light crossing an aperture. **A,** According to the corpuscular theory of light, a collimated beam should remain so after crossing an aperture that blocks the sides of the beam. **B,** Instead, the beam diverges. This phenomenon, called diffraction, violates the law of rectilinear propagation and suggests that light is a wave, not a series of particles (corpuscular). *(Illustration by Edmond H. Thall, MD.)*

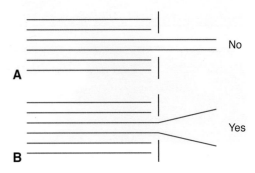

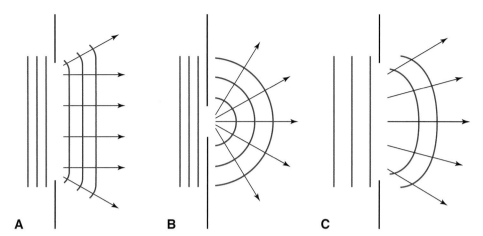

Figure 8-5 **A,** According to the law of rectilinear propagation, light should not change direction after traversing an aperture. **B,** In reality, apertures do cause light to change direction—a phenomenon called diffraction. **C,** The smaller the aperture is relative to the wavelength of incident light, the more pronounced is the diffraction. *(Illustration by Edmond H. Thall, MD.)*

corpuscular theory could explain diffraction. For the next 100 years, the nature of light—wave or particle—was an open question.

The Speed of Light

In 1687, Danish astronomer Ole Roemer noted an irregularity in the orbit of Jupiter's moon Io that he attributed to light having a finite speed. Later laboratory measurements confirmed that the speed of light is finite.

By international agreement, a meter had been defined by the length of a metal bar kept in Paris, France. Because this standard meter bar might be damaged or destroyed by war or natural disaster, the international community adopted a standard of measurement based on natural phenomena that are readily accessible and indestructible. Hence, the speed of light became the measurement standard, and the meter is defined as the distance light travels in a vacuum during 1/299,792,458 second. Thus, the speed of light is by definition exactly 299,792,458 m/s. A useful approximation for the speed of light in a vacuum is 3×10^8 m/s (approximately 1 ft/ns).

The Superposition of Waves

The superposition principle states that when 2 or more waves overlap, their amplitudes will add or cancel. The superposition of 2 waves of differing frequencies produces a changing "interference" pattern of reinforcement and cancellation that, in the case of light, is much too fast to be observed (Fig 8-6). However, the superposition of 2 waves of identical frequency produces a stable interference pattern (Fig 8-7).

The result of 2 particles striking the same place simultaneously is always additive, whereas 2 overlapping waves may reinforce or cancel each other, as just described. In

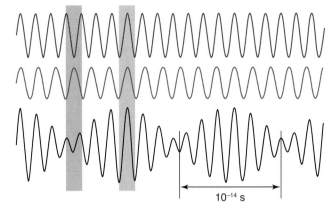

Figure 8-6 According to the principle of superposition, when 2 waves overlap, their amplitudes add, *producing a single resultant wave.* The 2 waves at top differ slightly in frequency and align peak to peak *(blue band)*, reinforcing each other in some places, and peak to trough *(red band)*, canceling each other in some places. In this example, complete cancellation does not occur because the waves differ in amplitude. In any case, the pattern alternates between reinforcement and cancellation about every 10^{-14} second—much too fast to be observed. *(Illustration by Edmond H. Thall, MD.)*

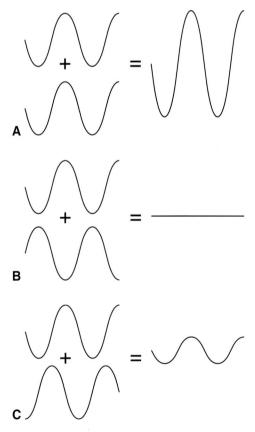

Figure 8-7 Overlapping waves of identical frequency and amplitude produce stable interference patterns. **A,** Waves overlap in phase—peaks coincide with peaks and troughs with troughs—producing a resultant wave of twice the amplitude. **B,** Waves overlap out of phase—the peak of one wave coincides with the trough of the other—and the waves cancel. **C,** Waves partially overlap—neither completely in nor out of phase—producing a wave of intermediate amplitude (between zero and twice the amplitude). *(Illustration developed by Edmond H. Thall, MD, and redrawn by C. H. Wooley.)*

1801, London physician Thomas Young demonstrated that light can produce patterns of cancellation and reinforcement, thus providing strong evidence that light is a wave phenomenon.

Coherence

Light from most sources consists of wave trains. Just as a train has many cars, a wave train consists of many sections, each having a dominant frequency (Fig 8-8). *Temporal coherence* is a function of the bandwidth of a light source (ie, the number of frequencies it is composed of). Wave trains from broadband light sources (ie, those radiating many frequencies) consist of short sections, whereas narrowband light sources consist of wave trains with longer sections. The length of one wave train section is the *coherence length*. The time required for light to travel one coherence length is the *coherence time*.

Consider a single section of a wave train from a broadband point source illuminating 2 small, closely spaced pinholes in an otherwise opaque screen (Fig 8-9A). Each section

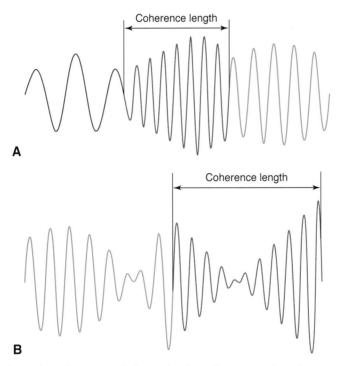

A

B

Figure 8-8 Each section of a wave train has a dominant frequency that changes randomly from one section to the next. The color of each section corresponds to its dominant frequency—eg, in **A,** the *red* section is lower in frequency, and the *blue* section is higher in frequency. The length of each section is the *coherence length*. **A,** Broadband wave trains have a short coherence length. **B,** Compared with **A,** the light represented in **B** has a narrower bandwidth and consequently a longer coherence length. *(Illustration by Edmond H. Thall, MD.)*

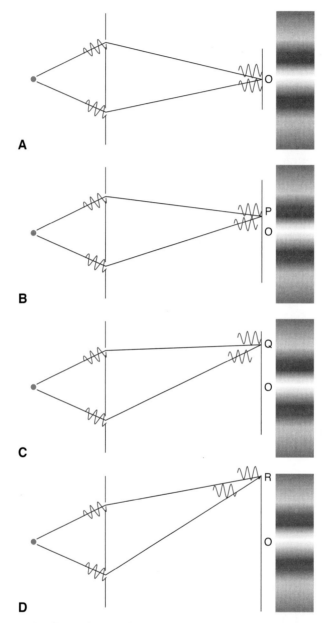

Figure 8-9 Schematic of Young's experiment demonstrating that light is a wave phenomenon. **A,** Wave train sections arrive at the pinholes simultaneously, then diffract and arrive simultaneously at point O. They constructively interfere, producing a bright spot. **B,** To reach point P, one section travels slightly farther than the other, which lags behind by half a wavelength. The 2 sections interfere destructively, and point P is dark. **C,** At point Q, one section lags behind the other by 1 full wavelength. The 2 sections interfere constructively, producing a reduced bright spot. **D,** At point R, one section lags the other by more than 1 coherence length so there is no interference, but a superposition of noncorresponding sections produces an average uniform illumination. *(Illustration by Edmond H. Thall, MD.)*

arrives at both pinholes simultaneously and is diffracted by the pinholes. The distance from each pinhole to point O is identical, so both sections produce a bright spot by constructive (ie, additive) interference.

At point P (Fig 8-9B), one section travels half a wavelength farther than the other, so the 2 sections cancel, producing a dark spot by destructive (ie, subtractive) interference. At point Q (Fig 8-9C), the sections differ by a full wavelength and again produce a bright spot by constructive interference. Alternating intervals of constructive and destructive interference produce a fringe pattern. However, as the distance from point O increases, the wave train sections overlap less and less, decreasing the degree of fringe contrast (ie, the difference in intensity between the brightest and darkest points). At point R (Fig 8-9D), one section lags the other by more than its coherence length, so the sections do not overlap at all. Because the superposition of nonidentical sections does not produce stable interference, fringes are no longer visible.

Sunlight (composed of numerous frequencies) has a coherence length of 1–2 μm, whereas laser light (composed of few frequencies) typically has a coherence length of several centimeters. If the point source in Figure 8-9 were to be replaced by a laser light source, many more fringes of much higher contrast would be generated.

Another aspect of coherence concerns a light source's physical size (ie, length or area). Consider a second point source illuminating 2 pinholes (Fig 8-10). Fringes produced by the second source are shifted slightly relative to the first. When the 2 fringe patterns are combined, the result is lower-contrast fringes. If the light source consists of many point sources distributed over a broad area, the net result will be a total loss of contrast and no fringes will be evident. *Spatial coherence* refers to the size of the light source, which must be small to produce visible fringes.

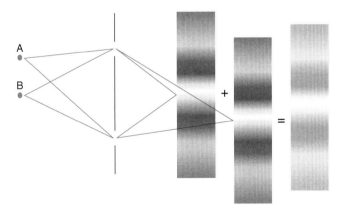

Figure 8-10 The effect of the size of a light source on spatial coherence. The interferometer fringe pattern produced by a second point source *(point B)* of light is shifted relative to the first point source *(point A)*. Superimposing both patterns results in a new pattern with decreased fringe contrast. A small light source has high spatial coherence and produces high-contrast fringes. If a light source is too large (ie, consists of numerous point sources), no fringes will be seen. *(Illustration by Edmond H. Thall, MD.)*

Electromagnetic Waves

The corpuscular theory of light was abandoned after Young provided strong evidence that light is a wave phenomenon. The next question is, What type of wave? James Clerk Maxwell developed equations describing the behavior of electric and magnetic fields. Maxwell discovered that oscillating electric fields (ie, those that rhythmically reverse polarity) are inextricably linked to oscillating magnetic fields and that such electromagnetic (EM) fields can radiate as waves. In 1862, Maxwell calculated the speed of EM waves and found that they moved at the speed of light, and he thus concluded that light is an EM wave. Several phenomena can be explained by the EM wave theory.

Polarization

The electric field of an EM wave oscillates perpendicularly to its magnetic field, and both oscillate perpendicularly to their direction of propagation (Fig 8-11). Because the electric and magnetic fields oscillate in lockstep, for simplicity only the electric field is shown in most illustrations. The EM plane of polarization is defined by the orientation of the electric-field oscillation (eg, vertical in Fig 8-11) and direction of propagation. In general, the plane of polarization of an EM wave may have any orientation (ie, horizontal, vertical, or oblique).

Note that there is no such thing as "unpolarized" light. Typically, the plane of polarization changes rapidly (about every 10^{-13} to 10^{-14} second) and randomly, resulting in light that is randomly polarized. *Linearly polarized light,* however, has a single unchanging plane of polarization. In *circularly polarized light,* the plane of polarization rotates, and the (maximum) electric-field vector traces a corkscrew pattern as the wave propagates. Viewed

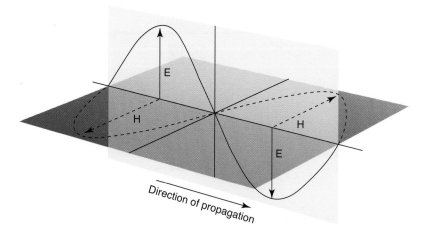

Figure 8-11 Light is polarized. The plane of polarization is specified with reference to the direction of propagation and the direction of the oscillating electric (E) or magnetic (H) field, which always oscillate perpendicularly to each other. In this view, the electric field is polarized vertically and the magnetic field horizontally, but they could be interchanged, or polarization could be in any oblique meridian. *(Illustration by Jonathan Clark.)*

head-on, the field vector traces a circle. In *elliptically polarized light,* which represents a more general case of circular polarization, the plane of polarization rotates as the wave propagates, but the (maximum) electric-field vector traces an ellipse instead of a circle.

Refractive Index and Dispersion

EM waves travel fastest in a vacuum and slower in any transparent material medium. All EM frequencies travel at the same speed in vacuum, but in any transparent medium, each frequency travels at a different speed—a phenomenon called *dispersion.* The refractive index *(n)* is the ratio of the speed of light in a vacuum divided by its speed in a given material. Dispersion is measured using the refractive index at 3 different wavelengths. This measurement, the Abbe number *(V),* is defined as

$$V = \frac{n_d - 1}{n_F - n_C}$$

where n_d, n_F, and n_C represent wavelengths (in a vacuum) of 587.6 nm, 486.1 nm, and 656.3 nm, respectively. Larger Abbe numbers indicate lower dispersion.

Reflection, Transmission, and Absorption

Consider light striking the interface between 2 materials such as air and glass (Fig 8-12). Some light is reflected according to the law of reflection and some transmitted (refracted) according to Snell's law.

The question is, How much light is reflected and how much transmitted? Applying electromagnetic wave theory, Fresnel demonstrated that the greater the difference in the refractive indices or the greater the angle of incidence, the greater the degree of reflection and, consequently, the less light transmitted. For an air–glass interface, typically about 4% of light is reflected at low angles of incidence. Tears have a lower refractive index than glass, so an air–tear-film interface reflects even less light—about 2%.

Light reflected at the front and back surfaces of the cornea and the crystalline lens produces the 4 Purkinje images. The reader should be able to rank the Purkinje images from brightest to dimmest in both phakic and pseudophakic eyes.

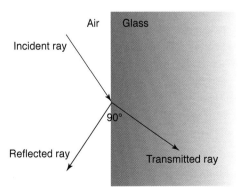

Figure 8-12 At the interface of 2 transparent media, some incident light is reflected and some is refracted (transmitted). The amount of reflected light increases as the angle of incidence increases, and the amount of light refracted decreases commensurately. When, as in this case, the reflected and refracted rays form a right angle, all the reflected light is linearly polarized parallel to the interface (ie, perpendicular to the plane of incidence). *(Illustration by Edmond H. Thall, MD.)*

Fresnel also showed that reflected light tends to be linearly polarized parallel to the interface. Reflected light is completely polarized if the angle of incidence equals the *Brewster angle:*

$$\text{Brewster Angle} = \tan^{-1} \frac{n_t}{n_i}$$

where n_t and n_i are the refractive indices of the transmitted and incident media, respectively. At the Brewster angle, all the reflected light is linearly polarized, but not all the linearly polarized light is reflected. Consequently, the *transmitted light* is a mixture of linearly and randomly polarized light.

When light moves from a higher to lower refractive index medium, it will be completely reflected *(total internal reflection [TIR])* if the angle of incidence exceeds the *critical angle:*

$$\text{Critical Angle} = \sin^{-1} \frac{n_t}{n_i}$$

Note that the critical angle always exceeds the Brewster angle. TIR is what prevents visualization of the anterior chamber angle during slit lamp examination. In rare cases, the cornea might be so distorted that the angle is visible without gonioscopy, but usually some method must be employed to prevent TIR and make the angle visible.

Absorption is usually expressed as an *optical density (OD).* An OD of 1 represents a transmittance of 10%; an OD of 2, a transmittance of 1% (0.01); and an OD of 3, a transmittance of 0.1% (0.001). In general, the expression for optical density is

$$\text{Optical Density} = \log_{10} \frac{1}{T}$$

where T is the transmittance. (See Chapter 3 for a discussion of absorptive lenses.)

The Electromagnetic Spectrum

All EM radiation is fundamentally the same phenomenon, but its manifestations strongly depend on frequency. The frequency of EM radiation has no specific upper or lower limit. The spectrum is divided into regions in which the radiation is produced and detected by similar techniques; thus, various EM regions partially overlap (Fig 8-13).

For instance, "light" generally refers to the very narrow portion of the electromagnetic spectrum that stimulates the retina. However, the limits of the visible spectrum are not well defined because the sensitivity of the retina approaches zero asymptotically. If the limits are taken (arbitrarily) as the points where the eye's sensitivity is 1% of maximum, then the visible spectrum spans the frequencies between 7.0×10^{14} Hz ($\lambda = 430$ nm) and 4.3×10^{14} Hz ($\lambda = 690$ nm). However, the eye can detect radiation, if sufficiently intense, beyond these limits.

Frequency and Color

Despite the use of terms such as *blue light* or *red light,* color is not a property of light but rather a phenomenon of perception. "Spectral colors" are perceived when an area of the retina is stimulated by a single frequency. The colors of the rainbow are spectral colors.

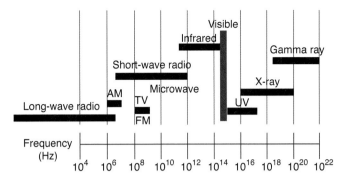

Figure 8-13 The electromagnetic (EM) spectrum. The spectrum is divided for practicality into regions in which the radiation is generated and detected by similar techniques and equipment; thus, various EM regions partially overlap. Notice the relatively small visible portion of the EM spectrum *(red bar)* compared with other portions. *(Illustration by Edmond H. Thall, MD.)*

Other color sensations not seen in the rainbow (eg, cyan, magenta) are perceived when multiple frequencies stimulate the same region of the retina simultaneously.

Energy in an Electromagnetic Wave

Light is both a form of energy and a means of conveying energy from one point to another. In EM wave theory, the energy carried by the wave is proportional to the square of its amplitude and does not depend at all on the frequency of the wave.

Quantum Theory

EM wave theory successfully explains "macroscopic" phenomena but fails to explain phenomena at the atomic and molecular levels. According to EM theory, electrons orbiting in an atom should constantly radiate EM waves, lose energy in the process, and ultimately crash into the nucleus—which, of course, does not happen. Thus, a new theory was required that would be capable of explaining the behavior of electrons in atoms and molecules.

The new theory—quantum theory—states that electrons in atoms (or molecules) exist in *nonradiating* states and that each state is associated with a specific energy level. The energy states possible for an atom differ from element to element, and those for a molecule differ from compound to compound. Each element or compound has a unique distribution of energy states (Fig 8-14).

When an electron "drops" from a higher energy state to a lower one, the difference in energy (E) is radiated as a "packet," called a photon, with a characteristic frequency (v) given by

$$E = hv$$

where h is the Planck constant. Similarly, an electron can "jump" to a higher energy state by absorbing a photon, with the resulting energy equal to the energy difference between states (Fig 8-15). According to EM theory, wave energy depends on amplitude only and

Figure 8-14 Energy levels for the electrons in a hypothetical atom. The vertical axis indicates the increasing energy associated with each successive energy state for an atom's electrons. Each element or compound has a unique distribution of energy levels. *(Illustration by Edmond H. Thall, MD.)*

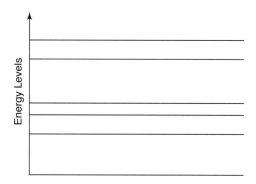

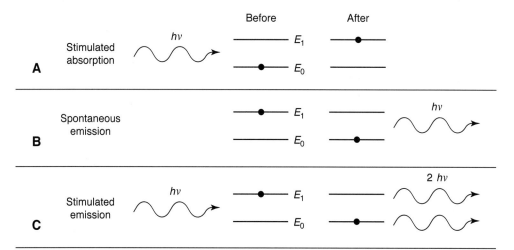

Figure 8-15 An electron moves between its lowest energy (ground) state (E_0) and an excited state (E_1) after absorbing a quantum of light energy ($\Delta E = E_1 - E_0 = h\nu$). **A,** Stimulated absorption. **B,** Spontaneous emission. **C,** Stimulated emission. *(Reproduced with permission from Steinert RF, Puliafito CA. The Nd:YAG Laser in Ophthalmology: Principles and Clinical Applications of Photodisruption. Philadelphia: Saunders; 1985. Redrawn by C. H. Wooley.)*

frequency does not matter, whereas according to quantum theory, energy depends on frequency only and amplitude does not matter.

Light Sources

Light sources convert nonlight forms of energy into light and may be categorized as thermal or luminescent.

Thermal Sources

The atoms in material warmer than absolute zero are thermally agitated and radiate EM waves as a result. As temperature increases, the amount of energy radiated increases, and a greater percentage of the total radiated energy occurs at higher frequencies. At body temperature (about 37°C, or 310 K), for instance, most of the radiated energy occurs in the infrared spectrum (eg, the thermal energy detectable by night-vision devices). At body temperature, however, a miniscule amount of visible light is produced well below the visual threshold.

As the temperature of an object increases, it begins to produce EM energy at visible frequencies, first glowing red and, with further increases in temperature, glowing brighter and bluer. The spectrum of all thermal sources of light is continuous; that is, thermal sources produce some EM radiation at every frequency. Planck showed that the energy radiated at any frequency can change only by discrete amounts (ie, multiples of hv).

Luminescent Sources

Luminescent sources produce light as a result of electron transitions between different energy states—a process different from thermal agitation. In a gas discharge tube, for example, a small amount of gas (eg, hydrogen, helium, or mercury vapor) well below atmospheric pressure is placed in an otherwise evacuated glass tube that is sealed with an electrode at each end. An electrical potential is applied across the electrodes, and the electrical energy raises the electrons of the gas to higher energy states. Almost immediately, the electrons drop to lower levels, emitting light.

The differences (ie, spacing) between energy states in each element are unique. Typically, electron transitions between only a few energy states will produce visible photons. Because every element (or molecule) has a unique set of energy levels, each produces a unique visible spectrum (Fig 8-16), a circumstance that is useful from a practical and scientific standpoint. For example, light produced at the center of the sun is absorbed by atoms at the cooler surface. Only the frequencies corresponding to specific transitions are absorbed, producing discrete dark lines in an otherwise continuous solar spectrum. The

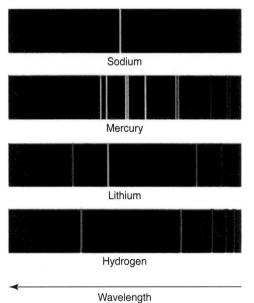

Sodium

Mercury

Lithium

Hydrogen

Wavelength

Figure 8-16 Discrete spectral lines produced by various elements. Every kind of atom has a different distribution of energy states. Each line in an atom's spectrum corresponds to an energy difference between 2 states.

pattern of dark spectral lines identifies the elements in the sun. Similarly, each frequency produced by a gas discharge tube can be isolated and used as a light source in its own right. Long before the advent of lasers, gas discharge tubes provided a practical source of monochromatic light.

Fluorescence

When an electron absorbs a photon and jumps to a higher energy level, usually it quickly drops back to the original level and emits a photon identical in frequency to the one it absorbed. However, atoms of some elements have 2 energy levels that are close together (Fig 8-17). When a photon is absorbed, the electron jumps to the highest energy level. Instead of dropping back to the original level, however, the electron transitions to the slightly lower level and emits nonvisible energy. Next, it drops to the initial energy level and emits a photon. The photon emitted is still visible but has less energy than the absorbed photon and, therefore, a lower frequency.

This phenomenon, called *fluorescence,* occurs only in materials possessing close spacing between energy levels. The essential feature is that the emitted photon has a lower frequency and, therefore, a different color from that of the stimulating photon. The clinical utility of this phenomenon (discussed later) derives from the difference in frequency between the absorbed and emitted photons. Fluorescence is the basis of fluorescein angiography, macular autofluorescence, and the Seidel test. In the Seidel test, the high concentration of fluorescein prevents fluorescence from occurring; only when the fluorescein is sufficiently dilute (eg, because of aqueous leaking from a lesion) is fluorescence seen.

Common fluorescent lights are gas discharge tubes containing mercury vapor. The discrete mercury spectrum is converted to a continuous spectrum by coating the inside of the glass tube with fluorescent materials, from which this light source gets its name.

Phosphorescence

In most cases, electrons remain in elevated energy states for very short periods. However, the elevated state is sometimes "metastable"; that is, the electron may remain in the elevated state for several seconds, minutes, or perhaps even days before dropping back down.

Figure 8-17 Light emission by fluorescence. In this example, an electron jumps from the lowest to highest energy level by absorbing a high-frequency (eg, blue) photon (1). The electron drops to a slightly lower, intermediate energy level through nonradiative processes or by emitting a low-energy (eg, infrared) photon (2). Eventually, the electron drops to its original energy level, emitting a photon of slightly lower frequency (eg, green) than the one it absorbed (3). *(Illustration by Edmond H. Thall, MD.)*

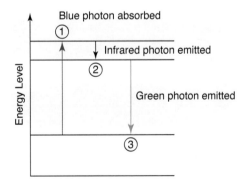

Such a process describes how light is produced by phosphorescence, which is essentially identical to fluorescence except that the transitions take longer. Light resulting from fluorescence stops immediately after removal of the exciting energy, whereas light resulting from phosphorescence persists long after the exciting energy ceases.

Lasers

An electron may stay in a metastable state for minutes or longer. However, a photon of appropriate frequency passing near such an electron will stimulate the electron immediately to drop to a lower state and radiate an identical photon (see Fig 8-15C). Such stimulated emission is the basis of the light emission in lasers. In fact, the word *laser* was initially an acronym for Light Amplification by Stimulated Emission of Radiation (LASER).

Lasers use an *active medium* with an appropriate metastable state. Energy is introduced into the active medium in a variety of ways. For example, *optical pumping* uses a bright incoherent light source to excite a large number of electrons into the metastable state. The active medium is inside a resonator cavity, which typically has a fully reflecting mirror on one end and a partially reflecting one on the other; this design causes light to make numerous passes through the active medium, producing more photons by stimulated emission with each pass (Fig 8-18).

Contrary to common belief, lasers are not very efficient light sources. Compared with the amount of energy required to power a laser, the amount of energy produced is modest. The light produced, however, has unique and useful characteristics. Laser light has a very narrow bandwidth (ie, it is nearly a single color or wholly monochromatic) and, consequently, it has high temporal coherence. The coherence length is relatively long—about half the length of the resonator cavity—typically a few centimeters. Lasers are the most intense sources of monochromatic light available.

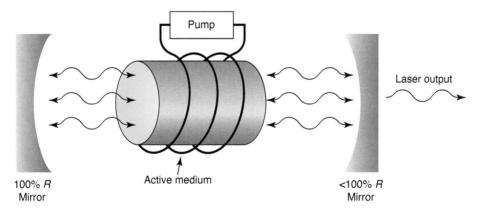

Figure 8-18 Simple schematic of a laser illustrating the active medium within the optical resonance cavity formed by the mirrors and the pump, which raises a majority of electrons to elevated states (population inversion) in the active medium. One mirror is fully reflective (100% *R*), whereas the other is partially transparent (<100% *R*). As drawn, the mirror is 66% reflective, and the average light wave makes 3 round-trips through the active medium before being emitted. *(Reproduced with permission from Steinert RF, Puliafito CA. The Nd:YAG Laser in Ophthalmology: Principles and Clinical Applications of Photodisruption. Philadelphia: Saunders; 1985. Redrawn by Jonathan Clark.)*

Although the total energy in laser light may be slight, it can be focused on a very small area to produce a very high energy density (ie, energy per square centimeter, or irradiance). Laser light is also highly directional and, depending on the design of the resonator, may also be polarized.

Lasers may operate continuously (eg, an argon laser photocoagulator) or in pulses (eg, a YAG laser for capsulotomy). Mode locking and Q-switching are 2 common methods of producing a pulsed output. The details of such methods are beyond the scope of this chapter.

Power is the amount of energy delivered in a given time period. A watt is 1 joule of energy delivered over 1 second, but the same joule delivered over a nanosecond has a power of 1 billion watts. Pulsing is a way of increasing the power of a laser's output by delivering a modest amount of energy over a very short time period.

Light–Tissue Interactions

Laser surgery involves 1 of 4 light–tissue interactions: photocoagulation, photoablation, photodisruption, or photoactivation.

Photocoagulation

Photocoagulation is the process by which heat generated by the absorption of light denatures proteins. Pigmented tissue absorbs light and converts it to heat, which denatures (coagulates) the pigmented and adjacent tissues.

Retinal photocoagulation was first performed by focusing sunlight onto the retina using a heliostat. Sunlight was replaced by a xenon light source, which was ultimately replaced by a variety of lasers. During retinal photocoagulation, laser light is absorbed by the retinal pigment epithelium (RPE), and the heat produced denatures (coagulates) the retinal proteins. The outer retinal layers are more affected than are the inner layers, a fact that has several clinical implications.

The more edematous the retina, the less heat reaches the inner layers and the less visible the laser burn. Accordingly, when photocoagulating an edematous retina, it is important to look for signs of photocoagulation occurring in the deeper retinal layers. The difficulty with coagulating the inner retinal layers is the reason laser photocoagulation is often ineffective in preventing the progress of retinoschisis, especially when only the innermost layers split. Controlling laser spot size and duration is crucial. Too much laser power concentrated into too small a spot and too short an exposure time can perforate the Bruch membrane, and choroidal neovascularization can result.

The cornea does not absorb enough visible light, even highly concentrated light, to produce a significant temperature increase. However, the cornea is opaque to some infrared wavelengths, so an infrared laser is used in laser thermokeratoplasty (LTK) to photocoagulate and shrink corneal collagen in the treatment of hyperopia.

Photoablation

Photoablation uses high-energy ultraviolet photons to break covalent chemical bonds. An excimer laser, for example, generates photons at a wavelength of 193 nm; these photons are absorbed by and break the covalent bonds in corneal collagen, thereby vaporizing the collagen molecules. Because the energy of photoablation is used only to break bonds, no heat is produced and the technique does not scar adjacent tissue. Presently, photoablation is used only for keratorefractive procedures.

Photodisruption

The posterior capsule is transparent to visible and near-infrared light, including the 1.06-μm wavelength produced by the Nd-YAG laser. This type of laser is pulsed, so the energy it produces is released in a very short time, producing a large momentary power. Also, the laser beam is focused, concentrating the power into a small area. In the vicinity of the focus, electrons are stripped from their atoms by ionization, but they quickly recombine, which produces a spark and an acoustic wave that mechanically disrupts the posterior capsule. (The spark is essentially a miniature lightning bolt, and the acoustic wave is analogous to thunder.) During a photodisruption procedure, it is the mechanical (acoustic) wave and not the laser light itself that breaks the capsule.

Photoactivation

Photoactivation is the conversion of a chemical from one form to another by light. Vision itself depends on the photoactivation (*cis–trans* isomerization) of rhodopsin in photoreceptor outer segments. A clinical application of photoactivation includes the use of verteporfin, a drug that remains chemically inert until activated by light, after which it destroys neovascular tissue.

Light Scattering

Molecules or small particles suspended in a medium disperse or scatter light. Light scattering by the ocular media increases with age; results include decreasing contrast of the retinal image, diminishing contrast sensitivity, and increasing glare sensitivity. Three mechanisms of light scattering—Rayleigh scattering, Mie scattering, and the Tyndall effect—influence the perception of light as well as the appearance of the eye.

Rayleigh Scattering

Rayleigh scattering is produced by particles that range in size from as small as molecules to as large as about one-tenth the wavelength of incident light. The degree of this form of light scattering varies inversely to the fourth power of the wavelength; thus, blue light (at 400 nm) is scattered about 9.4 times as much as red light (at 700 nm). The effect of Rayleigh scattering and the amount of melanin in the iris stroma determine iris color.

Mie Scattering

Mie scattering is caused by particles in a medium that are one or more wavelengths larger than the incident light. The effect varies with wavelength in a complex way, but the variation with wavelength is not very strong. In Mie scattering, forward scattering tends to be stronger than back scattering. Mie scattering accounts for the white color of the sclera and of clouds.

The Tyndall Effect

Light scattering from the Tyndall effect is due to light reflected by fairly large particles in a suspension. Anterior segment cells are visible during slit-lamp examination because of Tyndall-effect light scattering by cells (or proteins) in the aqueous humor.

Radiometry and Photometry

It is necessary at times to measure the amount of light produced by a source or illuminating a surface. For example, the bowl of a perimeter must be accurately illuminated in order for any comparisons of visual field measurements performed on different instruments or on the same instrument at different times to be meaningful.

Radiometry is the measurement of EM radiation occurring between 3×10^{11} Hz and 3×10^{16} Hz, a range corresponding to wavelengths between 10 nm and 1 mm. Therefore, radiometry spans the microwave, infrared, visible, ultraviolet, and soft x-ray regions of the EM spectrum. Often, such broad measurements are not necessary, and spectral radiometry is used instead to measure a narrower portion of the EM spectrum.

Photometry measures the human visual system's psychophysical response to light. Basically, photometry is a type of radiometry that takes into account the varying sensitivity of the eye to different wavelengths. Based on data from measurements of numerous people, weighting factors (presented graphically as luminous efficacy curves) have been developed for each wavelength across the visible spectrum. Different luminous efficacy curves are used to assess vision under photopic and scotopic lighting conditions.

In photometry, the spectral characteristics of a light source are determined by spectral radiometry. Then, each wavelength measured is multiplied by the appropriate luminous efficacy factor, and the responses are summed across the visible spectrum to estimate the response of the visual system. To give a simple example, a light source that produces only UV light has radiometric intensity but no luminous intensity.

To many clinicians, radiometric and photometric units of measurement are unfamiliar and confusing. For additional detail, a discussion of such units is provided in Appendix 8.1, at the end of this chapter.

Light Hazards

Although eyesight requires light, it has long been evident that exposure to excessive amounts of light, particularly at certain wavelengths, is hazardous to various parts of the eye, as indicated in the following:

- The cornea and lens are particularly susceptible to injury from UV light (180–400 nm), from which photokeratitis and cataract can result.
- The retina is susceptible to photochemical injury from blue light in wavelengths of 400–550 nm (310–550 nm for an aphakic eye). Such susceptibility to damage is

the basis for incorporating UV-blocking and blue-blocking chromophores in some intraocular lenses (IOLs).

- The retina is susceptible to thermal injury from optical radiation occurring from the visible to near-infrared wavelengths of 400–1400 nm.
- The lens of the eye is susceptible to thermal injury from near-infrared radiation in the wavelengths from 800 nm to 3000 nm.
- The cornea and lens of the eye are susceptible to thermal injury from radiation in the wavelengths from 400 nm to 1200 nm.
- The cornea is susceptible to thermal injury from optical radiation in the wavelengths from 1400 nm to 1 mm.

Clinical Applications

Polarization

Several stereopsis tests incorporate the use of linear polarizers. The well-known "stereo fly test" displays 2 slightly displaced images that linearly polarize light in perpendicular meridians. The person wears glasses containing linear polarizers, also at right angles to each other; each eye sees just one of the images, thus creating a 3-dimensional effect.

The cornea, retinal nerve fiber layer, and crystalline lens partially polarize light. Circularly polarized light entering the eye is reflected back and emerges elliptically polarized. The glaucoma diagnosis (GDx) test employs this effect to measure the thickness of the nerve fiber layer. However, because the cornea and crystalline lens also affect polarization, they may introduce artifacts into GDx nerve fiber layer measurements. A variable corneal compensator (VCC) may help mitigate such corneal polarization artifacts. However, even using the VCC, keratorefractive surgery can cause alterations in GDx measurements.

Reflected light is somewhat polarized parallel to the reflecting surface, and in most environments, reflecting objects tend to be horizontal. Accordingly, sunglasses incorporate vertically oriented linear polarizers to decrease glare from horizontal surfaces. To reduce glare from the corneal reflection, some direct ophthalmoscopes incorporate a circular polarizer.

Interference

Reflections from the front and back surfaces of a thin film interfere with each other, and depending on the film's thickness, certain wavelengths are reinforced while others are canceled (Figs 8-19, 8-20). The color swirls occasionally observed during slit-lamp examination of the tear film are produced by a thin layer of meibum and may indicate a tear-film abnormality. Interference filters composed of several thin layers are used in fluorescein angiography and autofluorescence imaging to produce very sharp boundaries between transmitted and blocked wavelengths, thus minimizing pseudofluorescence.

Optical coherence tomography (OCT) uses Michaelson interferometry to image the retinal layers. The coherence of the light source is crucial; a light source with high temporal coherence (eg, laser) actually decreases the accuracy of OCT thickness measurements.

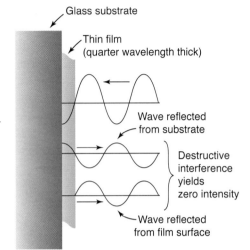

Figure 8-19 Destructive interference by an anti-reflection thin film. *(Redrawn by C. H. Wooley.)*

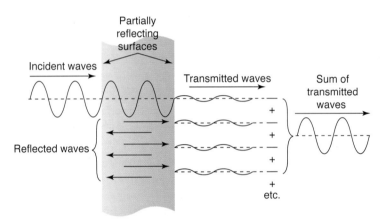

Figure 8-20 The interference filter transmits mainly those wavelengths for which the internally reflected waves are in phase with one another. *(Redrawn by C. H. Wooley.)*

However, a light source with too little coherence limits the thickness that can be measured. To measure the entire retina, OCT uses a superluminous diode, which operates in the near-infrared range and has a 50-nm bandwidth.

Diffraction

Some multifocal intraocular lenses use diffraction (and interference) to produce near and distance images simultaneously. Such lenses have at least one surface that is not smooth but that consists of circular steps that break wavefronts to produce diffraction. Such lenses rely for their effect on interference from the opposite side of each ring and, therefore, should be placed as well centered as possible with respect to the pupil. Consequently, eyes with irregular pupils may not be well suited for such lenses. Corneal astigmatism or IOL tilt also degrades the image quality of diffractive IOLs.

Imaging and the Point Spread Function

Two different but closely related approaches exist to understand the image formation process. (See Chapter 1 for discussions of image formation by lenses, mirrors, or pinholes.) The first approach is the basis for aberration theory, whereas the second is the basis for contrast sensitivity and the measurement of image quality. In the first approach, an object is regarded as a collection of point sources, each of which radiates light in all directions. Some of the light traverses the lens and focuses *at best* to a small, irregularly shaped region, *never* to a perfect point (Fig 8-21). The light from nearby point sources partially overlaps and causes a loss of detail in the formed image. Although *no* lens focuses perfectly, some focus better than others and produce more detail in the resulting image.

The point spread function (PSF) describes how light from a single point source is distributed in an image and completely describes the imaging characteristics of an optical system. During the design stage of a lens, calculating the PSF precisely is a complex matter that must account for not only refraction and reflection but also diffraction and characteristics such as interference, polarization, light scattering, and dispersion. Even using a computer, calculating a PSF that accounts for all optical variables is difficult. The PSF of a lens can be measured after it is manufactured, but doing so is a time-consuming and costly task requiring specialized equipment and expertise.

Fortunately, most image characteristics, such as location, size, orientation, and brightness, can be calculated or measured without considering PSF. The field of geometric optics greatly simplifies calculations of image characteristics by ignoring most of light's physical characteristics, especially diffraction. Using only the 3 laws of rectilinear propagation, refraction, and reflection, image characteristics can be determined with sufficient accuracy for most uses. Only when diffraction, interference, or some other physical property is a significant factor in image quality is it necessary to use calculations from physical optics.

The PSF is required only for the analysis of image quality, which in most cases is dominated by aberrations or diffraction. Sir George Airy calculated the PSF for an axial object point imaged by any *aberration-free* optical system with a circular aperture stop. Airy also assumed temporally coherent light, so the PSF contained interference rings. Airy found that the PSF consisted of a central bright spot (the Airy disc) surrounded by larger rings (Fig 8-22).

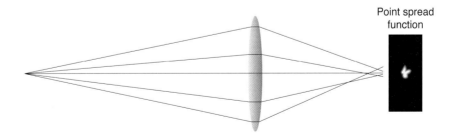

Point spread function

Figure 8-21 Light from a single object point never focuses to a perfect point. Even at best focus, it is usually distributed over a small, irregularly shaped region in the image. *(Illustration developed by Edmond H. Thall, MD, and Kevin Miller, MD, and rendered by C. H. Wooley.)*

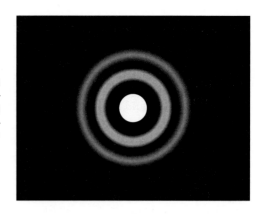

Figure 8-22 The point spread function of a single monochromatic axial object point produced by an aberration-free optical system with a circular aperture. *(From Campbell, CJ. Physiologic Optics. Hagerstown, MD: Harper & Row; 1974:20.)*

Most of the energy is in the central disc, so the outer rings are usually ignored. The diameter of the Airy disc is determined according to the equation

$$\text{Airy Disc Diameter} \approx 2.44\lambda\frac{f}{D}$$

where D is the exit pupil diameter and f is the focal length. For an eye with a 3-mm-diameter pupil, the PSF diameter is approximately 6 μm, encompassing the outer segments of roughly 7 photoreceptors.

As noted, the Airy disc diameter is the PSF produced solely by diffraction when no aberrations are present. Alternatively, the PSF can be calculated using only the 3 laws of geometric optics, entirely ignoring diffraction. As a rule, diffraction decreases as pupil size increases, but aberrations increase as pupil size increases.

If the geometric PSF value is much larger than the Airy disc diameter, then aberrations dominate and diffraction can be ignored, whereas if the geometric PSF is much smaller, then diffraction dominates and aberrations can be ignored. If values for the geometric PSF and the Airy disc diameter are about the same, then image quality is probably close to optimal for that optical system.

Image Quality—Modulation Transfer Function

Suppose an object is photographed using 2 different cameras. (Assume the photographs are gray scale to simplify discussion.) Even when conditions such as lighting, camera angle, and magnification are identical, the 2 resulting images will differ. Which one is better?

Because an image never perfectly duplicates its object, the image that comes closest to resembling its object could be considered the better image. Is it possible to say that one image contains 88% of the details in the object and that another image has 92%? Not quite, but it is possible to come close.

Just as sound is a mixture of frequencies, so are images. Whereas sound is a mixture of temporal frequencies, images are a mixture of spatial frequencies (Fig 8-23). An image of a single spatial frequency always has the same spatial frequency as the original but with lower contrast. In other words, the spatial frequency does not change from the original to the image, but the contrast does. A photograph will always have less contrast than the

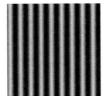 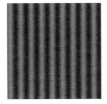 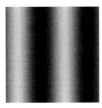

Figure 8-23 Spatial frequencies. The left and middle panels have identical frequencies, but the left has higher contrast. The left and right panels have the same contrast, but the right has a lower frequency. *(Illustration by Edmond H. Thall, MD.)*

original. One lens might image a single spatial frequency at 92% contrast, whereas another lens might image the same frequency at 88% contrast. The ratio of image contrast divided by object contrast (eg, the 88% and the 92% cited in the earlier example) is called the transfer factor because it measures how well the contrast of a single spatial frequency is transferred from the object to the image.

The transfer factor changes as the spatial frequency changes. As a general rule, the transfer factor decreases as spatial frequency increases. A graph plotting transfer factors on the vertical axis versus spatial frequency on the horizontal axis is called the *modulation transfer function (MTF)*. *Modulation* is another word for *contrast*. Every lens has a unique MTF, and by comparing the MTF of lenses, it is possible to determine which lens is better for an intended purpose.

Like the PSF, the MTF completely describes the imaging properties of a lens—in fact, the MTF and PSF are closely related. The MTF can be calculated from the PSF by employing Fourier transform mathematics. Further details of this process are beyond the scope of this discussion.

Chapter Exercises

Questions

8.1. Light in air is incident on glass ($n = 1.5$), making a 30° angle of incidence. What is the angle of transmission (refraction)? (*Hint:* Select the correct choice without using a calculator.)
   a. 11.2°
   b. 19.5°
   c. 20.0°
   d. 21.2°
   e. 29.5°

8.2. What is the Brewster angle when light travels from glass ($n = 1.5$) to air?
   a. 75.6°
   b. none
   c. 33.7°
   d. 56.7°
   e. 41.8°

8.3. What is the critical angle when light travels from air to glass?
   a. 75.6°
   b. none
   c. 33.7°
   d. 56.7°
   e. 41.8°

8.4. Which of the following statements is not true as the refractive index of a spectacle lens material increases?
   a. The velocity of light is increased in this material.
   b. Spectacle lenses made from this material can be thinner.
   c. Its value of n is higher.
   d. It has greater ability to refract light.

8.5. The Airy disc image on the retina is larger when
   a. the wavelength of light is shortened
   b. the focal length of the eye is shorter
   c. the pupil size decreases
   d. macular degeneration is present

8.6. Corneal haze secondary to corneal edema is primarily caused by
   a. reflection
   b. light scattering
   c. refraction
   d. diffraction

Answers

8.1. **b.** The question illustrates a way to use the small-angle approximation of Snell's law, the complete form of which is

$$n_1 \sin \theta_1 = n_2 \sin \theta_2$$

The approximate form of Snell's law that is valid for small angles is

$$n_1 \theta_1 = n_2 \theta_2$$

The approximate form is usually accurate only for angles of less than 5°. For larger angles, the approximate form overestimates the angle of transmission (refraction), but only by a small amount. Using 30° as an example you can do in your head:

$$1(30°) = 1.5(\theta_2)$$

$$\theta_2 = \frac{30°}{1.5} = 20°$$

The actual angle of refraction is slightly smaller than 20°, but not by much. Options **c, d,** and **e** are too large, and although **a** is smaller than 20°, it is much too small. Option **b** is correct, which can be proved using the exact form of Snell's law on a calculator.

8.2. **c.** The formula is

$$\text{Brewster Angle} = \tan^{-1} \frac{n_2}{n_1}$$

$$= \tan^{-1} \frac{1}{1.5}$$

$$= 33.7$$

8.3. **b.** There is no critical angle when light travels from a material with a lower index of refraction to one with a higher index of refraction.

8.4. **a.** The index of refraction *(n)* of a transparent medium is the ratio of the speed of light in vacuum to the speed of light in the given material. Each transparent medium (eg, lens material) has a unique index of refraction determined by the velocity with which light travels through it. The more light slows in a transparent (lens) material, the higher the material's *n* value and the greater its ability to refract light, thereby allowing for thinner spectacle lenses.

8.5. **c.** The Airy disc is the central portion of a pattern of light and dark rings formed when light from a point source passes through a circular aperture and is diffracted. The size of the Airy disc increases with smaller pupil size (especially pupil diameter <2.5 mm), longer wavelengths of light, and longer focal lengths. Retinal conditions such as macular degeneration have no effect on the size of the Airy disc.

8.6. **b.** Light scattering occurs when small particles suspended in a transparent medium interfere with the transmittance of light and cause photons to deviate from a straight path. Short wavelengths of light are scattered more strongly than are longer wavelengths. Larger particles scatter light more intensely than do smaller particles. In a healthy cornea, the tightly arranged and regularly spaced collagen molecules minimize the effects of scattering. When a cornea becomes edematous, excess fluid in the stroma disrupts the regular collagen structure, causing light scattering.

Appendix 8.1

Radiometric and Photometric Units

Understanding radiometry is a matter of not simply knowing the definitions of various units of measurement but also knowing how to use them appropriately. Every radiometric (or photometric) unit of measurement has a specific purpose.

In studying radiometry, it is helpful to think of light as a collection of photons. Broadband light consists of photons at many frequencies, whereas narrowband light consists of photons at just a few frequencies. For the purposes of this discussion, imagine it is possible to count every photon and identify its frequency.

Radiometry counts every photon—not just visible ones but also those at infrared and UV wavelengths, and all photons at wavelengths between 10 nm and 1 mm. Radiometric units are identified by the subscript ($_e$). Spectral radiometry counts photons within a more limited range—whatever frequencies are of interest in a specific situation. Spectral radiometric units are identified by the subscript ($_\lambda$).

Radiant energy (Q_e)

Radiant energy (Q_e) is the total energy produced, typically expressed in joules. Every photon produced by a source is counted, and its energy is calculated using $E = h\nu$. For example, an incandescent lightbulb produces not only visible light but also infrared and even some UV light, and photons from each of these spectra need to be included to determine the value for Q_e. Also, Q_e is a cumulative measurement; that is, it is taken over time. The Q_e value for an incandescent bulb operating for 2 hours is twice that for the same bulb operating for 1 hour.

Q_e (or Q_λ) is the appropriate quantity when cumulative exposure is important. For instance, there is some evidence that cases of post–cataract-extraction cystoid macular edema are related to microscope illumination. Investigators should consider Q_e (as well as other parameters) in evaluating light hazards.

Fluence (H_e)

Fluence (H_e) is a measure of energy density and is defined as radiant energy (Q_e) divided by area. For example, 6 J of radiant energy applied to an area of 2 cm^2 equals a fluence of 3 J/cm^2. Fluence measurements are often used clinically in association with laser ablation and photodynamic therapy (PDT).

Photoablation breaks chemical bonds, and in laser in situ keratomileusis (LASIK) or photorefractive keratectomy (PRK), the number of chemical bonds to be broken by a single laser pulse is proportional to the area of the laser beam. If the pulse energy is low in comparison with the beam area, too few bonds will be broken and the resulting ablation will be uneven. Similarly, in PDT the number of verteporfin molecules to be activated depends on the area of the lesion. Fluence is the appropriate radiometric unit to employ for calibrating lasers used for these procedures.

Radiant flux (Φ_e)

The word *flux* means flow, and radiant flux (Φ_e) is the amount of radiant energy emitted by a source or striking a surface per unit of time. It is a measure of power, typically expressed in joules per second, or watts. A source radiating 60 J for 1 minute produces a radiant flux of 1 W (60 J/60 s).

Irradiance (E_e) or exitance (M_e)

Irradiance (E_e) is radiant energy divided by area and time, and it is typically expressed in watts per square meter or watts per square centimeter. For example, a 0.25 cm^2 surface illuminated by 2 W has an irradiance of 2 W/0.25 cm^2 = 8 W/cm^2. *Irradiance* is used for surfaces illuminated by an external source, but the term *radiant exitance* (M_e) may be used instead when the surface itself is the light source (eg, a light box used to view x-rays). However, irradiance and radiant exitance both have the same units (W/cm^2), so some authorities use *irradiance* in both cases. Clinically, irradiance is the appropriate unit of measurement for photocoagulation equipment.

Radiant intensity (I_e)

Measurements of radiant intensity account for the directional properties of a light source. For example, a flashlight beam diverges somewhat but propagates in the same direction. Some flashlight beams are more narrowly divergent than others, whereas laser beams are extremely directional. It is therefore necessary to incorporate an angular measurement in the description of such light sources, a function served by radiant intensity (I_e), expressed as the radiant flux per unit solid angle or watts per steradian (W/sr).

Radiance (L_e)

The measurement of radiance (L_e) takes into account irradiance and radiant intensity, and it is the radiometric unit most closely related to brightness. Radiance is radiant flux per unit area per steradian (sr), typically expressed as $W/m^2 \cdot sr$.

Photometry

Photometry measures the human visual system's psychophysical response to light; it is essentially radiometry that takes into account the varying response of the eye to light of different wavelengths. Based on data from measurements of people, weighting factors (presented as luminous efficacy curves) have been developed for each wavelength of the visible spectrum. There are luminous efficacy curves for photopic and scotopic conditions.

Photometry is a straightforward extension of radiometry—each photon and its frequency are counted. Each photon's energy is calculated and multiplied by the luminous efficacy for its frequency. (To cite a trivial example of the difference between radiometry and photometry, a source that emits only UV light has radiometric intensity but no luminous intensity.) Photometric units are analogous to radiometric units and are indicated by the same symbols but subscripted with ($_v$) (for *visual*) instead of ($_e$). Table 8-1 compares radiometric units with analogous photometric units.

There are many ways to measure photometric quantities. For clinical use, SI units are often not the most convenient. Table 8-2 lists alternative units commonly used to measure illuminance and luminance and their conversion factors. To develop a "feel" for photometric units, Table 8-3 lists photometric values associated with visual functions.

The troland (Td) is a unit that estimates retinal illuminance based on source luminance. A source with a luminance of 1 nit produces a retinal illuminance of 1 Td when viewed through a 1 mm^2 pupil. If the pupil area is 10 mm^2, then the retinal illuminance is 10 Td.

Table 8-1 Comparison of Radiometric and Photometric Units

Radiometric Quantity	SI Unit	Photometric Quantity	SI Unit
Radiant energy, Q_e	joule (J)	Luminous energy, Q_v	lumen second (lm · s)
Fluence, H_e	joules per meter^2 (J/m^2)	Luminous exposure, H_v	lumen second per meter^2 (lm · s/m^2)
Radiant flux, Φ_e	watt (W)	Luminous flux, Φ_v	lumen (lm)
Radiant intensity, I_e	watts per steradian (W/sr)	Luminous intensity, I_v	candela (cd)
Irradiance, E_e	watts per meter^2 (W/m^2)	Illuminance, E_v	lux (lx)
Radiance, L_e	watts per meter^2 per steradian (W/m^2 · sr)	Luminance, L_v	nit (cd/m^2)

Table 8-2 Various Photometric Units and Their Conversion Factors

Photometric Quantity	SI Unit	Alternative Units and Conversion Factors (Some Are Obsolete)
Illuminance, E_v	lux	1 lux = 1 lm/m^2 = 1 m · cd
		1 phot = 1 lm/cm^2 = 10,000 lux
		1 milliphot = 10 lux
		1 foot-candle = 1 lm/ft^2 = 10.76 lux
Luminance, L_v	nit	nit = 1 cd/m^2
		Stilb = 1 cd/cm^2 = 10,000 nits
		Apostilb = $(1/\pi)$ cd/m^2 ≈ 0.32 nits
		cd/ft^2 = 10.76 nits
		cd/in^2 = 1550 nits

Table 8-3 Luminance Levels Associated With Various Visual Functions

Visual Function	Luminance (nits)
Best acuity	1000
Cone threshold	10^{-4}
Damage	10^8
Limit of rod sensitivity	10^{-7}
Mesopic range	10^{-4}–10
Photopic range	10–10^8
Rod saturation	10
Scotopic range	10^{-7}–10^{-4}

Basic Texts

Clinical Optics

Albert DM, Miller JW, Azar DT, Blodi BA, eds. *Albert & Jakobiec's Principles and Practice of Ophthalmology.* 4 vols. 3rd ed. Philadelphia: Elsevier/Saunders; 2008.

Campbell CJ. *Physiological Optics.* Hagerstown, MD: Harper & Row; 1974.

Corboy JM. *The Retinoscopy Book: An Introductory Manual for Eye Care Professionals.* 5th ed. Thorofare, NJ: Slack; 2003.

Duke-Elder S, Abrams D. *Ophthalmic Optics and Refraction.* St Louis: Mosby; 1970. *System of Ophthalmology;* vol 5.

Michaels DD. *Visual Optics and Refraction: A Clinical Approach.* 3rd ed. St Louis: Mosby; 1985.

Milder B, Rubin ML. *The Fine Art of Prescribing Glasses Without Making a Spectacle of Yourself.* 3rd ed. Gainesville, FL: Triad; 2004.

Rubin ML. *Optics for Clinicians.* Gainesville, FL: Triad; 1993.

Stein HA, Slatt BJ, Stein RM, Freeman MI. *Fitting Guide for Rigid and Soft Contact Lenses: A Practical Approach.* 4th ed. St Louis: Mosby; 2002.

Tasman W, Jaeger EA, eds. *Duane's Ophthalmology on DVD-ROM.* Philadelphia: Lippincott Williams & Wilkins; 2012.

Yanoff M, Duker JS. *Ophthalmology: Expert Consult Premium Edition.* 3rd ed. St Louis: Mosby; 2009.

Related Academy Materials

The Academy is dedicated to providing a wealth of high-quality clinical education resources for ophthalmologists.

Print Publications and Electronic Products

For a complete listing of Academy products related to topics covered in this BCSC Section, visit our online store at http://store.aao.org/clinical-education/topic/comprehensive .html. Or call Customer Service at 866.561.8558 (toll free, US only) or +1 415.561.8540, Monday through Friday, between 8:00 AM and 5:00 PM (PST).

Online Resources

Visit the Ophthalmic News and Education (ONE®) Network at www.aao.org/clinical -education to find relevant videos, online courses, journal articles, practice guidelines, self-assessment quizzes, images, and more. The ONE Network is a free Academy-member benefit.

Access free, trusted articles and content with the Academy's collaborative online encyclopedia, EyeWiki, at www.aao.org/eyewiki.

Requesting Continuing Medical Education Credit

The American Academy of Ophthalmology is accredited by the Accreditation Council for Continuing Medical Education to provide continuing medical education for physicians.

The American Academy of Ophthalmology designates this enduring material for a maximum of 15 *AMA PRA Category 1 Credits*™. Physicians should claim only the credit commensurate with the extent of their participation in the activity.

The American Medical Association requires that all learners participating in activities involving enduring materials complete a formal assessment before claiming continuing medical education (CME) credit. To assess your achievement in this activity and ensure that a specified level of knowledge has been reached, a posttest for this Section of the Basic and Clinical Science Course is provided online. A minimum score of 80% must be obtained to pass the test and claim CME credit.

To take the posttest and request CME credit online:

1. Go to www.aao.org/cme-central and log in.
2. Click on "Claim CME Credit and View My CME Transcript" and then "Report AAO Credits."
3. Select the appropriate Academy activity. You will be directed to the posttest.
4. Once you have passed the test with a score of 80% or higher, you will be directed to your transcript. *If you are not an Academy member, you will be able to print out a certificate of participation once you have passed the test.*

CME expiration date: June 1, 2017. *AMA PRA Category 1 Credits*™ may be claimed only once between June 1, 2013, and the expiration date.

For assistance, contact the Academy's Customer Service department at 866-561-8558 (U.S. only) or 415-561-8540 between 8:00 AM and 5:00 PM (PST), Monday through Friday, or send an e-mail to customer_service@aao.org.

Study Questions

Please note that these questions are not part of your CME reporting process. They are provided here for self-assessment and identification of personal professional practice gaps. The required CME posttest is available online (see "Requesting CME Credit"). Following the questions are a blank answer sheet and answers with discussions. Although a concerted effort has been made to avoid ambiguity and redundancy in these questions, the authors recognize that differences of opinion may occur regarding the "best" answer. The discussions are provided to demonstrate the rationale used to derive the answer. They may also be helpful in confirming that your approach to the problem was correct or, if necessary, in fixing the principle in your memory. The Section 3 faculty thanks the Self-Assessment Committee for reviewing these self-assessment questions and discussions.

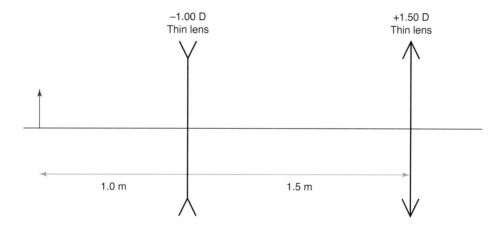

Questions 1–6 refer to the figure above. An object is 1.0 m to the left of a –1.00 D thin lens. The –1.00 D lens is, in turn, 1.5 m to the left of a +1.50 D thin lens.

1. Where is the (intermediate) image formed by the first lens?
   a. 2.0 m to the right of the lens
   b. 0.5 m to the right of the lens
   c. 0.5 m to the left of the lens
   d. 2.0 m to the left of the lens

2. What are the characteristics (eg, real or virtual, upright or inverted, and transverse magnification) of the intermediate image?
   a. upright, real, enlarged
   b. inverted, real, reduced
   c. upright, virtual, enlarged
   d. upright, virtual, reduced

3. What is the size of the intermediate image compared with the object?

    a. one-fourth the size

    b. one-half the size

    c. same size

    d. twice the size

4. What is the location of the final image?

    a. 1.0 m to the left of the second lens

    b. 1.0 m to the right of the second lens

    c. 4.0 m to the right of the second lens

    d. at optical infinity

5. What are the characteristics (eg, orientation, real or virtual, and transverse magnification) of the final image compared with the original object?

    a. upright, real, enlarged

    b. upright, real, reduced

    c. inverted, real, enlarged

    d. inverted, real, reduced

6. What is the size of the final image compared with the original object?

    a. one-fourth the size

    b. one-half the size

    c. same size

    d. twice the size

7. An object is placed 50 cm in front of a concave spherical mirror with a radius of curvature of 2.0 m. What is the transverse magnification of the image, and is it real or virtual?

    a. virtual with a transverse magnification of +2×

    b. virtual with a transverse magnification of –2×

    c. real with a transverse magnification of –0.5×

    d. real with a transverse magnification of +0.5×

8. Which of the following statements is true about the derivation of intraocular lens (IOL) formulas using geometric optics?

    a. The index of refraction of the IOL is ignored because it does not differ significantly from that of the aqueous and vitreous.

    b. The refractive contribution of the cornea may be neglected because the light reaches the IOL plane after it has already passed through the corneal surface.

    c. The formula for change of vergence with change in implant location must be modified because of the index of refraction of the aqueous.

    d. The anterior chamber depth may be neglected because studies have shown a negligible increase in accuracy if it is included in power calculations.

9. Which of the following statements is correct regarding the segment choice when prescribing bifocals for a patient with hyperopia?

    a. The practitioner should leave the choice of the segment type to the optician.

    b. A round-top segment is preferred because it lessens image jump.

    c. A flat-top segment is preferred because of its thin upper edge, which causes less prismatic effect.

    d. The use of a round-top segment reduces the prismatic displacement effect and increases image jump.

10. A child has a cycloplegic refraction OD +6.00 D, OS +2.00 D. What is the best way to manage the anisometropia?

    a. full correction

    b. partial correction

    c. pleoptic therapy

    d. occlusion therapy

11. If a cornea has an anterior radius of curvature of 7.7 mm, a posterior radius of curvature of 6.8 mm, and a center thickness of 0.5 mm, what will its dioptric power be if it is submerged in water? Assume index of refraction of water = 1.333; index of refraction of cornea = 1.376; index of refraction of aqueous = 1.336.

    a. −5.89 D

    b. −0.30 D

    c. +32.00 D

    d. +37.60 D

12. Why is there no anterior chamber depth term in the SRK equation?

    a. The formula was specifically designed to eliminate the need for this measurement.

    b. Regression analysis did not show increased accuracy when anterior chamber depth was included in the IOL formula.

    c. Modern IOLs are all designed to have about the same anterior chamber depth.

    d. The postoperative anterior chamber depth is not necessarily the same as the measured preoperative anterior chamber depth.

13. The ability of a light wave from a laser to form stable interference fringes with another wave from the same beam, separated in time, is an illustration of what property?

    a. temporal coherence

    b. spatial coherence

    c. dispersion

    d. intensity

14. Proper medical management of a patient with bilateral dry macular degeneration and recent visual deterioration to the "legal blindness" level (20/200) should include which of the following options?

   a. a 10× magnifier for reading

   b. referral to an orientation and mobility specialist

   c. a spectacle prescription for prismatic half-glass readers

   d. a 10.00 D magnifier for reading

15. How much does a 15Δ prism bend light, in degrees?

   a. 5.55°

   b. 8.53°

   c. 15.00°

   d. 30.00°

16. The anterior and posterior focal points of a thin lens are located at different distances from the lens. Additionally, the nodal points of the lens do not correspond with the principal points. Which of the following statements is true?

   a. This situation is not possible as described.

   b. The optical characteristics described are found only in thick-lens or multi-element systems.

   c. Media of different refractive indices bound the lens.

   d. Two separated principal planes must be used to define the lens mathematically.

17. Which of the following characteristics is a property of all ophthalmic lasers?

   a. a plasma active medium

   b. high efficiency

   c. stimulated emission

   d. continuous wave operation

18. Which of the following properties of light is used by the scanning laser polarimeter to measure nerve fiber layer thickness?

   a. focal spot size

   b. power level

   c. pulse duration

   d. polarization

19. Which of the following statements about dispersion and chromatic aberration is correct?

   a. In the human eye, blue rays focus behind red rays.

   b. Red print appears nearer than blue print when both are displayed against a black background.

   c. Image sharpness is improved by chromatic aberration in the eyes of patients with achromatopsia.

   d. Blue-blocking and red-blocking sunglasses improve image sharpness by eliminating part of the chromatic interval, thereby reducing chromatic aberration.

20. A Snellen visual acuity of 20/20 is equivalent to which of the following logMAR values?

    a. 1.00

    b. 0.00

    c. 10.00

    d. 0.10

21. A cycloplegic streak retinoscopy is performed on a nonverbal, adult patient at a testing distance of 67 cm. The result for the right eye is as follows:

    +3 D sphere neutralizes the reflex when the streak is horizontal (180°);

    +4 D sphere neutralizes the reflex when the streak is vertical (90°).

    Which of the following refractions is correct for the right eye?

    a. +1.50 sphere +1.00 × 90

    b. +1.50 sphere −1.00 × 90

    c. +3.00 sphere +1.00 × 90

    d. +3.00 sphere −1.00 × 90

22. Which of the following statements correctly describes the relationship between intraocular lens (IOL) implant power, axial length, and corneal power?

    a. The IOL power should be increased as the power of the cornea increases and the axial length increases.

    b. The IOL power should be increased as the power of the cornea decreases and the axial length increases.

    c. The IOL power should be increased as the power of the cornea increases and the axial length decreases.

    d. The IOL power should be increased as the power of the cornea decreases and the axial length decreases.

23. Which of the following statements about astronomical telescopes is true?

    a. The astronomical telescope always produces an inverted image.

    b. The principal planes of an astronomical telescope coincide with the objective lens and eyepiece.

    c. The tube length of an astronomical telescope with a +4.00 D objective and a +10.00 D eyepiece is 35 cm.

    d. The angular magnification of an astronomical telescope with +4.00 D objective and a +10.00 D eyepiece is 4×.

24. Which of the following statements about keratometers is true?

    a. They measure the radius of curvature of the central cornea.

    b. The size of the mires depends on the corneal refractive index.

    c. They measure the dimensions of a virtual image in specific meridians.

    d. They measure the refractive power of the cornea.

25. Which of the following statements about the prescription of visual aids is true?

    a. The Kestenbaum rule provides an endpoint to determine the addition required to read 1 M type.

    b. Base-in prisms increase effective magnification for binocular patients using reading spectacles.

    c. Illuminated stand magnifiers help overcome stability and lighting problems associated with higher-power magnification.

    d. Optical magnification is sufficient for patients with severely reduced contrast sensitivity.

26. Which of the following conditions best characterizes a person with low vision?

    a. a bitemporal hemianopia

    b. best-corrected visual acuity of 20/70 or worse

    c. myopia greater than –20 D

    d. a disability related to visual dysfunction

27. Which of the following components is part of an optical coherence tomography (OCT) system?

    a. laser light source

    b. beam splitter

    c. double pinhole

    d. split prism

28. Which of the following adjustments can improve binocular visualization when examining an eye with small pupils using a head-mounted, binocular indirect ophthalmoscope?

    a. moving the ophthalmoscope's mirror away from the observer

    b. narrowing the observer's effective interpupillary distance

    c. diverging the examiner's eyes slightly

    d. reducing the distance between the observer's head and the patient

29. A 92-year-old patient with dry age-related macular degeneration reports deteriorating vision in 1 eye. Best-corrected visual acuity 12 months earlier was 20/30. With the same spectacle correction, it is now 20/100. Attempted refinement of the manifest refraction using ±0.50 D spherical lenses and a ±0.50 D Jackson cross cylinder elicits no change in the refraction. What is the next step?

    a. Perform a darkroom pinhole test.

    b. Repeat the manifest refraction using larger step changes in sphere and cylinder (eg, a ±0.75 D or ±1.00 D change in sphere and a ±0.75 D or ±1.00 D Jackson cross cylinder).

    c. Perform a slit-lamp examination for cataract or other media opacity.

    d. Dilate the pupil and examine for a choroidal neovascular membrane.

30. Which of the following statements describes the nodal points of the reduced schematic eye?

a. They represent the points through which light rays enter or leave the eye undeviated.

b. They are equivalent to the posterior focal point of the cornea.

c. They allow the size of a retinal image to be calculated if the object height is known.

d. The nodal points of the reduced schematic eye coincide, and they are located 6.5 mm posterior to the corneal surface.

31. Which of the following statements correctly describes the far point of the nonaccommodated –4.00 D myopic eye?

a. The far point and the fovea are conjugate points.

b. The far point is 25 cm posterior to the eye.

c. The far point is 20 cm in front of the eye.

d. The far point is nearer to the eye than is the point of focus of the fully accommodated eye.

32. Which of the following statements describes the near point of a fully accommodated young hyperopic eye in which the amplitude of accommodation is greater than the amount of hyperopia?

a. The near point is beyond plus infinity.

b. The near point is between plus infinity and the cornea.

c. The near point is behind the eye.

d. The near point is beyond minus infinity, optically speaking.

33. Which of the following pairs is matched correctly?

a. diopter—meter

b. prism diopter—meters per centimeter

c. refractive index—meters per second

d. wavelength—nanometers

34. Which of the following statements about irregular astigmatism is true?

a. Manifest refraction and automated refraction rarely differ significantly in the presence of large amounts of irregular astigmatism.

b. Irregular astigmatism is best treated with soft contact lenses.

c. Irregular astigmatism may be induced by a decentered refractive surgical procedure, pellucid marginal degeneration, or keratoconus.

d. Best-corrected visual acuity is usually better with spectacles than with rigid gas-permeable contact lenses in patients with large amounts of irregular corneal astigmatism.

35. Which of the following factors increases the risk of infection in a patient using extended-wear contact lenses?

    a. switching to daily-wear lenses

    b. exposure to smoke

    c. normal eyelid function

    d. intact corneal epithelium

36. Which of the following statements concerning a patient with a central scotoma is true?

    a. Most patients will fixate using the central foveal location, the preferred retinal locus (PRL).

    b. The location, shape, and number of scotomata variably affect visual function.

    c. Eccentric fixation and PRL training are of no value in helping a patient improve coordination, tracking, and scanning.

    d. Reading is usually not possible because central macular function is required to read.

37. Which of the following conditions typically affects central vision more than the peripheral visual field?

    a. retinitis pigmentosa

    b. age-related macular degeneration

    c. retinal detachment

    d. panretinal photocoagulation

38. Which of the following statements about the entrance pupil of the eye is true?

    a. It is the pupil we see when we look at a patient's eye.

    b. It is the image formed by the lens of the anatomic pupil.

    c. It is located 0.5 mm posterior to the anatomic pupil.

    d. It is 10%–15% smaller than the anatomic pupil.

39. What is the Brewster angle when light travels from air to glass ($n = 1.500$)?

    a. 65.7°

    b. 47.6°

    c. 56.3°

    d. 41.8°

40. What is the critical angle for light traveling from glass ($n = 1.500$) to air?

    a. 65.7°

    b. 47.6°

    c. 56.7°

    d. 41.8°

Answer Sheet for Section 3
Study Questions

Question	Answer	Question	Answer
1	a b c d	21	a b c d
2	a b c d	22	a b c d
3	a b c d	23	a b c d
4	a b c d	24	a b c d
5	a b c d	25	a b c d
6	a b c d	26	a b c d
7	a b c d	27	a b c d
8	a b c d	28	a b c d
9	a b c d	29	a b c d
10	a b c d	30	a b c d
11	a b c d	31	a b c d
12	a b c d	32	a b c d
13	a b c d	33	a b c d
14	a b c d	34	a b c d
15	a b c d	35	a b c d
16	a b c d	36	a b c d
17	a b c d	37	a b c d
18	a b c d	38	a b c d
19	a b c d	39	a b c d
20	a b c d	40	a b c d

Answers

1. **c.** Vergence is the ratio of refractive index, n, divided by the distance from the object or to the image. Vergence (in diopters) = n/distance (in meters). Vergence is negative for divergent light and positive for convergent light. In this case, the lenses are in air, for which the refractive index, n, is 1.000. Light diverges from the object so the vergence is negative. The object is 1.0 m from the lens and therefore has a vergence of -1.00 D = $-1.000/1.0$ m = -1.00 D. The first lens adds an additional -1.00 D of vergence. Light leaving the lens, therefore, has a vergence of -2.00 D. Light rays with a vergence of -2.00 D appear to be coming from a point 0.5 m to the left of the lens.

2. **d.** The terms *anterior focal point* and *posterior focal point* can be confusing because, for minus lenses, the anterior focal point is actually behind the posterior focal point. The anterior focal point, F_a, is always in object space, and the posterior focal point, F_p, is always in image space. By convention, primed letters indicate image space and unprimed letters, object space. Often, the anterior focal point is designated F and the posterior focal point, F′. For a -1.00 D thin lens in air, F is 1.0 m behind the lens, and F′ is 1.0 m in front of the lens. For all thin lenses, the principal planes coincide. Likewise, the nodal points coincide. The image features can be determined graphically, as shown in the figure below. A ray from the tip of the object directed to F exits the lens parallel to the optical axis. A ray from the tip of the object parallel to the axis exits the lens divergent, as if it had come from F′. A ray from the tip of the object directed to the nodal points exits undeviated and, in this case, undisplaced, as shown in black below. The image characteristics—upright, virtual, and reduced—are apparent from this graphical approach.

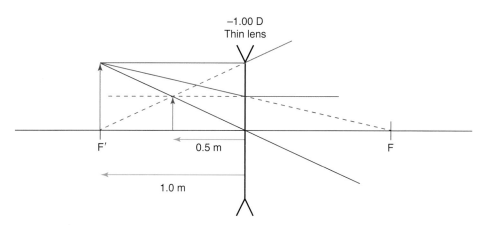

3. **b.** Using only the ray traversing the nodal points and similar triangles, the height of the intermediate image is found to be one-half the height of the object (see figure on the next page). The transverse magnification is +0.5×.

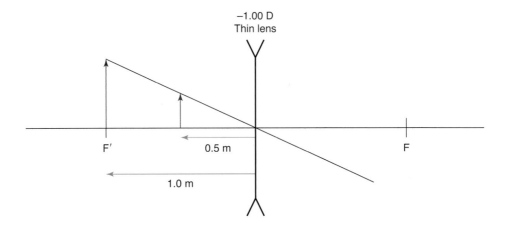

4. **b.** To answer questions 4–6, we treat the intermediate image as the object for the second lens. From this point on, the first lens can be ignored. The intermediate image is 2.0 m to the left of the second lens. The vergence of light entering the second lens is, therefore, –0.50 D. The lens adds +1.50 D of vergence. Therefore, the light exiting the lens has a vergence of +1.00 D. Light rays with a vergence of +1.00 D come to a focus 1.0 m to the right of the second lens.

5. **d.** For the second lens F′ is 2/3 m (0.66 m) to the right of the lens, and F is 0.66 m to the left of the lens. Rays can be traced as before. A ray passing from the object tip parallel to the axis emerges as a ray going through F′. A ray through F emerges parallel to the axis. A ray through the coincident nodal points is undeviated and undisplaced. The image is inverted compared with both the intermediate object and the original object, is real, and is half the size of the intermediate image and therefore is also smaller than the original object.

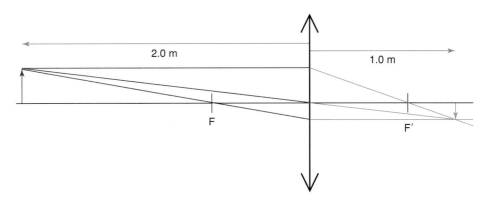

6. **a.** By similar triangles, the image is half the size of the intermediate image. The intermediate image is half the size of the object. Consequently, the final image is (1/2)(1/2) = 1/4 the size of the original object.

7. **a.** The power of a mirror is 2/r, or in this case, +1.00 D. The object vergence is –2.00 D, so the image vergence is –1.00 D. Therefore, the image is virtual and 1.0 m behind the mirror. The image is upright, and the transverse magnification is +2×, as shown in the figure on the next page.

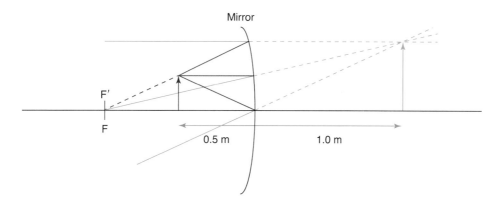

8. **c.** The intraocular lens (IOL) must, of course, have an index of refraction different from that of the aqueous and vitreous for it to have any significant refractive effect. The refractive contribution of the cornea must not be neglected; in fact, it must be specifically considered. The IOL must provide only the vergence that is still required at the IOL plane, which is the total vergence required minus that already provided (at the IOL plane) by the cornea. Although the anterior chamber depth appears to have little importance in regression-derived formulas, it is essential in formulas based on geometric optics. The formula for the change in vergence with change in location is the familiar $P/(1 - Pd)$, where a vergence of power P is moved a distance d. If the refractive index, n, of the material is not 1, a "reduced distance" of d/n must be substituted.

9. **d.** In general, patients perceive image jump as more of a problem than they do image displacement. Flat-top segments minimize image jump because the optical center is near the top. In patients with hyperopia, round-top segments reduce prism displacement because the base-up effect of the distance portion is reduced by the base-down effect of the segment.

10. **a.** In children still developing binocularity, a little anisometropia can lead to a large amblyopia. Anisometropic amblyopia is a fairly common entity and easily missed because the strabismic cosmetic defect is often absent. Full correction of the anisometropia may lead to improvement of visual acuity. Treatment of amblyopia after full correction is total occlusion of the better eye. Better yet, amblyopia should be prevented by providing the best optical focus for each eye and the best potential for binocular vision. The younger the child, the more likely that full correction will prevent amblyopia. In large anisometropia, particularly in older children, contact lenses are necessary to overcome the large image-size difference. Pleoptics has no place in the treatment of anisometropia per se.

11. **b.** The power of any rotationally symmetric refracting surface is given by the equation

$$P = \frac{n_2 - n_1}{r}$$

where r is the radius of curvature at the vertex.

For the anterior corneal surface, n_2 is 1.376 (cornea) and n_1 is 1.333 (water). P_1, the power of the anterior surface under water, is

$$P_1 = \frac{1.376 - 1.333}{0.0077} = +5.58 \text{ D}$$

For the posterior corneal surface, n_2 is 1.336 (aqueous humor) and n_1 is 1.376 (cornea). P_2, the power of the posterior corneal surface, is

$$P_2 = \frac{1.336 - 1.376}{0.0068} = -5.89 \text{ D}$$

The total power of a cornea of thickness $t = 0.0005$ m submerged in water is calculated using the equation for the total power of 2 optical systems separated by distance t:

$$P = P_1 + P_2 - \left(\frac{t}{n}\right) P_1 P_2$$

$$= 5.58 + (-5.89) - \left(\frac{0.0005}{1.376}\right)(5.58)(-5.89)$$

$$= -0.30 \text{ D}$$

It is apparent from this calculation that the cornea has a slight diverging (negative) refracting power under water. In this environment, the crystalline lens has more converging power than the cornea in the average eye. This explains why things appear blurry when you open your eyes under water if you are not wearing goggles.

12. **b.** No optical principles were used to derive the SRK formula. Rather, it was derived using only statistical methods, specifically by using linear regression based on a large number of cases with anterior chamber IOL implants. During development, the formula included terms for (preoperative) axial length, average K readings, and anterior chamber depth (ACD). The statistical correlation between preoperative ACD and IOL power was very weak, so the ACD term did not significantly enhance accuracy, and it was dropped from the final formula. The SRK formula was not intended to eliminate the need for an ACD measurement; the measurement was simply found to be unnecessary. With the introduction of posterior chamber IOLs, it was found that the SRK formula still worked well provided that the A constant was modified for different implant designs. Although adjusting the A constant is perhaps not the best way to adjust for variations in ACD, it is sufficiently accurate for clinical purposes. Option c is incorrect because, clearly, all IOLs are not intended to have the same ACD. Option d is not the best choice for subtle reasons. The preoperative ACD certainly differs from the postoperative ACD, but the question is not whether the measurements differ, but rather whether the preoperative ACD statistically correlates with IOL power. The preoperative and postoperative ACDs can differ and yet the preoperative ACD may still correlate statistically with IOL power. The reason the SRK formula contains no ACD term is not because the preoperative and postoperative ACDs differ but because preoperative ACD does not correlate with IOL power.

13. **a.** To observe stable interference patterns, it is necessary for the 2 interfering wavefronts to have a stable phase relationship. Light consists of a series of wave trains, and each wave train has a dominant frequency. Stable interference can be achieved as long as 2 identical wave trains partially overlap. For instance, in the Michaelson interferometer, light travels slightly different path lengths, and therefore the 2 interfering wavefronts arise from the same beam but at different times. If the time difference is small, identical wave trains still partially overlap and stable interference is observed. If the time difference is too large, different wave trains overlap and no interference is observable. *Spatial coherence* refers to the physical extent of the light source and the presence or absence of a fixed phase relationship between different parts of a light source. *Dispersion* refers to the variation of

refractive index with frequency and is unrelated to interference. *Intensity* refers, roughly speaking, to the brightness of a source and again is unrelated to interference.

14. **d.** In the United States and Canada, legal blindness is defined as visual acuity in the better eye of 20/200 or worse. This level corresponds to severe low vision, in which the patient's reading speed is slowed despite use of monocular reading aids (not binocular prismatic glasses). Using the Kestenbaum rule, the dioptric power of the add is the reciprocal of the visual acuity fraction. Thus, a 10.00 D lens, not a 10× magnifier (a 40.00 D lens), would be the most appropriate aid. Referral to an orientation and mobility specialist is usually not needed until the profound low vision range (20/500–20/100) is reached.

15. **b.** A useful rule of thumb is that for small angles, a prism diopter produces a little more than half a degree of deviation. Thus, a 15Δ prism produces slightly more than 7.5° of deviation, so the only reasonable choice is option b. Alternatively, the exact value can be calculated. A 15Δ prism deflects light 15 cm at a distance of 100 cm. The tangent of the angle of the deflection is 15/100; the angle, therefore, is arctan (0.15) = 8.53°.

16. **c.** Although a thick-lens or multi-element lens system could have the features described, the lens in the question is thin. By definition, the principal planes and nodal points coincide when media with different refractive indices surround a lens; however, the anterior and posterior focal lengths are different. The nodal points shift in the direction of the medium with the higher refractive index.

17. **c.** Laser light is created when atoms of an active medium are exposed to a source of energy (the pumping source). This introduction of energy causes most of the active medium's electrons to rise to a higher energy state, a condition called *population inversion.* Some of these high-energy electrons undergo spontaneous emission, generating photons. If these photons first encounter low-energy electrons, they are merely absorbed. However, if they encounter other high-energy electrons, *stimulated emission* occurs. In order to maintain the chain reaction of stimulated emissions, mirrors are placed at each end of the cavity, an optical feedback arrangement. One mirror reflects totally and the other partially. Most of the coherent light generated is reflected back into the cavity to produce more stimulated emissions. The relatively small amount of light that is allowed to pass through the partially reflecting mirror produces the actual laser beam.

18. **d.** The nerve fiber layer is birefringent, meaning it polarizes light or changes the polarization of incident light that passes through it. The scanning laser polarimeter uses this property to measure nerve fiber layer thickness. The cornea also polarizes light, so a corneal compensator is necessary to eliminate the cornea's polarization effects.

19. **b.** Because red rays focus behind blue rays, the eye must make an accommodative effort to focus on red print after looking at blue print. It must relax accommodation to focus on blue print after looking at red print. The brain therefore perceives that the red print is in front of the blue print when both are displayed against the same background. Achromatopsia or any other color defect affects the way the retinal image is converted into nerve impulses but has no effect on the quality of the retinal image, which is determined solely by the ocular media.

20. **b.** LogMAR is calculated by taking the logarithm of the reciprocal of the Snellen fraction. For instance, if the Snellen visual acuity is 20/200, then the reciprocal is 200/20, or 10, and the logarithm of 10 is 1. Likewise, for a 20/20 eye, the reciprocal of the Snellen visual acuity is also 20/20, or 1, and the logarithm of 1 is 0.

21. **a.** If the retinoscopy streak is horizontal, the axis of the cylindrical lens is also horizontal (180°). Thus, the spherocylindrical lens combination for this patient (before subtracting the working distance adjustment) is +3.00 +1.00 × 90. The working distance (67 cm, or 0.67 m) must be subtracted from the final refraction. Thus, subtracting 1/0.67 m, or 1.50 D, yields the correct answer: +1.50 +1.00 × 90. Note that the cylindrical power acts 90° from the axis. If the retinoscopy streak is horizontal, the axis of the cylindrical lens is 180°, but the actual power is at 90°. Accordingly, the powers (after subtracting the working distance) are +1.50 D at 90° and +2.50 D at 180°.

22. **d.** A certain vergence of light is necessary to focus incoming light on the retina. As the power of the cornea decreases, a corresponding amount of IOL vergence power (corrected for the different location of the refractive element) must be added. Similarly, as the eye becomes shorter, more IOL vergence power is needed to bring the light into focus on the now-less-distant retina.

23. **c.** There are basically 2 types of telescopes: the Galilean, or terrestrial, telescope and the Keplerian, or astronomical, telescope. Each consists of a fairly low-power, positive objective (front) lens and a high-power eyepiece. The Galilean telescope has a minus-power eyepiece, and the astronomical telescope has a plus-power eyepiece. The Galilean telescope produces an upright image and has a shorter distance between the objective and eyepiece (tube length) than does an astronomical telescope. The astronomical telescope produces an inverted image unless prisms or mirrors are incorporated to invert the image. The image produced by an astronomical telescope is brighter than the image produced by a Galilean, which is a major advantage. However, the prisms or mirrors necessary for an astronomical telescope to render an upright image add weight and expense. Spectacle-mounted visual aids utilize the Galilean design, but other instruments such as hand-held binoculars use the Keplerian approach. Both telescope designs are afocal. An object ray parallel to the axis emerges as an image ray parallel to the axis. Consequently, there are no focal points or principal planes. The angular magnification is the negative of the ratio of the eyepiece's power divided by the objective's power. In this case (ignoring the minus sign), the angular magnification is 10.00 D/4.00 D = 2.5×. Tube length is the sum of the focal lengths of the eyepiece and objective, so option c is correct.

24. **c.** Keratometers estimate the refractive power of the cornea. An object of known size is placed in front of the eye. The tear film—acting as a convex mirror—produces a virtual image of the object. The keratometer *measures* the linear dimensions in a few meridians of the virtual image. The first assumption in the estimation is that, in the measured meridian, the tear film's cross-section is circular. In fact, the cross-section is closer to hyperbolic. A hyperbola does not have a single radius of curvature but rather has a different curvature at each point. Assuming a circular cross-section greatly simplifies matters because a circle has a single, constant curvature at each point; however, this assumption can also introduce inaccuracy. Nevertheless, under the circular assumption, the "power" can be estimated using the formula $r = 2u(I/O)$, where r is the radius of curvature of the tear film's assumed circular cross-section, u is the distance from the object to the cornea, I is the size of the image in a specific meridian, and O is the size of the object.

Once the radius of the assumed circular cross-section has been calculated, the power in the meridian of the assumed circular cross-section can be calculated using the formula $P = (n-1)/r$, where n is the tear-film refractive index ($n = 1.333$). Because the tear film is quite thin, the power of the anterior corneal surface can be calculated by replacing the refractive index of the tear film with the refractive index of the cornea. The power of the anterior corneal surface, based on the circular cross-section assumption, is calculated using the refractive index of the cornea ($n = 1.376$). The power of the anterior corneal surface exceeds the power of the entire cornea because the posterior corneal surface has a negative power of about –6.00 D. Therefore, the power of the entire cornea can be calculated using a refractive index that is less than the true refractive index of the cornea. Several modified refractive indices have been suggested, but most keratometers use $n = 1.3375$. A reasonable estimate of total corneal power is produced, not only through use of this value of 1.3375, but also because a radius of 7.5 mm converts to exactly 45.00 D.

Clinically, it is important to remember that the keratometer *estimates* corneal power based on a series of assumptions. For certain purposes, such as contact lens fitting, K readings are sufficiently accurate. However, for other purposes, such as calculating IOL implant power in patients who have undergone corneal refractive surgery, the underlying assumptions are invalid and the K readings are unreliable.

25. **c.** The Kestenbaum rule provides a starting point not an endpoint for the required add. Base-in prisms should be incorporated into high-power reading spectacles to assist accommodative convergence in patients who have similar visual function binocularly, but they do not affect magnification. Magnification alone does not enhance contrast and therefore would not suffice by itself for patients with low contrast sensitivity.

26. **d.** A person is considered to have low vision when a visual deficit significantly affects his or her activities. Visual disability is related to the interaction of a number of factors, including the complexity of the task, the skill of the person, the individual's response to reduced vision, and other aspects of visual function, including contrast sensitivity. A visual field deficit (such as bitemporal hemianopia) or a specific level of visual acuity (such as less than 20/70) does not in and of itself qualify as low vision if it does not significantly affect that person's particular activities or if he or she is able to adequately compensate. Conversely, a patient who performs relatively well on a Snellen test may be considered to have low vision if he or she is not able to perform necessary tasks because of loss of vision.

27. **d.** Optical coherence tomography (OCT) is used to create cross-sectional images of the living eye. Rays from a light source consisting of a superluminescent diode—not a laser—are split by a beam splitter into a reference beam, which is directed to a movable mirror, and an object beam, which is directed to one of the reflective interfaces within the tissue being examined. The 2 reflected beams are then superimposed by the same beam splitter and transmitted together to a light detector. By correlating the resulting interference patterns with the position of the movable mirror, information about the reflectivity of the internal structure of the cornea, lens, or retina can then be constructed.

28. **b.** When looking through a small pupil, the observer can improve visualization by narrowing his or her effective interpupillary distance. This can be accomplished by several means. Moving the ophthalmoscope's mirror closer to the observer (the "small-pupil feature" available on some ophthalmoscopes) decreases the distance between the light paths to the observer's left and right eyes, effectively narrowing the observer's interpupillary distance. If the examiner can slightly converge, it will narrow the observer's effective interpupillary distance. Increasing the distance between the observer and the patient decreases the angle formed by the observer's 2 eyes and the patient's eye, thereby allowing the light paths from the observer's eyes to "squeeze through" a smaller pupil.

29. **b.** Changes of ±0.25 D and ±0.50 D in sphere and cylinder are likely to be below the "just noticeable" threshold for a patient with 20/100 visual acuity. Because the first issue to rule out when vision changes is a change in refraction, an additional attempt should be made to refine the refraction using larger-step changes in sphere and cylinder. The darkroom pinhole test is a test of potential vision. It should be performed after the refraction has been optimized.

30. **a.** An optical system's nodal points are the points through which light rays entering or leaving the system are undeviated (but not necessarily undisplaced). In the reduced schematic eye, the nodal points coincide and are located 5.6 mm posterior to the corneal surface. Because all light rays passing through this point are undeviated, a light ray that leaves the tip of an object will pass through the nodal point and strike the retina undeviated. Retinal image size can be calculated by similar triangles if both the image height and distance are known.

31. **a.** The far point of the eye and the fovea are always corresponding points when accommodation is relaxed. All the other statements are false. The far point is 25 cm in front of the eye and is farther away from the near point of the fully accommodated eye.

32. **b.** The nonaccommodated hyperopic eye has a far point behind the eye. A virtual image of the retina forms at this location. As the eye begins to accommodate, the point of focus recedes to minus infinity. Minus infinity and plus infinity are essentially the same optically. As the eye continues to accommodate through optical infinity, the point of focus moves in front of the eye to a point between plus infinity and the cornea. The near point of the eye, in diopters, is equal to the far point location, in diopters, plus the amplitude of accommodation. Because we are told that the amount of hyperopia is less than the amplitude of accommodation, we conclude that the near point is in front of the eye (between infinity and the cornea).

33. **d.** A diopter is the reciprocal of distance in meters. A prism diopter measures the deviation in centimeters at 1 m, or centimeters per meter. Refractive index is the ratio of the speed of light in a vacuum to the speed of light in the medium and, therefore, is dimensionless. Wavelength can be measured in any unit of length. For optical wavelengths, the nanometer is convenient. Frequency is measured in cycles per second, or hertz.

34. **c.** Irregular astigmatism is a general term that encompasses most higher-order aberrations. Irregular astigmatism caused by an irregular corneal surface is best corrected by a rigid gas-permeable (RGP) contact lens that replaces the anterior corneal surface with a smooth air–lens interface. Soft contact lenses are not as effective in creating a smooth surface because they conform somewhat to the irregular corneal surface, although they may correct an irregular corneal surface to some extent. If spectacles could be manufactured to compensate for higher-order aberrations, they would work in 1 gaze direction only. For this reason, RGP contact lenses provide the best visual acuity for patients with irregular astigmatism produced by an irregular cornea.

35. **b.** There are many risk factors associated with even the most current extended-wear contact lenses, including swimming with the lenses, previous history of eye infection, any exposure to smoke, abnormal eyelid function, severe dry eye, and corneal neovascularization.

36. **b.** Patients with central scotomata can still read by using eccentric fixation, along with appropriate magnification and enhanced contrast, if necessary. Reading speed is usually decreased, but reading ability can often be improved with training and practice.

37. **b.** Loss of peripheral visual field makes it difficult to navigate unfamiliar territory and may cause the patient to bump into objects or people. Retinitis pigmentosa, panretinal photocoagulation, and retinal detachment typically affect the peripheral visual field, whereas age-related macular degeneration typically affects central visual acuity.

38. **a.** The entrance pupil of the eye is the pupil we see when we look at a patient's eye. For a refractive index of $n = 4/3$ and a cornea with a power of +43.00 D, the entrance pupil is the image of the anatomical pupil formed by the cornea. The crystalline lens does not contribute to the formation of the entrance pupil. The entrance pupil is located about 0.5 mm in front of the anatomical pupil and is about 13%–15% larger.

39. **c.** The formula is

$$\text{Brewster Angle} = \tan^{-1} \frac{n_2}{n_1}$$

$$= \tan^{-1} \frac{1.500}{1}$$

$$= 56.3°$$

40. **d.** The formula is

$$\text{Critical Angle} = \sin^{-1} \frac{1}{n_2}$$

$$= \sin^{-1} \frac{1}{1.500}$$

$$= 41.8°$$

Index

(*f* = figure; *t* = table)